Psychology
for Health Professionals

Second edition

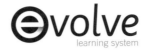
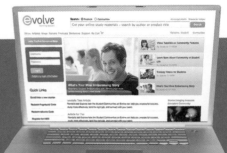

Psychology
for Health Professionals

Second edition

Patricia Barkway

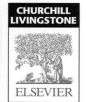

Sydney   Edinburgh   London   New York   Philadelphia   St Louis   Toronto

Churchill Livingstone
is an imprint of Elsevier

Elsevier Australia. ACN 001 002 357
(a division of Reed International Books Australia Pty Ltd)
Tower 1, 475 Victoria Avenue, Chatswood, NSW 2067

ELSEVIER

This edition © 2013 Elsevier Australia

First edition © 2009.

eISBN: 9780729581561

National Library of Australia Cataloguing-in-Publication Data

Barkway, Patricia.

Psychology for health professionals / editor, Patricia Barkway.

2nd ed.
9780729541565 (pbk.)
Includes index.

Clinical health psychology.
Medical care–Psychological aspects.
Medicine and psychology.

610.19

Publisher: Libby Houston
Developmental Editor: Elizabeth Coady
Project Managers: Natalie Hamad and Nayagi Athmanathan
Edited by Matt Davies
Proofread by Gabrielle Challis
Permissions Editor: Sarah Johnson
Cover and internal design by Georgette Hall
Cover image © jhorrocks/iStockphoto
Index by Robert Swanson
Typeset by Toppan Best-set Premedia Limited
Printed in China by 1010 Printing Int'l Ltd.

Dedication

To Mike and our children: Matt, Steve and Catherine, whose love, support and encouragement contributes to my resilience and wellbeing.

Contents

Foreword

We are living in a time of rapid change in the way in which health and illness are understood and healthcare services are organised and provided. New treatments, better ways of providing health services, greater use of evidence to guide practice, the emergence of a health consumer movement – these trends and many others have had a significant impact on health policy and practice and on the education of health professionals. Such developments have undoubtedly made the complex business of healthcare even more complicated. If undergraduate students of medicine, midwifery, nursing, paramedic, psychology and the allied health professions are to be prepared for effective practice in the health services of the 21st century, careful thought needs to be given to what will be taught and how the learning material will be delivered. A judicious selection of topics, authors and learning/teaching approaches is evident in this compilation edited by Patricia Barkway.

The main purpose of the volume is to introduce psychology to undergraduate health professional readers. However, the text goes beyond what one would typically expect of an introductory psychology text and herein is its novelty and strength. The initial chapters provide a clear overview of theories of individual personality, human behaviour and lifespan development. This is followed by consideration of how health and health outcomes might be influenced by the complex interaction of biological, psychological and social factors, contextualising this in relation to key national and global concerns and priorities (Chapter 4). Chapter 5 crosses over into health sociology to examine the social context within which people live, work, maintain health or become unwell – the social determinants of health. If this is a departure for a psychology text, it is one to be applauded. Increasingly, healthcare is being seen as a shared responsibility involving health professionals from a range of disciplines, communities, families and individuals. Examining the personal alongside the social and individual troubles in the context of public issues will contextualise the learning for students and foster interdisciplinary consideration of encounters with consumers, models of care and communication between health professionals. This is at the leading edge of developments in health policy and practice and health professional education.

The chapter introducing health research (6) is primarily concerned with establishing the basics for becoming an effective consumer of research to guide practice: how to access and appraise the quality of research findings; approaches for systematically critiquing research reports; and the application of evidence-based findings to healthcare practice. The remaining chapters address the psychological and social aspects of a range of encounters, issues and interventions relevant to health professional students. Chapter 7 examines theories and models informing understandings of behaviour and techniques of health behaviour change. The role of communication problems in healthcare failures highlight the importance of the material covered in Chapter 8. The requirements for effective communication are examined in relation to cultural difference, power imbalances, advocacy and interpersonal relationships. The impact of information communication technology, including social media, has made it even more important that health professionals are thoroughly grounded in the requirements for effective communication. The chapter on partnerships (9) raises a number of contemporary concerns arising out of the changing nature of encounters between health professionals and consumers. The very practical treatment of recovery-oriented practice provided is likely to demystify a concept that students and qualified practitioners understand to be important but often find elusive. The next three chapters, addressing stress and coping (10), loss (11) and pain (12), touch on topics of considerable relevance to all health professional students. The final chapter revisits much of the content of the previous chapters, demonstrating how health promotion has shifted over time from a largely individualised focus to also include the social determinants of health and a population focus.

The carefully selected combination of foundational and clinically relevant content delivered in a lucid and lively style, combined with a range of learning objectives, illustrative case studies, critical thinking prompts, classroom activities and extensive reference lists, will ensure the book has a shelf life extending well beyond the student years.

Mike Hazelton
Professor of Mental Health Nursing
Head of Nursing and Midwifery
The University of Newcastle, Australia

Preface

The first edition of *Psychology for Health Professionals* was designed to introduce healthcare students to psychological and other theories to assist them in developing an understanding of the complex and interactive nature of the factors that influence health behaviours and health outcomes. In this second edition we have maintained the original focus while updating the materials with evidence-based research, references and clinical examples to ensure the content remains relevant to contemporary healthcare practice. Students can apply the material in the text to the health behaviours of the people they care for, their colleagues and themselves. It is written for, but is not limited to, undergraduate students of medicine, midwifery, nursing, paramedic, psychology, social work and the allied health professions.

Unlike many health psychology textbooks *Psychology for Health Professionals* examines individual personality and psychological theory within the social context of people's lives. This approach is taken because of the increasing awareness that a person's behaviour is not only influenced by internal biological and psychological factors but also by external factors within the person's social and physical environment. There is abundant evidence to support this hypothesis, for example, the report of the World Health Organization Commission of the Social Determinants of Health *Closing the gap in a generation: Health equity through action on the social determinants of health*. In keeping with a social determinants theme the book takes into account the social, political and cultural contexts of healthcare in Australia and New Zealand. Nevertheless, despite the theories and practices outlined in the book being situated in these two countries, they are also relevant to other countries and contexts.

The book also includes material that is not always found in undergraduate health psychology texts, such as an introduction to psychological theory and healthcare research. Furthermore, in order to reflect the current interdisciplinary focus of tertiary healthcare education and practice, contributors to the book were recruited from and represent a range of healthcare disciplines including psychology, nursing, sociology and physiotherapy. All contributors are currently engaged as health professionals or academics in their respective fields.

The first half of the book outlines psychological and other relevant theory and, in the second half, those theories are applied to health issues and healthcare practice.

Chapters 1–5 present psychological, lifespan and social theory; Chapter 6 addresses the role and contribution of research to healthcare practice; and Chapters 7–13 cover the psychological aspects of specific health encounters, issues and interventions. Throughout the book critical thinking questions, case studies and examples of research are included to encourage students to reflect on the application of theory to practice. Activities are provided for lecturers to use in the classroom.

Psychology for Health Professionals is intended to assist future health professionals to understand the diversity of human responses, particularly in relation to health behaviours, and to develop the knowledge, skills and disposition required to care for the patients and clients they will encounter in their chosen career. I trust that readers will find the content to be engaging, interesting and professionally relevant.

Pat Barkway
May 2013

About the editor

PATRICIA BARKWAY

RN, CMHN, FACMHN, BA (Psychology/Education), MSc (PHC)

Pat is a Senior Lecturer at Flinders University, Adelaide where she teaches health psychology to nursing, paramedic and allied health undergraduate students, and mental health nursing to postgraduate students. She is a credentialled mental health nurse and a Fellow of the Australian College of Mental Health Nurses.

Pat has always been interested in and fascinated by people and human behaviour. This led to her undertaking a degree majoring in psychology, followed by a career in mental health nursing and academia. Pat's professional experience was gained in acute mental health settings, psychiatric liaison nursing, community mental health and through 25 years experience in tertiary healthcare education and academia.

Throughout her career Pat has become increasingly aware that individual explanations, on their own, are insufficient to provide insights into human behaviour. This is reflected in her choice of postgraduate study in primary healthcare. Consequently, her approach to understanding human behaviour and to healthcare clinical practice is situated within a social determinants framework, and takes account of psychological theory while recognising the social and political contexts in which people live their lives.

Contributors

PATRICIA BARKWAY
RN, CMHN, FACMHN, BA (Psychology/Education), MSc (PHC)
Senior Lecturer, Mental Health Nursing, Flinders University, Adelaide, SA

MICHAEL A BULL
BSW, MSW
Senior Lecturer (Social Work), Flinders University, Adelaide, SA

MARIA DE SOUSA
MScMed (PainMgt), BSc, GDip Phty
Senior Physiotherapist, Pain Management and Research Centre, Royal North Shore Hospital, St Leonards, NSW

BERNARD GUERIN
BA (Hons), PhD
Professor of Psychology, University of South Australia, Adelaide, SA

PAULINE GUERIN
PhD
Psychology Program Coordinator, Pennsylvania State University, Brandywine Campus, Media, PA, USA
Associate Professor, Academic Status, School of Nursing and Midwifery, Flinders University, Adelaide, SA

DEB O'KANE
RN, ENB603, GradDip CN, MN, GradCert Higher Education
Lecturer, School of Nursing and Midwifery, Flinders University, Adelaide, SA

SARAH OVERTON
BA (Hons), MPsychol (Clin), PhD
Senior Clinical Psychologist, ADAPT Program, Pain Management and Research Centre, Royal North Shore Hospital, St Leonards, NSW
Clinical Lecturer, Faculty of Medicine, The University of Sydney, Sydney, NSW

YVONNE PARRY
RN, BA (Psychology & Public Policy), MHSM, GradCertEdu (Higher Education), PhD
Lecturer, School of Nursing and Midwifery, Flinders University, Adelaide, SA

EILEEN WILLIS
BEd, MEd, PhD
Deputy Dean, School of Medicine, Flinders University, Adelaide, SA

Reviewers

MURRAY BARDWELL
DipAppSc, BN, MN, Credentialled Mental Health Nurse
Mental Health Clinician, St John of God Hospital, Ballarat, VIC

ANNA CHUR-HANSEN
BA (Hons Psychology), PhD, FAPS, FHERDSA
Professor, Discipline of Psychiatry, School of Medicine, The University of
Adelaide, Adelaide, SA

MAIRWEN JONES
BA (Hons), PhD
Senior Lecturer, Psychology, Faculty of Health Sciences, The University of
Sydney, Sydney, NSW

JASON LANDON
BSc, MSc (1st), PhD
Senior Lecturer, Department of Psychology, Gambling and Addictions Research
Centre, University of Technology, Auckland, New Zealand

JAN LAWRENCE
MNurs (MntlHlth)
Senior Lecturer, Nursing, Eastern Institution of Technology, Hawkesbay,
New Zealand

CHRIS SPENCER
RN, MA
Senior Lecturer, School of Nursing, Otago Polytechnic, Dunedin, New Zealand

Acknowledgements

The writing of this book has been a collaborative effort and I wish to acknowledge the many people who contributed.

First, the contributors who agreed to revise and update one or more chapters for the second edition – I appreciate your willingness to again share your insights about your area of specialty. To the patients, clients and students with whom I have worked over the years – I thank you for challenging my thinking and sharpening my understanding of psychological theory applied to real life. To my colleagues, who have contributed to my professional development, I am indebted to you all for generously sharing your wisdom, particularly Lesley Meredith, Michael Crotty, Judith Condon, Mary Luszcz and Eimear Muir-Cochrane, who have been significant mentors. To the publishing team at Elsevier – you did a fantastic job keeping me and the project on track, especially Libby Houston (publisher), Liz Coady (developmental editor) and Matt Davies (copyeditor). And thank you to the reviewers for your critical and constructive feedback.

And finally, it is impossible to name you all, but I sincerely appreciate the interest and support of all my family, friends and colleagues who sought updates and encouraged me throughout the writing phase – I thank you all.

Chapter 1
Psychology: An introduction

PATRICIA BARKWAY

Learning objectives

The material in this chapter will help you to:

- understand the psychological theories that provide explanations of human behaviour and personality
- describe and critique biomedical, psychological and sociological theories of human behaviour
- apply your knowledge of psychological theory to understand the behaviour of yourself and others
- describe how psychological theory informs interventions in healthcare practice
- explain the nature versus nurture debate
- understand the interrelationship between psychological, biological and social influences on human behaviour.

Key terms

- Psychological theories
  - Psychoanalytic
  - Behavioural (learning)
  - Cognitive
  - Cognitive behavioural
  - Humanistic
- Biomedical theory
- Sociological theory
- Eclectic/holistic approach
- Nature versus nurture

Introduction

Who are you? How have you come to be who you are? What influences how you think, feel and act? Are your personality and behaviour determined by your genetic makeup and biological events, by thoughts and feelings, by your experiences in the world, or by an interrelationship between some or all of these? Most of us, at one time or another, have thought about these questions. Through attempting to understand why humans behave as they do, a further question arises: Are human behaviour and personality determined by genetics and biology (nature) or shaped by one's upbringing, experiences and environmental factors (nurture)?

These questions have long engaged the interest and passion of philosophers, healers and health professionals and, in more recent times, psychologists and scientists. Investigation of these questions has resulted in various theories being proposed to explain normal and abnormal thoughts, feelings and behaviours, as well as mental health and mental illness. These concepts – the theories that attempt to explain and provide understandings of behaviour – will be examined in this chapter. The nature versus nurture debate will also be explored.

Psychology

Psychology is a theoretical and applied discipline that emerged in the 19th century in Europe and North America from the established disciplines of physiology and philosophy. Its principal focus is the scientific study of behaviour. To achieve this psychologists study how organisms (primarily humans but not exclusively) act, think, learn, perceive, feel, interact with others and understand themselves. Nevertheless, given that psychological theory originated in a Western context, caution is recommended when applying psychological theory to people from other cultures such as New Zealand Māori or Australian Aboriginal and Torres Strait Islanders.

The discipline of psychology focuses on behavioural responses (including affective and cognitive) to certain sets of conditions. Psychology is both a natural and a social science that attempts to determine the laws of nature at a cellular level (as in bioscientific enquiry) and also to explain human behaviour in individuals and groups. Within the discipline professional psychologists practise in two broad areas: theoretical (research or academic) and applied (clinical practice or organisational psychology).

The major theoretical perspectives (also called paradigms) that attempt to explain and predict specific behaviours include psychoanalytic, behavioural (learning), cognitive and humanistic. At times these theories can be complementary, but at other times they can be contradictory. Finally, other theoretical perspectives that are outside the field of psychology are recognised for the role they play in influencing behaviour. These paradigms include the biomedical model and sociological theories.

Theories of personality and human behaviour

Personality theories propose psychological models to explain human behaviours. They emerged from curiosity about and philosophical enquiry into the human condition. The theories also place particular emphasis on identifying the causes of abnormal behaviour so as to develop models for understanding, prevention or treatment of health problems with a behavioural or lifestyle component such as physical activity or tobacco smoking. Explanations of human behaviour can be broadly divided into three paradigms:

- biomedical or biological/physical models
- psychological models, including psychoanalytic, behavioural, cognitive and humanistic approaches
- sociological models.

Within these paradigms are a number of major viewpoints that offer a theory of personality development or an explanation of human behaviour. They are listed below.

- *Biomedical model* – proposes that behaviour is influenced by physiology, with normal behaviour occurring when the body is in a state of equilibrium and abnormal behaviour being a consequence of physical pathology.

- *Psychoanalytic theory* – asserts that behaviour is driven by unconscious processes and influenced by childhood/developmental conflicts that have either been resolved or remain unresolved.

- *Behavioural psychology* – presents the view that behaviour is influenced by factors external to the individual. Behaviours are learned depending on whether they are rewarded or not, by association with another event or by imitation.

- *Cognitive psychology* – acknowledges the role of perception and thoughts about oneself, one's individual experience and the environment in influencing behaviour.

- *Humanistic psychology* – focuses on the development of a concept of self and the striving of the individual to achieve personal goals.

- *Eclectic approach* – (also called holistic) draws on the theory and research of several paradigms to obtain an overall understanding or provide a more comprehensive explanation than would be achieved by using one theoretical model alone. For example, in clinical practice cognitive behavioural therapy (CBT) is a frequently used counselling approach; in research a mixed-methods approach may be utilised.

- *Sociological theories* – shifts the emphasis from the individual to the broader social forces that influence people. This model challenges the notion of individual pathology and acknowledges the responsibility of society for the health of its citizens.

Each of these seemingly disparate perspectives makes a substantial contribution to the understanding of how and why humans think, feel and behave as they do, and thereby identifies opportunities for prevention and treatment of health problems with a behavioural component. Nevertheless, as a comprehensive theory of human behaviour, each also has major shortcomings, hence the practice of using an eclectic approach that utilises more than one theory.

BIOMEDICAL MODEL

Also known as psychobiology or the neuroscience perspective, the biomedical model asserts that *normal* behaviour is a consequence of equilibrium within the body and that abnormal behaviour results from pathological bodily or brain function. This is not a new notion; in the fourth century BC the Greek physician Hippocrates attributed mental disorder to brain pathology. His ideas were overshadowed, however, when throughout the Dark Ages and later during the Renaissance, thinking and explanations shifted to witchcraft or demonic possession (Butcher et al 2011, Kring et al 2010). In the 19th century, a return to biophysical explanations accompanied the emergence of the public health movement.

In recent times, advances in technology have led to increased understanding of organic determinants of behaviour. Research and treatment have focused on four main areas:

- *Nervous system disorders, in particular neurotransmitter disturbance at the synaptic gap between neurons* – more than 50 neurotransmitters have been identified, four of which are implicated in mental illness. These are acetylcholine (Alzheimer's disease), dopamine (schizophrenia), noradrenaline (mood disorder) and serotonin (mood disorder).

- *Structural changes to the brain* – perhaps following trauma or in degenerative disorders such as Huntington's disease.

- *Endocrine or gland dysfunction, as in hypothyroidism* – this has a similar presentation to clinical depression and hormonal changes are considered to be a contributing factor in postnatal depression.

- *Familial (genetic) transmission of mental illness* – twin studies reviewed by Irving Gottesman found the following lifetime risks of developing schizophrenia: general population 1%, one parent 13%, sibling 9%, dizygotic (non-identical) twin 17%, two parents 46% and monozygotic (identical) twin 48% (Butcher et al 2011, Cando & Gottesman 2000).

Although genetic studies demonstrate a correlation between having a close relative with schizophrenia and the likelihood of developing the disorder, a shared genetic history alone is not sufficient. If genetics were the only aetiological factor, the concordance rate for monozygotic twins could be expected to be 100%. Gottesman's (1991, 1997) research is important because it supports the diathesis-stress hypothesis, a widely held explanation for the development of mental disorder that proposes that constitutional predisposition combined with environmental stress will lead to mental illness (Kring et al 2010).

Critique of the biomedical model

Among treatments that emerge from the biomedical model are medications that alter the function, production and reabsorption of neurotransmitters in the synaptic gap. However, evidence that a particular intervention is an effective treatment is not proof of a causal link with the illness. For example, consider a person with type 1 (insulin-dependent) diabetes mellitus. Because this person lacks insulin to metabolise glucose, the condition is managed with regular insulin injections. However, the lack of insulin is a symptom of the disease, not the cause. Whatever caused the pancreas to cease producing insulin is not known, despite the treatment being effective. Similarly, with schizophrenia, the relationship between taking antipsychotic medications (which are dopamine antagonists), dopamine levels and symptom management is correlational, not causal. Therefore, although antipsychotic medication affects dopamine receptors and hence dopamine levels, and can be an effective treatment to manage the symptoms of schizophrenia, this does not provide evidence that elevated dopamine levels cause the disorder.

PSYCHOANALYTIC THEORY

Sigmund Freud developed the first psychological explanation of human behaviour – psychoanalytic theory – in the late 19th century. He placed strong emphasis on the role of unconscious processes (not in the conscious mind of the individual) in determining human behaviour. Central tenets of the theory are that intrapsychic (generally unconscious) forces, developmental factors and family relationships determine human behaviour. According to psychoanalytic theory normal development results when the individual satisfactorily traverses each developmental stage and mental illness is seen as a consequence of fixation at a particular developmental stage or conflict that has not been resolved.

Sigmund Freud

Freud (1856–1939) was an Austrian neurologist who, in his clinical practice, saw a number of patients with sensory or neurological problems for which he was unable to identify a physiological cause. These patients were mainly middle-class Viennese women. It was from his work with these patients that Freud hypothesised that the cause of their illnesses was psychological. From this assumption he developed an explanation of personality development, which he called psychoanalytic theory. According to Freud the mind is composed of three forces:

- *The id* – the primitive biological force comprising two basic drives: sexual and aggressive. The id operates on the pleasure principle and seeks to satisfy life-sustaining needs such as food, love and creativity, in addition to sexual gratification.

- *The ego* – the cognitive component of personality that attempts to use realistic means (the reality principle) to achieve the desires of the id.

- *The superego* – the internalised moral standards of the society in which one lives. It represents the person's ideal self and can be equated to a conscience.

Freud's theory proposes that personality development progresses through five stages throughout childhood. At each stage the child's behaviour is driven by the need to satisfy sexual and aggressive drives via the mouth, anus or genitals. Failure of the child to satisfy these needs at any one of the stages will result in psychological difficulties that are carried into adulthood. For example, unresolved issues at the oral stage can lead to dependency issues in adulthood; problems in the anal stage may lead to the child later developing obsessive-compulsive traits. Freud's stages of psychosexual development are:

1. *oral* – from birth to about 18 months, where the primary focus of the id is the mouth
2. *anal* – from approximately 18 months to three years, where libido shifts from the mouth to the anus and primary gratification is derived from expelling or retaining faeces
3. *phallic* – from approximately three to six years, where gratification of the id occurs through the genitals
4. *latent* – Freud proposed that from approximately six to 12 years, the child goes through a latency phase in which sexual urges are dormant
5. *genital* – once the child passes through puberty, sexual urges re-emerge but now they are directed towards another person, not the self as they were at an earlier stage of development (Butcher et al 2011, Kring et al 2010).

Defence mechanisms

An important contribution of psychoanalytic theory to the understanding of behaviour has been the identification of defence mechanisms and the role they play in mediating anxiety. Defence mechanisms were first described by Freud and later elaborated on by his daughter, Anna (Freud 1966). They are unconscious, protective processes whereby anxiety experienced by the ego is reduced. Commonly used defence mechanisms include:

- *repression* – the primary defence mechanism and an unconscious process whereby unacceptable impulses/feelings/thoughts are barred from consciousness (e.g. memories of sexual abuse in childhood)
- *regression* – the avoidance of present difficulties by a reversion to an earlier, less mature way of dealing with the situation (e.g. a toilet-trained child who becomes incontinent following the birth of a sibling)
- *denial* – the blocking of painful information from consciousness (e.g. not accepting that a loss has occurred)
- *projection* – the denial of one's own unconscious impulses by attributing them to another person (e.g. when you dislike someone but believe it is the other person who does not like you)
- *sublimation* – an unconscious process whereby libido is transformed into a more socially acceptable outlet (e.g. creativity, art or sport)
- *displacement* – the transferring of emotion from the source to a substitute (e.g. a person who is unassertive in an interaction with a supervisor at work and 'kicks the cat' on arriving home)
- *rationalisation* – a rational excuse is used to explain behaviour that may be motivated by an irrational force (e.g. cheating when completing a tax return, with the excuse that 'everyone does it')
- *intellectualisation/isolation* – feelings are cut off from the event in which they occur (e.g. after an unsuccessful job interview the person says, 'I didn't really want the job anyway')
- *reaction formation* – developing a personality trait that is the opposite of the original unconscious or repressed trait (e.g. avoiding a friend's partner because you are attracted to that person).

Being aware of defence mechanisms and the role they play in managing anxiety can assist health professionals to understand that a person's seemingly irrational behaviour may have an unconscious cause. For example, the child who regresses following a serious illness is not attention seeking, but reverting to behaviours from a time when they felt safe.

Critique of psychoanalytic theory

Although the notions of unconscious motivations and defence mechanisms are helpful in interpreting behaviours, Freud's version of psychoanalytic theory has not been without its critics. Fellow psychoanalyst Erik Erikson disagreed with Freud's theory of psychosexual stages of development and proposed instead a psychosocial theory in which development occurred throughout the lifespan not just through childhood as in Freud's model (e.g. Erikson 1963, Santrock 2009). (See Chs 2 and 3 for more detail on developmental theories.)

The unconscious nature of Freud's concepts and stages renders them difficult to test and therefore there is little evidence to support Freudian theory. Feminists also object to Freud's interpretation of the psychological development of women, arguing that there is scant evidence to support the hypothesis that women view their bodies as inferior to men's because they do not have a penis (Kring et al 2010). Nevertheless, despite these criticisms, psychoanalytic theory does provide plausible explanations for seemingly irrational behaviour.

CASE STUDY: HAYLEY

Hayley is a 15-year-old high school student who is a member of the national Olympic swimming team. She currently holds the national title for the 100 and 200 metres breaststroke events. She is an only child and her mother has recently resigned from work to support Hayley's strenuous training regimen.

Two weeks ago Hayley suffered a seizure and collapsed at training. When she woke up in hospital she was paralysed on her left side. Subsequent investigations identified an inoperable brain tumour. Hayley and her parents were told that the life expectancy for this particular type of tumour is three to six months.

Jake is a physiotherapist who has been assigned Hayley in his caseload. The referral from the neurosurgeon requests that Hayley be assisted to mobilise and taught how to use a walking stick prior to her discharge home. She will attend the hospital daily for radiotherapy, but this treatment is considered to be palliative not curative.

Hayley welcomed Jake warmly when she met him and said, 'Am I pleased to see you? I want to get moving again so that I can return to my swimming training. The Olympic selections are only three months away'. Jake was puzzled by Hayley's statement because he read in the notes that Hayley had been informed of her diagnosis and prognosis.

Critical thinking

- Which defence mechanism is Hayley using?
- What purpose might this defence mechanism serve Hayley at the moment?
- How useful is this coping strategy in the longer term?
- How might Jake respond to Hayley when she talks about returning to training for the Olympics?

BEHAVIOURAL PSYCHOLOGY

Behavioural psychology (also called behaviourism) is a school of psychological thought founded in the United States by J B Watson in the early 20th century with the purpose of objectively studying observable human behaviour, as opposed to examining the mind, which was the prevalent psychological method at the time in Europe. The model proposes a scientific approach to the study of behaviour, a feature that behaviourists argue is lacking in psychoanalytic theory (and in humanistic psychology, which developed later).

Behaviourism opposes the introspective, structuralist approach of psychoanalysis and emphasises the importance of the environment in shaping behaviour. The focus is on observable behaviour and conditions that elicit and maintain the behaviour (classical conditioning) or factors that reinforce behaviour (operant conditioning) or vicarious learning through watching and imitating the behaviour of others (modelling).

Three basic assumptions underpin behavioural theory. These are that personality is determined by prior learning, that human behaviour is changeable throughout the lifespan and that changes in behaviour are generally caused by changes in the environment. The following people were prominent figures in the development of behavioural psychology.

Ivan Pavlov

Russian physiologist Ivan Pavlov (1849–1936) was the first to describe the relationship between stimulus and response. Pavlov demonstrated that a dog could learn to salivate (respond) to a non-food stimulus (a bell) if the stimulus was simultaneously presented with the food. His discovery became known as learning by association or classical conditioning. Phobias and fear, for example, can be explained by classical conditioning. See Table 1.1 for an explanation of how fear or phobia of a rabbit (an animal that is not normally feared) can develop.

Table 1.1		
CLASSICAL CONDITIONING OF FEAR		
Before conditioning		
Neutral stimulus Rabbit	No reaction	
During conditioning		
Neutral stimulus Rabbit	Unconditioned stimulus Loud noise	Unconditioned response Fear response
After conditioning		
Conditioned stimulus Rabbit	Conditioned response Fear of the rabbit	

Critical thinking

- Consider how classical conditioning can explain why a patient receiving chemotherapy injections commences vomiting when the chemotherapy nurse enters the patient's room.
- Identify which of the following is the neutral stimulus, unconditioned stimulus, conditioned stimulus, conditioned response and enter them into the table below:
  - » nurse
  - » chemotherapy injection
  - » vomiting
  - » vomiting at the sight of the nurse.

Before conditioning		
Neutral stimulus	No reaction	
During conditioning		
Neutral stimulus	Unconditioned stimulus	Unconditioned response
After conditioning		
Conditioned stimulus	Conditioned response	

John B Watson

Watson (1878–1958), who is attributed as being the founder of behaviourism, changed the focus of psychology from the study of inner sensations to the study of observable behaviour. In his quest to make psychology a true science Watson further developed Pavlov's work on stimulus–response learning and experimented by manipulating stimulus conditions. In the classic 'Little Albert' experiment Watson and his colleague Rayner (1920) conditioned a young child to fear a white rat by producing a loud noise at the same time that Albert touched the rat (which he initially did not fear). Albert's fear reaction also generalised to other furry objects such as a fur coat and a white rabbit.

Watch it on YouTube! For a short video of the 'Little Albert' experiment see <http://www.youtube.com/watch?v=9hBfnXACsOI>.

Furthermore, Watson believed that abnormal behaviours were the result of earlier faulty conditioning and that reconditioning could modify these behaviours. His work heralded the introduction of psychological approaches to treat problem behaviours.

B F Skinner

Skinner (1904–1990) formulated the notion of instrumental or operant conditioning in which reinforcers (rewards) contribute to the probability of a response being either repeated or extinguished. Skinner believed that behaviour was the result of an interaction between the individual and the environment and, because the environment was more readily amenable to change, this was the most appropriate place to intervene to bring about change. His research demonstrated that by changing contingencies that were external to the person, behaviour could be altered. This is an underlying principle in interventions using an operant conditioning or learning by consequence approach (Skinner 1953).

Critique of behavioural psychology

Behaviourism provided the first scientifically testable theories of human development, as well as plausible explanations of how behaviours are learned and, in the clinical arena, how conditions such as addictions, depression, phobias and anxiety develop. Behavioural principles underpin many approaches to behaviour change (these are discussed more fully in Ch 7). Behavioural explanations are less convincing, however, when applied to complex human emotions (e.g. compassion) or behaviours (e.g. altruism), or the behaviours of a person with a medical condition like dementia. Furthermore, most behavioural research has been conducted on animals under laboratory conditions, so to extrapolate findings from this research to humans is mechanistic and does not allow for intrinsic human qualities like creativity or altruism. Finally, behavioural theory falls short in explaining the success of an individual brought up in an adverse environment or why a person whose environment is apparently healthy and advantaged engages in deviant or antisocial behaviour.

COGNITIVE PSYCHOLOGY

Since the 1950s, interest in the cognitive or thinking processes involved in behavioural responses has expanded. Cognitive psychological theory proposes that people actively interpret their environment and cognitively construct their world. Therefore, behaviour is a result of the interplay of external and internal events. External events are the stimuli and reinforcements that regulate behaviour and internal events are one's perceptions and thoughts about oneself and the world, as well as one's behaviour in the world. In other words, how you think about a situation will influence how you behave in that situation. The following people are prominent figures in the development of cognitive psychology.

Albert Bandura

According to Bandura (b. 1925) it is not intrapsychic or environmental forces alone that influence behaviour. Rather, human behaviour results from the interaction of the environment with the individual's perception and thinking. Self-efficacy, or the belief that one can achieve a certain goal, is the critical component in the achievement of that goal. Bandura also proposed that consequences do not have to be directly experienced by the individual for learning to occur – learning can occur vicariously through the process of modelling or learning by imitation (Bandura 2000, 2006, 2012).

Aaron T Beck

Problem behaviour, says Beck (b. 1921), results from cognitive distortions or faulty thinking. For example, a depressed person will selectively choose information that maintains a gloomy perspective. Depression is experienced when one has a negative schema about oneself or one's situation. According to Beck, depression is a behavioural response to an attitude or cognition of hopelessness, as opposed to hopelessness being a symptom of depression. Anxiety, he says, is experienced when the person has a distorted anticipation of danger. Treatment within Beck's model involves changing the person's views about themselves and their life situation (Beck 1972, Beck et al 2005).

Martin Seligman

Seligman (b. 1942) first proposed his theory of learned helplessness as an explanation for depression. The theory suggests that if an individual experiences adversity, and attempts to alleviate the situation are unsuccessful, then depression follows. Seligman later expanded his model to include learned optimism (Seligman 1994): a process of challenging negative cognitions to change from a position of passivity to one of control. He currently conducts research to investigate factors and circumstances that enable humans to *flourish*. Seligman's theoretical approach is called positive psychology (Seligman 2004, 2011).

Critique of cognitive psychology

The therapeutic techniques derived from cognitive (and cognitive behavioural) theory are practical and effective, and can be self-administered by the client under the direction of a therapist. These therapies have an established record in changing problem behaviours such as phobias, obsessions and compulsions, and in stress management (Butcher et al 2011). They also make a contribution in the treatment of depression and schizophrenia, though whether the treatment result is more effective than other interventions is inconclusive in the literature (Lynch et al 2010, Turkington et al 2004). Furthermore, cognitive theory is criticised as being unscientific (as are psychoanalytic and humanistic theories) because mental processes cannot be objectively observed and subjective reports are not necessarily reliable (Kring et al 2010). Additionally, the insight that one's thinking is the cause of one's problems will not in itself bring about behaviour change.

Finally, contrary to the proposal that *thoughts* influence *feelings*, which in turn influence *behaviour* (a notion that underpins the cognitive approach), research conducted by Kearns and Gardiner (2010) into procrastination and motivation among postgraduate university students suggests that if the behaviour is changed first – that is, the student starts working on their study – then the student will feel more motivated and procrastination will be reduced. These findings can be explained by the relational model of Ivey, Ivey and Zalaquett (2010) in which thoughts, feelings and behaviour interact with each other and with meaning, in contrast to the linear unidirectional explanation of cognitive psychology (see Ivey et al 2010 Fig 8.1). The thrust of the interactive model is that a change in any one part of the system may result in a change in other parts as well (Ivey et al 2010 p 294). So while cognitions play an integral part in behavioural outcomes, they may not necessarily be the initiating factor as proposed by cognitive theory.

HUMANISTIC PSYCHOLOGY

Following disenchantment with the existing psychological theories of the time, Charlotte Bühler, Abraham Maslow, Carl Rogers and their colleagues in the United States established the Association for Humanistic Psychology in 1962. Humanistic psychology has its intellectual and social roots in philosophical humanism and existentialism, which brought psychology back to a close relationship with philosophy (Bühler & Allen 1972). This school of psychology, which became known as the Third Force, arose in response to dissatisfaction at the time with the mechanistic approach of psychoanalysis and behaviourism and the negative views of humankind that were implicit in both these theoretical perspectives.

Humanist psychologists objected to the determinism of the two prevailing theories: psychoanalysis, with its emphasis on unconscious drives; and behaviourism, which saw the environment as central in shaping behaviour. Humanistic psychology rejected the reductionism of explaining human behaviour, feelings, thinking and motivation merely in terms of psychological mechanisms or biological processes. It also opposed the mechanistic approach of behaviourism and psychoanalysis for the way in which they minimised human experience and qualities such as choice, creativity and spontaneity.

Humanistic psychologists focused on the intrinsic human qualities of the individual, such as free will, altruism, self-esteem, freedom and self-actualisation, qualities which, they asserted, distinguished humans from other animals. Humanistic psychology therefore differed from its predecessors in its emphasis on the whole person, human emotions, experience and the meaning of experience, the creative potential of the individual, choice, self-realisation and self-actualisation. The theory also opposed dualistic (subject/object–mind/body splits), deterministic, reductionistic and mechanistic explanations of human behaviour.

The humanistic movement also reflected a historical trend in Western industrialised cultures at that time, namely an interest in the worth of the individual and the meaning of life and to be concerned about the rise of bureaucracy, the threat of nuclear war, the growing emphasis on scientific/positivist paradigms, alienation of the individual and consequent loss of individual identity in mass society. This led to humanistic psychology being aligned with the philosophical school of existentialism, as well as being associated with the human potential movements of the 1960s and 1970s, the legacy of which can be seen today in individual and group counselling approaches. Humanistic psychology also played a part in the growing interest in qualitative research methods (see Ch 6) that seek to understand the experience of the individual and the meaning of the experience, such as phenomenology. The following people were prominent figures in the development of humanistic psychology.

Charlotte Bühler

Bühler (1893–1974) distinguished her theory from Freudian psychoanalysis with the thesis that development was lifelong, goals were personally selected and that the individual was searching for meaning in life beyond their own existence. She maintained that self-fulfillment was the key to human development and that this was achieved by living constructively, establishing a personal value system, setting goals and reviewing progress to thereby realise one's potential. Throughout the lifespan, according to Bühler, individuals strive to achieve four basic human tendencies, which are to:

- satisfy one's need for sex, love and recognition
- engage in self-limiting adaptation in order to fit in, belong and feel secure
- express oneself through creative achievements
- uphold and restore order so as to be true to one's values and conscience (Bühler & Allen 1972, Ragsdale 2003).

Carl Rogers

Rogers (1902–1987) proposed a more hopeful and optimistic view of humankind than that of his psychoanalytic and behaviourist contemporaries. He believed that each person contained within themselves the potential for healthy, creative growth. According to Rogers, the failure to achieve one's potential resulted from constricting and distorting influences of poor parenting, education or other social pressures. Client-centred therapy is the counselling model that Rogers developed to assist the individual to overcome these harmful effects and take responsibility for their life (Rogers 1951, 1961).

Abraham Maslow

As a frequently cited author in the healthcare literature, Maslow (1908–1970) is renowned for his theory of human needs. Maslow, like Bühler and Rogers, premised his theory on the notion that human beings are intrinsically good and that human behaviour is motivated by a drive for self-actualisation or fulfillment. Maslow (1968) identifies three categories of human need:

- fundamental needs
    - physiological (hunger, thirst and sex)
    - safety (security and freedom from danger)

- psychological needs

    - belongingness and love (connection with others, to be accepted and to belong)

    - self-esteem (to achieve, be competent, gain approval and recognition)

- self-actualisation needs

    - to achieve one's innate potential (Gething et al 2004, Maslow 1968).

Typically, Maslow's needs are represented in a hierarchical pyramid with fundamental needs at the base of the triangle and self-actualisation at the top, although Maslow did not describe his model in this way, nor did he suggest that progression through the hierarchy was in one direction (i.e. ascending) as his model is often depicted. For example, one may have a positive sense of self (self-esteem needs met) but be vulnerable regarding safety needs during a natural disaster like a tsunami.

Critique of humanistic psychology

Intuitively, humanistic psychology appeals as a positive, optimistic view of humankind with its focus on personal growth, not disorder. However, this can also be a criticism in that, as a theory, humanistic psychology is naïve and incomplete. If humans are driven by a need to achieve their best and to live harmoniously with others as Bühler, Rogers and Maslow suggest, how does this account for disturbed states like depression or antisocial behaviour like assault? Humanistic concepts can be difficult to define objectively, thereby posing a challenge for scientific investigation of the theory. Finally, there is little recognition of unconscious drives in explaining behaviour, which limits the ability of the theory to contribute to an understanding of abnormal, deviant or antisocial behaviour.

ECLECTIC APPROACH

An eclectic or holistic approach is used in both psychological research and clinical practice. For example, initially Seligman's theory of learned helplessness (to explain depression) was underpinned by cognitive principles (Seligman 1974). However, as Seligman (2004, 2011) broadened his theory to seek explanations for *happiness and wellbeing*, and to establish a branch of psychology, which he called positive psychology, he integrated theoretical principles from cognitive psychology (e.g. focus on strengths, setting of achievable goals), humanistic psychology (e.g. the seeking of meaning) and sociology (e.g. the importance of relationships). Joseph, an advocate of such an approach states '[t]he convergence of interests between humanistic and positive psychology promises to provide new avenues for research and theory development' (Joseph 2008 p 223). Furthermore, in healthcare practice settings, biomedical and psychological interventions are frequently used concurrently to achieve better outcomes, as demonstrated in the following *Research focus*.

Research focus

Schramm, E., Schneider, D., Zobel, I., et al., 2008. Efficacy of interpersonal psychotherapy plus pharmacotherapy in chronically depressed inpatients. Journal of Affective Disorders 109 (1–2), 65–73.

ABSTRACT

Background

Clinical guidelines recommend the combination of pharmacotherapy and psychotherapy for treating chronic depression, although there are only a few studies supporting an additive effect of psychotherapy.

Methods

Forty-five inpatients with a chronic major depressive disorder were randomised to five weeks of either interpersonal psychotherapy (IPT) modified for an inpatient setting (15 individual and eight group sessions) plus pharmacotherapy or to medication plus clinical management (CM). The 17-item Hamilton rating scale for depression was the primary outcome measure. The study included a prospective naturalistic follow-up, three and 12 months after discharge.

Results

Intent-to-treat analyses revealed a significantly greater reduction of depressive symptoms, as well as better global functioning of patients treated with IPT compared with the CM group at week 5. Response and sustained response rates differed significantly between the two treatment conditions, favouring the IPT group. Remission rates were considerably higher for IPT patients who completed the treatment (67% compared with 32%). Patients who initially responded to IPT exhibited greater treatment gains at 12 months, since only 7% of these subjects relapsed compared with 25% of the CM subjects. In the long term additional IPT led to a lower symptom level and higher global functioning.

Limitations

The study uses data of a subset of patients from a larger trial. Both treatment groups did not receive comparable amounts of therapeutic attention. Extrapolating the data from this inpatient study to chronically depressed outpatients may not be possible.

Conclusions

Intensive combined treatment provides superior acute and long-term effects over standard treatment in chronically depressed inpatients.

SOCIOLOGICAL THEORIES

Sociological and psychological theories differ in that sociological theories do not seek explanations for individual behaviour; rather, they examine societal factors for their influence on the behaviour of its members (see Ch 5). Sociologists propose that the origin of behaviour (both normal and abnormal) lies not in the individual's mind but in the broader social forces of the society in which the individual lives. For example, demographic factors for which patterns of mental illness are observed include:

- *age* – the elderly are more likely to suffer from depression
- *gender* – the suicide rate for men is higher than for women, although the rate for attempted suicide is higher for women than for men
- *socioeconomic status* – poverty is associated with poorer physical and mental health outcomes
- *marital status* – depression and alcohol problems are two to three times more prevalent in people who have never married or are divorced than among people who are married (AIHW 2012, NZ Ministry of Health 2010).

The following social commentators propose interpretations of mental illness that challenge the notion of individual pathology.

Emile Durkheim

Durkheim's (1858–1917) classic study of suicide led him to postulate a societal rather than an individual explanation for this phenomenon. He argued that suicide was not an individual act but that it could be understood in terms of the bonds that exist between the person and society or the regulation of the individual by social norms. Durkheim's analysis of suicide statistics found that suicide was more prevalent in groups where the bond between the individual and the group was overly weak or strong, or where the regulation of individual desires and aspirations by societal norms was either inadequate or excessive. According to Durkheim there are four types of suicide:

- *egoistic* – where the social bonds of attachment are weak and the individual is less integrated into the social group and therefore not bound by its obligations (e.g. unmarried men)
- *altruistic* – where the social bonds of attachment are overly strong and the individual's sense of self is not distinguished from the group; the individual may be driven to suicide by a commitment to the group (e.g. suicide bombers)
- *anomic* – where regulation of the individual's desires and aspirations is not adequate: this can occur in a society undergoing rapid change, which dislocates social norms, as has been the experience of farmers who have had to adjust to the change in their economic circumstances as a result of the rural economic downturn
- *fatalistic* – where there is over-regulation by society that renders a sense of powerlessness in the individual and predisposes the person to suicide (e.g. deaths in custody) (Durkheim 1951).

Thomas Szasz

Since the 1960s prominent psychiatrist Thomas Szasz (1920–2012) challenged the concept of mental illness, arguing that disease implies a pathology that often cannot be objectively identified (Szasz 1961, 2000). He attacked the biomedical model, claiming that its purpose was to give control over people's lives to psychiatrists and argued that psychiatrists exercised coercive domination in the guise of protecting the public and the 'mad from their madness' (Szasz 2000 pp 44–45). Contrary to the illusion that psychiatry was coping well with society's vexing problems, Szasz claimed that social problems were in fact being obfuscated and aggravated by the disease interpretation of psychiatry (Szasz 2000 p 53).

Critique of sociological models

Sociological models identify social determinants of health (WHO 2008), vulnerable populations and health promotion opportunities (Navarro 2009), as well as biases that influence diagnosis and treatment. It is important to note, however, that although social determinants are associated with better or poorer health outcomes, the relationships are correlational and cannot be assumed to be in themselves causative. Nevertheless, the contribution of population statistics and social demographic data remains significant. By identifying social determinants that are associated with protective factors for mental health and risk factors for mental illness, potential areas for prevention and intervention are thereby identified. For example, the Australian Government's suicide prevention plan *Mental health: Taking action to tackle suicide* was developed in response to the Senate Committee's report, *The hidden toll: suicide in Australia*, which identified at risk population groups as 'Indigenous Australians; men; young people; gay, lesbian, bisexual and intersex communities; those bereaved by suicide; those living with mental health disorders and people living in rural areas' (Commonwealth of Australia 2010 p 1).

Personality theories and explanations of human behaviour

Table 1.2 outlines the key features of the major biomedical, psychological and sociological theories that propose explanations of human behaviour. These theories inform our understanding of ourselves and others and underpin interventions for health promotion, health behaviour change and treatments for mental illness.

Personality and behaviour: nature versus nurture

Who or what is responsible for personality and human development: heredity or the environment? Philosophers have long debated this issue, though scientific interest is more recent, dating from the work of Galton. Galton was a 19th-century British pioneer in the study of individual differences and is reportedly credited with proposing the immortal phrase *nature versus nurture* (Gottesman 1997, Schaffner 2001). The ensuing debate resulted in a proliferation of philosophical discussion about, and scientific investigation into, the effects of biological phenomena and inheritance (nature) and the individual's environment and experiences in the world (nurture).

Table 1.2

PERSONALITY THEORIES AND EXPLANATIONS OF HUMAN BEHAVIOUR

	Focus	Stage theory	Motivation	Individual control	Development explanation	Intervention
Biomedical	Physiological homeostasis/ pathology	No.	Physiological homeostasis	Internal Biological	Genetics Biological homeostasis/ pathology	Medication Physical treatments
Psychoanalytic	Unconscious processes	Yes. e.g. Freud, Erikson	Internal drives Seek pleasure	Internal Psychological	Stage progression Ego development	Psychoanalysis Insight therapy
Behavioural	Learning Environment	No. e.g. Pavlov, Skinner	Seek reinforcement Avoid punishment	External Psychological	Behaviours are learned through reinforcement, association or observation	Learn new behaviours Extinguish unwanted behaviour
Cognitive	Thinking Perception	Some no. e.g. Seligman, Bandura Some developmental e.g. Piaget	Thoughts and beliefs	Internal Psychological	Thoughts and beliefs influence feelings and behaviour	Cognitive restructuring/therapy including cognitive behavioural therapy, dialectical behavioural therapy
Humanistic	Self concept Self-actualisation	No. e.g. Maslow, Rogers	Meet needs Set goals Self-actualisation	Internal Psychological	Seek meaning Achieve goals Accomplishments	Find meaning or set achievable goals Client-centred therapy
Sociological	Social determinants Power Inequities	No. e.g. Marmot, Durkheim, Szasz	Social influences Power	External Social	Societal determinants influence health outcomes Notion of mental illness challenged	Social justice Economic and political reform

THEORETICAL PERSPECTIVES ON NATURE VERSUS NURTURE

The theories discussed in this chapter place varied emphasis on whether hereditary or environmental factors play a more important role in personality development, human behaviour and mental illness. Behavioural and cognitive psychology advocate for the environment and factors external to the individual being more influential, as does the sociological perspective, though for different reasons. The biomedical model argues for a nature explanation, while psychoanalytic theory and humanistic psychology acknowledge the contribution of both. The psychoanalytic concept of the id, for instance, is biological but it interacts with the environment in personality development. In humanistic psychology the need to achieve one's potential is considered to be innate, but the eventual outcome is influenced by the person's experiences in the world.

NATURE OR NURTURE?

There is an abundance of evidence to support an interactive explanation of nature and nurture rather than the answer being found in the either/or proposal (Gottesman 1991, Gottesman & Shields 1976, Hunter & Woodroofe 2005). Despite this, some commentators and theorists continue to advocate for the relative importance of one over the other, notably exponents of the biomedical model for nature and behaviourism for nurture.

Evidence to support a genetic or nature position can be found in family, twin and adoptee studies. Research over the past 20 years demonstrates that human behaviour, personality and mental illness do have a genetic component (Gottesman 1991, Gottesman & Shields 1976, Keshavan et al 2005). Findings from studies into the heritability of intelligence (IQ) offer the most convincing nature evidence. An American, British and Swedish study of 240 octogenarian twins found the heritability of IQ to be 62% (Gottesman 1997). In the Colorado Adoption Project a correlation was found between the IQ of adopted adolescents and their birth parents but no relationship was found between the IQ of adopted adolescents and their adoptive parents. The researchers concluded that the environment in which the young person was reared had little impact on cognitive ability.

In the case of schizophrenia, however, heredity accounts for less than 50% of the predictability of the disorder. Genetic inheritance is only a partial influence, with the environment accounting for the rest. Gottesman's research found that even when an identical twin had schizophrenia, the likelihood of the other twin not developing schizophrenia was 52% (Gottesman 1991). In addition, 63% of people with schizophrenia do not have a first- or second-degree relative with the condition (Schaffner 2001). It is clearly evident, therefore, that factors in addition to one's genetic inheritance influence whether the disorder manifests. Such factors, it is assumed, can be found in the environment.

Gottesman's research assumes that siblings reared together share the same environment. Schaffner (2001) recommends caution in presuming this, as different siblings in the same family do not necessarily experience exactly the same environment. Siblings do share many experiences, such as the same parents, social class and home environment; however, other experiences are unique to the individual and not shared by siblings. This non-shared environment can include such experiences as birth trauma, illness and different schooling. Significantly, it appears that it is the non-shared environment that accounts for most of the environmental influence on children's personality and mood (Santrock 2009) and that behaviour is a result of the interplay between the inherited characteristics and the environment rather than either/or (Rutter 2006).

NATURE AND NURTURE

An individual's personality does not develop without a genetic inheritance, nor can it develop in the absence of influences from experience and the environment. How, then, can the nature versus nurture debate be resolved?

Gestalt psychology, founded by Fritz Perls (1893–1970) in the 1960s, comprises humanistic and existentialist elements and offers a model for understanding the nature versus nurture debate – that is, to view personality development as a gestalt. There is no exact English equivalent for this German term but it loosely translates as 'a meaningful, organised whole' that is more than the sum of its parts (Perls et al 1973 p 16). Consider a cake, for example: flour, eggs, milk and sugar are its basic ingredients, but the product or gestalt bears no resemblance to any of the original ingredients. Yet each of the ingredients is vital to the final product, as is the process of cooking. Leave out the sugar and it will not taste like a cake; omit the heating process and it will not have the texture of a cake.

Considering human personality development as a gestalt means that neither nature nor nurture can be considered in isolation from the other. The process of their interaction and the context in which they interact are significant. Attributing a relative value of one over the other serves no purpose. Both nature and nurture are vital, inseparable, interdependent components of personality and human development that also influence human behaviour and health outcomes.

Conclusion

The theoretical perspectives discussed in this chapter provide complementary, overlapping and, at times, contradictory theories of human behaviour and personality development. Yet despite individual theories being able to provide plausible explanations for specific human behaviours, no theory alone is sufficient to explain all human behaviour or a single behaviour in all circumstances. Additionally, the theories must be used cautiously when being applied to people from non-Western cultures.

Some psychological theories offer a nature, others a nurture, explanation, and yet others incorporate both. Even when a specific theory provides convincing evidence to support a nature or nurture explanation, such evidence is generally correlational and therefore cannot be considered to be causative. Consequently, in seeking to identify factors that influence personality development and human behaviour, it is evident that the answer will not be found in asking the nature or nurture question; rather, in investigating how the nature is nurtured.

In conclusion, although psychological theories do have limitations, they nonetheless provide insightful understandings of human behaviour and explanations of personality in many contexts. These theories can be used by health professionals to understand the motivations and behaviours of the people they care for and to plan appropriate interventions and care. Furthermore, humans are biological beings who exist in a social context therefore psychological theories must be utilised within a biopsychosocial framework that also acknowledges these other influences.

Note: This chapter is an adaptation of Barkway P 2012 Ch 8, Beyond theory: Understanding theories of mental health and mental illness. In: Elder R, Evans K, Nizette D (eds) Practical perspectives in psychiatric and mental health nursing, 3rd edn. Elsevier, Australia.

REMEMBER

- Psychology is the scientific study of behaviour – particularly, but not exclusively, the study of human behaviour.
- Psychological theories offer competing and, at times, complementary explanations for human behaviour.
- Psychological theories are effective in explaining specific behaviours in specific circumstances but have limitations regarding global explanation for human behaviour.
- Psychological theory underpins therapeutic interventions in healthcare practice.
- Often human behaviour can be best understood by utilising an eclectic/holistic approach – that is, by taking into consideration biomedical, psychological and sociological factors (a biopsychosocial approach).

Classroom activity

1. Prior to beginning of the tutorial divide students into three groups. Ask students to find and bring to the tutorial articles that report on biomedical, psychological or combined (eclectic) approaches to managing one of the following health problems:
   - pain
   - chronic fatigue syndrome
   - anxiety.
2. Identify and discuss the key findings of the research.
3. Identify and discuss how theory informs the intervention.
4. Relate the discussion to the students' clinical practice experiences.

Classroom activity

1. For this activity, students should:
   - stand at the front of the class
   - move to the left if you think personality and human behaviour is most influenced by nature (genetics, biology) and move to the right if you think personality and human behaviour is most influenced by nurture (learning and experiences in the world)
   - pair up with a student holding the opposite view and explain your view to your partner.

2. Repeat this activity regarding your views about whether you think personality and human behaviour are:
   - constantly changing or essentially unchanging
   - influenced by past (history and experiences) or future events (goals and aspirations)
   - personal decisions (own values and ambitions) or social influences (family and societal values).

3. Reflection questions for the class:
   - What did you learn from this activity?
   - What was surprising about this activity?
   - What are the implications of
     » Working with other health professionals who hold different explanatory views to your own?
     » Caring for patients who hold different explanatory views to your own?

Further resources

Bandura, A. (Ed.), 2006. Psychological modeling: conflicting theories, second ed. Aldine Transaction, New Jersey.

Carducci, B., 2009. The psychology of personality: Viewpoints, research and application, second ed. Wiley-Blackwell, New York.

Germov, J. (Ed.), 2009. Second opinion: an introduction to health sociology, forth ed. Oxford University Press, Melbourne.

Kring, A., Johnson, S., Davison, G., et al., 2010. Abnormal psychology, eleventh ed. Wiley, New York.

Seligman, M., 2011. Flourish: a new understanding of happiness and well-being. Free Press, New York.

van Lange, P., Kruglanski, A., Higgins, E., 2012. Handbook of theories of social psychology, Vol. 1. Sage, London.

Weblinks

About.com: psychology theories

http://psychology.about.com/od/psychology101/u/psychology-theories.htm

This website provides an overview of the major psychological and developmental theories.

American Psychological Association

www.apa.org

This website contains useful information about psychology topics, publications and resources.

Authentic happiness

http://www.authentichappiness.sas.upenn.edu/Default.aspx

This website contains information about positive psychology, which focuses on the empirical study of wellbeing, positive emotions, strengths-based research.

The Australian Psychological Society

www.psychology.org.au

The Australian Psychological Society is the peak professional association for psychologists in Australia. The society's website contains information relevant to psychologists and health professionals and provides academic resources, publications and community information.

The New Zealand Psychological Society

www.psychology.org.nz

The New Zealand Psychological Society is the premier professional association for psychologists in New Zealand. The society's website contains information about the society, membership, services and publications, as well as acting as a gateway to psychology in New Zealand.

References

Australian Institute of Health and Welfare (AIHW), 2012. Australia's health 2012. AIHW, Canberra.

Bandura, A., 2012. Social cognitive theory, Ch 17. In: van Lange, P., Kruglanski, A., Higgins, E. (Eds.), 2012. Handbook of theories of social psychology, Vol. 1. Sage, London.

Bandura, A. (Ed.), 2006. Psychological modeling: conflicting theories, second ed. Aldine Transaction, New Jersey.

Bandura, A., 2001. Social cognitive theory. Annual Review of Psychology 52, 1–26.

Beck, A., 1972. Depression: causes and treatment. University of Pennsylvania Press, Philadelphia.

Beck, A., Emery, G., Greenberg, R.L., 2005. Anxiety disorders and phobias: a cognitive perspective. Basic Books, New York.

Bühler, C., Allen, M., 1972. Introduction to humanistic psychology. Brooks/Cole, California.

Butcher, J., Mineka, S., Hooley, K., 2011. Abnormal psychology: care concepts. Allyn & Bacon, Boston.

Cando, A., Gottesman, I.I., 2000. Twin studies of schizophrenia: from bow-and-arrow concordances to Star Wars Mx and functional genomics. American Journal of Medical Genetics 97 (1), 12–17.

Commonwealth of Australia, 2010. Commonwealth response to: The hidden toll: suicide in Australia. Commonwealth of Australia, Canberra. Online. Available: http://www.health.gov.au/internet/main/publishing.nsf/content/mental-pubs-c-commresp-suicide 24 Sep 2012.

Durkheim, E., 1951. Suicide: a study in sociology. The Free Press, New York.

Erikson, E., 1963. Childhood and society, second ed. WW Norton, New York.

Freud, A., 1966. The ego and the mechanisms of defence. International Universities Press, New York.

Gething, L., Papalia, D., Olds, S., 2004. Lifespan development, second Australian ed. McGraw-Hill, Sydney.

Gottesman, I., Shields, J., 1976. A critical review of recent adoption, twin and family studies of schizophrenia: behavioral genetics perspectives. Schizophrenia Bulletin 2 (3), 360–401.

Gottesman, I.I., 1991. Schizophrenia genesis: the origins of madness. Freeman, New York.

Gottesman, I.I., 1997. Twins: en route to QTLs for cognition. Science 277 (5318), 1522–1523.

Hunter, M., Woodroofe, P., 2005. History, aetiology and symptomatology of schizophrenia. Psychiatry 4 (10), 2–6.

Ivey, A., Ivey, M., Zalaquett, C., 2010. Intentional interviewing and counselling: facilitating client development in a multicultural society, seventh ed. Thompson Brooks/Cole, Pacific Grove.

Joseph, S., 2008. Humanistic and integrative therapies: the state of the art. Psychiatry 7 (5), 221–224.

Kearns, H., Gardiner, M., 2010. Waiting for the motivation fairy. Nature 472, 127.

Keshavan, M., Diwadkar, V., Montrose, D., et al., 2005. Premorbid indicators and risk for schizophrenia: a selective review and update. Schizophrenia Research 79 (1), 45–57.

Kring, A., Johnson, S., Davison, G., et al., 2010. Abnormal psychology, eleventh ed. Wiley, New York.

Lynch, D., Laws, K., McKenna, P., 2010. Cognitive behaviour therapy for major psychiatric disorders: does it really work? A meta-analytical review of well-controlled trials. Psychological Medicine 4, 9–24.

Maslow, A., 1968. Towards a psychology of being. Van Nostrand, New Jersey.

Navarro, V., 2009. What we mean by social determinants of health. International Journal of Health Sciences 39 (3), 423–441.

New Zealand Ministry of Health, 2010. Data and statistics. Online. Available: http://www.moh.govt.nz/moh.nsf/indexmh/dataandstatistics 24 Sep 2012.

Perls, F., Hefferline, R., Goodman, P., 1973. Gestalt therapy now: experiment and growth in the human personality. Pelican, London.

Ragsdale, S., 2003. Charlotte Malachowski Bühler, PhD (1893–1974). Online. Available: http://www.webster.edu/~woolflm/charlottebuhler.html 24 Sep 2012.

Rogers, C., 1951. Client-centered therapy. Houghton Mifflin, Boston.

Rogers, C., 1961. On becoming a person: a therapist's view of psychotherapy. Houghton Mifflin, Boston.

Rutter, M., 2006. Genes and behaviour: nature–nurture interplay explained. Blackwell, Boston.

Santrock, J., 2009. Life-span development, twelfth ed. McGraw-Hill, New York.

Schaffner, K., 2001. Nature and nurture. Current Opinions in Psychiatry 14 (5), 485–490.

Seligman, M., 1974. Depression and learned helplessness. In: Friedman, J., Katz, M. (Eds.), The psychology of depression: theory and research. Winston-Wiley, Washington.

Seligman, M., 1994. Learned optimism. Random House, Sydney.

Seligman, M., 2004. Authentic happiness: using the new positive psychology to realize your potential for lasting fulfillment. Free Press, New York.

Seligman, M., 2011. Flourish: a new understanding of happiness and well-being. Free Press, New York.

Skinner, B.F., 1953. Science and human behaviour. Macmillan, New York.

Szasz, T., 1961. The myth of mental illness. Harper & Row, New York.

Szasz, T., 2000. The case against psychiatric power. In: Barker, P., Stevenson, C. (Eds.), The construction of power and authority in psychiatry. Butterworth–Heinemann, Oxford.

Turkington, D., Dudley, R., Warman, D., et al., 2004. Cognitive-behavioral therapy for schizophrenia: a review. Journal of Psychiatric Practice 10, 5–16.

Watson, J., Rayner, R., 1920. Conditioned emotional reactions. Journal of Experimental Psychology 3 (1), 1–14.

World Health Organization (WHO), 2008. Closing the gap in a generation: health equity through action on the social determinants of health. WHO, Geneva. Online. Available: http://www.who.int/social_determinants/thecommission/finalreport/en/index.html 24 Sep 2012.

Chapter 2
Lifespan: The early years (birth to adolescence)

BERNARD GUERIN & PAULINE GUERIN

Learning objectives

The material in this chapter will help you to:

- describe some of the major developmental changes of infants, children and adolescents
  - » describe and critique the main theories of child development (Freud, Erikson, Piaget, Vygotsky)
  - » describe the main parenting styles and the influences on parenting
  - » describe how health professionals can adapt their practice when working with children at different ages and why this is important.

Key terms

- Lifespan development – early years
- Developmental theories
- Psychoanalytic theory
- Behaviourist theory
- Cognitive theory
- Sociocultural theory
- Parenting styles

Introduction

Numerous theories and stage models have been proposed to describe the years of life from birth to adolescence (e.g. Erikson 1959, 1963, Freud 1917, Piaget 1952, 1954, 1962, Vygotsky 1978). Rather than learn these exhaustively, it is more important to understand the broad changes that can be observed across these years. These observable changes are important for health professionals to consider when working with children.

If we were to compare a two-year-old child with a 12-year-old child we would find enormous differences in almost everything about their life situation and their behaviour. Researchers and theorists observe the changes in activities and processes that occur as children develop and then describe and explain them in various ways. The patterns that are thought to occur between these monumental differences prompt researchers to develop and propose their theories, and when they observe patterns of change they propose stage models.

Clearly, there are many changes taking place as a child develops including physical, emotional, cognitive, social and psychological changes. All of these changes ('developments') occur within historical and cultural contexts that also influence development. While this may seem obvious, it was not that long ago that children were viewed as 'little adults' with the same cognitive, emotional and psychological abilities of adults, although without all the physical abilities (Aries 1962). Theorists have attempted to simplify the many details of changes throughout childhood and adolescence and to describe and explain how the changes take place. How these theorists have attempted to do this has varied because they have focused on different aspects of development.

In this chapter the focus is on the social and psychological aspects of development. The biological or physical development of children is a large field that, due to improvements in technology, is changing drastically and is therefore not discussed in this chapter. Students with particular interest in biological development might like to read Gottesman and Hanson's review article (2005) or Stiles' (2011) article that discusses the nature versus nurture debate and contemporary understandings of brain development.

When learning about developmental theories, avoid focusing solely on learning the theories; it is important to learn what the theorists were observing, reacting to and trying to describe or explain in their theories. To help with this, complete *Classroom activity, Exercise 1*.

Classroom activity

Before reading about the various theories of child development, sit down in groups and pool your knowledge from everyday life of what children are able to accomplish. Try dividing your collective experience into categories of:

- birth to 1 year old
- 1–3 years old
- 3–6 years old
- 6–10 years old
- 10–15 years old.

EXERCISE 1

Each person considers their own experiences with children and identifies for each age group:

- what children are able to accomplish (what they can do at this age)
- what children cannot accomplish (what they can't do at this age)
- what main patterns and activities change as children get older
- what triggers or brings about the changes
- in what ways children rely on others around them to do what they do.

EXERCISE 2

If you need more structure, consider that theorists have often broken behaviour patterns into:

- physical changes of the body
- physical skills or behaviours
- thinking and talking (cognitive) skills
- social skills
- emotional or interpersonal influence skills.

Outline the changing patterns you have observed across age groups in these five domains.

EXERCISE 3

For this book we are especially interested in health. Think again about each age group and discuss:

- What are the main health challenges at this age?
- What healthy and unhealthy patterns might children have at this age?
- What health knowledge or discussions about health would this age group have?
- From where would children get this health knowledge?
- Who would usually take responsibility for the child's health at this age?

Theorising about development

Having completed *Classroom activity, Exercise 1* you are hopefully devising your own ideas and theories about what changes between these age groups. There are many ways to categorise theories: reductionistic, mediational, deterministic, essentialistic, causal, contextual, explanative or descriptive. A *reductionistic theory*, or *reductionism*, is a theory in which complex things are reduced or understood in terms of basic, simplified elements. For example, risk-taking behaviour among adolescents would be understood in terms of brain development in a reductionistic theory. Specifically, research has shown that the prefrontal cortex, which is considered to be the site of higher order cognitive functioning (i.e. the ability to think things through), is not yet fully developed in adolescents (Nelson & Guyer 2011).

A *mediational theory* is similar to reductionism but the key element in mediationism is that a behaviour or concept is *mediated* by something else. Using again the example of adolescent risk taking, a mediationist would say that brain development *mediates* risk-taking behaviour. Another example would be that an adolescent who is observed to be sleeping excessively, lacks interest in things they used to enjoy and spends a lot of time alone, might then be considered to be depressed, such that depression is then the mediator of these behaviours. This is an important distinction because it influences how we then go about intervening or what we do to change the behaviour. Do we change the sleeping, lack of interest, the time spent alone, or the depression?

Determinism is a theoretical approach in which the behaviour we observe is determined by past history: history of relationships (e.g. parental relationships in the case of Freud) or the history of consequences of behaviours (in the case of the behaviourism of B F Skinner, discussed later). Using the above examples, risk-taking behaviour may be explained in a deterministic way by referring to the history of consequences of behaviour, specifically that risk-taking behaviour has been positively reinforced, perhaps by getting attention. In contrast, *essentialism* views characteristics of groups (e.g. groups based on ethnicity, gender or age) as fixed or unchangeable, therefore risk taking by adolescents would be seen as an *essential quality* or characteristic among adolescents that is not changeable or influenced by context.

Causal and *contextual* theorising can be understood by contrasting them. Causal theories look to understand exactly what it is that *causes* what we observe while a contextual theory looks to understand the *contexts* in which those behaviours emerge. Again, for adolescent risk-taking behaviour, we could say that brain development causes risk taking or, contextually, that risk-taking behaviour is more likely to occur in groups of youth in unsupervised situations, for example.

Finally, *explanative* or *descriptive* theories can also be understood by contrasting them. They are similar to causal and contextual theorising, with an explanative theory similar to causal explanations and descriptive theories similar to contextual explanations. Using the depression example, we could refer to physiological deficits (e.g. low serotonin levels) to *explain* why an adolescent is depressed, or we could describe the contexts (especially social ones) in which depressive behaviours are more or less likely to occur, such as a lack of social support.

These theoretical approaches are not mutually exclusive and refer to different perspectives. Most theorists develop a view based on their own experiences and understandings in the same way you did in your first *Classroom activity*.

In this chapter we will refer to only one major difference between theories: whether changes that arise with age are explained by something *within* the person and their body (reductionism, mediationism, essentialism) or by forces *outside* of the person (contextualism or determinism). While many theorists today combine theories and do not rely exclusively on one or the other, this distinction will help to understand what the original theorists observed and were trying to explain.

DEVELOPMENTAL THEORISTS

Sigmund Freud is probably best known for his theories of psychoanalysis, but he also developed a theory of psychosexual development where he suggested that events that occurred in childhood *determined* behaviour patterns later in life (Freud 1917, also see Ch 1). In his clinical practice, Freud talked extensively with many hundreds of people and believed that there was a pattern in which particular events in people's early history contributed to the kind of person they would become. Freud believed that key events in childhood, such as learning to control eating, drinking and defecating ('potty training'), learning about genitals and learning the rules about them ('you will be punished if you touch them'), and learning about family control were the most important factors contributing to personality development. Specifically, Freud suggested five stages of psychosocial development: oral, anal, phallic, latency and genital, and that these stages corresponded with age, from birth to death.

Very simply put, Freud's experience with people suggested that these key events in childhood could lead to various peculiarities that he could detect when talking to people with serious clinical issues later in life. For example, Freud suggested that an adult who was very obsessive would have had trouble relating to 'potty training'. If a person's obsessiveness became serious to a clinical extent then Freud's psychoanalysis would involve talking about obsessiveness as well as their early childhood history (including 'potty training') in therapy sessions.

Freud's theorising about adult behaviour, and that it was influenced by earlier childhood experiences, was actually quite revolutionary at that time. While the particulars of Freud's theories have not been supported with rigorous research, there is no doubt that Freud's theories have had a huge impact on Western society. Consider the popularised use of phrases like 'anal retentive' to label someone with obsessive qualities as described above, or even the use of 'Freudian slip' to describe verbal faux pas usually with sexual connotations. As we will see later, Erik Erikson also followed through with psychoanalytic theory but made the social dimension much larger than just the family circle.

Burrhus Frederick Skinner (Fred) (1938, 1957, 1969) was a famous psychologist who mainly worked with animals. What he found fascinating was that changing minute details of an animal's environment or context (primarily its cage and the lights and switches in its cage) could control how the animal behaved. Skinner's theory, known as *radical behaviourism*, includes and elaborates on the basic concepts of antecedents (environments, contexts or stimuli), behaviour and consequences (what

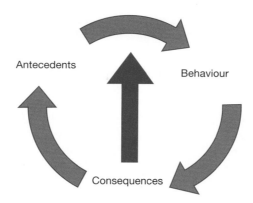

Figure 2.1 How antecedents (or the environment) can influence behaviour, leading to consequences

happens when a behaviour occurs). For example, rats that had to press a lever (behaviour) more than once to get food (consequences) when a light was on (antecedent or stimuli) would persist in pressing the lever longer when the food supply was stopped compared with those rats that received food on every press they made. Skinner was impressed that small and not easily observed changes in an animal's environment could make a large difference to its behaviour. Figure 2.1 illustrates how antecedents (or the environment/context) can influence behaviour that then leads to a consequence. These consequences contribute to both changing the environment, and changing behaviour in a circular pattern.

These observations led Skinner to advocate a theory that almost all behaviour was determined or controlled by factors in the environment rather than something that seemed to be 'stored' inside the body or that was 'made into your personality' (i.e. Freud's approach or mediationism). Skinner found that he could change the environment for his animals and watch their behaviour change subtly and in precise and predictable ways. This means that for any behaviour changes observed, we need to examine and describe the environment or context very carefully for the details that might be controlling that change or influencing the behaviours observed.

When applying this to humans, opinions are divided. One perspective is that such environmental factors do not apply to humans since we often complete actions although nothing can be found in the environment that might have changed. The other perspective says that we are not looking hard enough for these factors and that they might be observable but have occurred in the earlier history. For example, using the depression example above, we might not be able to see anything in the immediate environment that can explain the behaviour, so we say that the person is 'depressed', but it may be that past events contributed to the development of depression and that other factors then contribute to the maintenance of the behaviours we then call 'depression'. According to Skinner, it would be possible (although often very difficult) to discover environmental changes that contribute to all human behaviour.

Skinner's work and observations with children and humans was mostly in relation to his own children. Perhaps his best known work with children was his development of an air crib for his own child. Skinner believed that a highly controlled environment would eliminate the mundane tasks of baby care such as keeping them warm and clean. In this way, parents could more effectively (and would have more time to) engage in other aspects of parenting such as playing and reading.

The original testing ground for Skinner's ideas about human behaviour involved looking at what controls our talking and use of language (Skinner 1957). While some researchers stated that no observable environmental changes could be seen when children start talking or using language Skinner's response was that they had not been looking in the right places. His ideas about environmental influences on language development and use were not well received (e.g. Chomsky 1959); however, newer versions of Skinner's ideas have been developed (Andresen 1990, Catania 1997, Hayes et al 1994).

Watch it on YouTube! See a short video about B F Skinner at <http://www.youtube.com/watch?v=mm5FGrQEyBY>.

Jean Piaget (1952, 1954, 1962) was the most famous psychologist to consider how children think (cognition) and speak (language). In contrast to Skinner, he was not looking for environmental influences but was more interested in theoretical ideas of 'information processing' centres and 'cognitive processes' in the brain.

Like both Freud and Skinner, Piaget spent a lot of time observing behaviour, particularly by participating in thinking games with children, which contributed to the development of his theories. Regardless of the theory or issue under consideration, understanding children requires spending a lot of time systematically observing and participating with them.

Piaget observed that children of different ages think in very different ways from each other. What he saw was not a continuum of thinking from simple to complex but a set of stages (see Table 2.1 for a summary). For example, he observed that very young children did not seem to be able to think in terms of causality – that one event can cause another event. It was not that the children had different causes for the same event but, rather, they did not seem to be able to think in terms of causes at all. He surmised that causality was *not thinkable* below a certain age. Piaget observed

Table 2.1		
PIAGET'S STAGES OF COGNITIVE DEVELOPMENT		
Approx. age	**Stage**	**Description**
Birth–2 years	Sensorimotor	An infant understands the world through senses (sensori) and movement (motor)
2–7 years	Preoperational	A child begins to use words and symbols to make sense of the world
7–11 years	Concrete operational	Reason is used to logically make sense of concrete events in the world and to classify objects
11–15 years through adulthood	Formal operational	Reasoning becomes more abstract, logical, and idealistic

that older children start to explain what caused events, naming events and objects that might have caused something else and trying to justify the way things occurred the way they did.

These observations led Piaget to argue for a stage model in which children learn more and more complex ways of thinking whereby they are not able to think in one level until they have achieved the level before that in the sequence. He also argued that once a certain stage of thinking was reached this had consequences for what the child could accomplish and would lead to new ways of communicating or thinking. For example, once a child could think in terms of causality, then they could think in terms of making excuses and getting themselves out of trouble. 'I only did it because Giles told me to' requires a level of causal thinking before it can be thought at all.

While Piaget described a number of stages and substages of cognitive development, we focus here on the broader overall changes he described and not the complex details of these stages. Table 2.1 shows the basic stages, the approximate ages associated with those stages and a brief description. (You may like to refer to a developmental psychology textbook such as Peterson 2009 for more detailed versions.) The first broad stage Piaget called *sensorimotor* because children at this age think, as it were, through their senses and their physical movements. Something like, 'If I can't see it, taste it or touch it then it does not exist and I cannot think it!'. Children explore and learn only what they physically interact with through their senses. At this stage, children cannot 'think' about a cat being somewhere else if it is not in front of them, or they are not touching it, or they do not have its tail in their mouth.

CASE STUDY: SOPHIE

Four-year-old Sophie is brought to the paediatric plastic surgery clinic by her mother after being referred by her GP for a cyst under her right eyebrow that has been present for approximately four months. The referral letter indicates Sophie's anxiety in attending medical appointments and the GP and nurses' inability to examine the cyst as a result (she kicks and screams when approached). When the mother and Sophie are called in to see the specialist, he addresses the mother and asks her to tell him about why they are there. While the mother explains about the cyst, Sophie begins to get upset. He tries to look at the cyst, telling the mother to hold Sophie still, and Sophie's discomfort escalates, such that he cannot examine her. The specialist tells the mother that she will need to reschedule the appointment and 'have a talk' with Sophie about how to behave when she comes to see the doctor. The specialist has not looked at the cyst above Sophie's eye, nor has he communicated with Sophie during the consultation.

Critical thinking

- Consider:
  - » Sophie's age and her social and emotional development and how the social, emotional and cognitive domains influence her behaviour
  - » the contextual factors that may influence the mother and how she does or does not respond in the situation.
- What factors are influencing the specialist and his behaviour?
- How might you approach working with Sophie and her mother in a consultation that considers the social, emotional, and cognitive elements?
- Are there other factors that influence the people in this scenario?

At the *preoperational* stage children begin to attribute words to the things around them and use those words, but this stage is 'pre' operational, with 'operational' referring to 'logic'. This is not just being able to reliably say a sound when something is there, as even very young children can say 'caaa' when a cat is presented. It is the beginning of 'representing' things by words so that the child can also say 'caaa' when the cat's box is there or 'caaa' when a parent gets the cat's food out of the cupboard.

One interesting thing Piaget found for children at an early age was that if, say, a cat was hidden under a blanket, the child would act as if the cat had gone for good and was no longer in existence – 'out of sight, out of mind'. However, as a child developed, they began to look under the blanket for the cat – that is, the object has permanence even if it cannot be seen. Piaget called this developmental aspect *object permanence*. Around the same time children would also begin using the word 'caaa' in the preoperational sense explained above. These were the sorts of real changes Piaget noted from his extensive observations and that he was trying to capture in his theories and stages.

From this preoperational stage of beginning to 'see things that are not immediately there' and being able to talk about things not in front of them, children then develop the ability to reason and to classify and code. In the *concrete operational* stage children begin to use logical forms of reasoning (note that there are several main systems of logic, not just one) and to classify things into groups based on characteristics. However, these processes are only for concrete things and events, such as 'my trucks' or 'Gracie got an ice cream, why can't I have one?' rather than anything more abstract.

The ability to complete complex tasks or abstract ways of thinking arise in the *formal operational* stage in which abstract thinking is possible and can be used in reasoning and logical processes. Piaget, as well as other child development researchers, devised a number of tests to determine development at this stage and it is not so much the resolution to these tests that is important but, rather, how children come up with the resolution. For example, to combine a yellow solution with a blue solution to create a green solution, a child in the concrete operational stage may, through trial and error, mix the solutions together. However, a child in the formal operational stage may use logic to come up with the answer before using trial and error.

Typically, the ages associated with these stages are: *sensorimotor* 0–2 years, *preoperational* 2–7 years, *concrete operational* 7–11 years and *formal operational* 11–adulthood. However, these have been found to vary depending upon the education system and the context of the child and, indeed, not everyone may reach every stage. What is important is that vast changes are taking place in the very way children think and talk about things through these ages and this is what Piaget observed through intense observations and then tried to put into a formal theoretical structure. For us, whether the latter is exactly correct or not is not so important and learning the real changes is what matters most.

Piaget consistently focused his observations and theorising on individual children and the ways that they were thinking and talking about events. He treated the stages he saw as changes in internal information processing or the 'structure' of cognition. Later theorists spent more time in those same situations but focused on how the children's social interactions influenced the 'individual cognitive' abilities (Bruner 1973). As we will see Vygotsky, Bruner and others showed there was a 'social scaffold' that supported 'cognitive' development.

Box 2.1 Children talking about health

It is worth learning about the limitations of children's talk and thinking since we often attribute too much logic to what children say. Children can talk as if they are saying complicated and wise things, but they often have no real conception of the meaning or consequences.

This might be keywords they have picked up before they really know how to use them. As an example, a doctor might ask if the child has 'constipation' and the child knows the word means something and answers either yes or no. Further questioning will show whether or not the child actually knows the meaning of constipation. You can even ask fictitious concepts to check out how likely the child will answer something when they are not sure: 'And have you been feeling soppid pains?'.

Once the child gets to an *operational* stage in Piaget's framework, another problem occurs. In those stages (and into adulthood) the words become more abstract and disconnected from any sort of reality. While this is good, for example, in that we can talk about a cat without it being present, the problem when talking about health is that what a child says can be determined by social influences as much as the so-called reality of what is being talked about. So the answer to a question such as whether there has been constipation, even if understood properly, is now subject to a variety of influences. In the extreme, imagine the child answering that question in front of a group of peers, or their parents, or just alone with a doctor. Regardless of the truth, we would get strategically different answers even if the answers are all basically saying yes: 'Sort of…', 'Just a little', 'A little but it was quickly over', 'Not really', or 'Would that be normal?'.

So when working with children at early ages, health professionals need to be very careful about how and when questions are asked, in the earlier case because the child might respond quite happily without really knowing the

Cont… ▶

answer, and in the later case because of extraneous but strong influences over what they say since it is no longer fully determined by concrete objects.

In all cases, the best strategy for the health professional is to ask questions more than once in very different ways, and ask in different contexts if that seems to be a problem.

Lev Vygotsky (1978), a Russian theorist in the early 1900s, was the first of a series of theorists who, like Skinner, explored the environmental or external factors that control the changes that appeared to occur 'within' the child. However, it is interesting that Vygotsky was not familiar with Skinner's work even though it came earlier and that Vygotsky's work was not known in English-speaking countries until much later.

The important contribution that Vygotsky made to our understanding of human development was that the 'hidden' environmental factors that bring about developmental changes but that are hard to see are *social* ones. That is, he suggested that the internal cognitive changes and stages depend upon social relationships – hence, his theory is known as a *sociocultural* theory or a constructivist theory. The idea was that the 'mind' and the 'cognitive processes' were in fact controlled by social factors that were very subtle and not easy to observe unless you observed closely and over a long period. According to this line of thinking, the mind is not inside the body but, rather, it is a name for processes of social interaction that cannot be directly seen and that occur over time.

Watch it on YouTube! You can hear a brief description of Vygotsky's theory:

Vygotsky's developmental theory: An introduction at <http://www.youtube.com/watch?v=hx84h-i3w8U&feature=related>.

Vygotsky did not theorise about children 'having' or 'possessing' skills (whether physical or cognitive), nor did he talk or theorise about children learning to think in 'stages' set apart from their social interactions, conversations, modelling and other social experiences. Instead, Vygotsky wrote about how children think in the context of development, especially in the social context. This idea of considering the social influences on what seem to be purely 'internal' thinking events has been developed in various ways. For example, some researchers have looked for patterns in social relationship thinking that facilitate thinking about causality or mathematics. Researchers have also looked at how social support, encouragement or training facilitates cognitive thinking. Psychologists still have some way to go in describing the finer details of these approaches (see Guerin 2001, 2004).

Vygotsky's ideas often become clearer to people in the context of his notion of Zone of Proximal Development (ZPD). Rather than conceiving of children reaching new stages of cognition as a result of changes taking place inside them somewhere, Vygotsky proposed that the changes occur within interactions with other people, through processes of imitation, cooperation, support, guidance and enrichment. If children act totally alone then there are many things they cannot do and cannot easily learn to do – this is the lower limit to the ZPD. If children act with other people in concert, or with support, they can do a lot of things by accepting the other person's responsibility and help – this is the upper limit of the ZPD.

Therefore, there are skills children learn through others and, perhaps, when they are not present, they can no longer do those skills. For example, a child may learn how to turn on the computer and open the program to play their favourite game when she is with her older brother and in response to his prompting, but later she may not be able to recall all the necessary steps to play the game when he is not there. Eventually, as people get older, they can do more without other people's direct involvement. But this Vygotskian way of thinking means that skills are not absolute, all-or-none possessions that once gained cannot be lost. We lose skills as well as develop them and we have a variable set of skills that we sometimes have and sometimes do not have.

We can apply these ideas to children and physical activity, and how behaviour can change depending on the people the children are with and the contexts. For example, learning to ride a bike may develop with help from parents or older siblings. Riding without training wheels may start with someone holding onto the seat and letting go when the rider is not aware, but this skill may depend on the presence of others until the skill refines. Eventually, riding a bike may develop into very complex skills such as riding with friends at a bike park. But, after not riding a bike for a long time, a child would not be able to go straight back to the bike park and perform all the tricks again. Even though we may be able to ride a bike even after a long period of not riding one, some of the finer skills would require practise to re-learn.

The Vygotskian answer to the question of 'What cognitive stage is that child up to?' is: 'Well, it depends on who that child has been interacting with and has been supported by. By themselves they might not be showing too many thinking skills, but when interacting with a parent or a favourite carer or teacher they might show remarkable cognitive prowess'. In essence, the answer is in the environment (social environment), not inside the child.

Some recent approaches to describing human development have set similar ideas within *multidimensional* approaches. This means that human biology, social factors, psychological factors, spirituality, structural issues and culture are all considered when trying to understand human development (Harms 2005). Some call these approaches biopsychosocial models, ecological approaches or contextual approaches. What they all try to encapsulate is that human development is obviously made up of lots of changes, that most of the determinants of these changes are difficult to observe easily and that the changes all involve the body, the environment and the social world. Psychologists do not yet know how these elements might all fit together, but these approaches suggest that all of these elements are necessary ingredients.

OVERALL DEVELOPMENT

Much of the theorising and research discussed in this chapter revolves around the development of thinking and social relationships. Others have characterised the whole development sequence through the use of stages. Sometimes this is called *lifespan development* (e.g. Santrock 2008). In this regard it is worth looking at the model of **Erik Erikson**, since he also proposed a very different and interesting stage theory of development.

Instead of proposing a series of stages that all people purportedly travel through, Erikson suggested a series of life conflicts, tasks or issues that are dealt with at

Box 2.2 How health professionals can utilise Piaget and Vygotsky

Piaget's observations might suggest that the health professional be cautious about asking too much of children in thinking through issues about health. Until the *operational* stages children are unlikely to have the reasoning skills to understand causes of health and illness, or the classificatory skills to position various symptoms or illnesses. As mentioned earlier, children can give the impression of performing these skills when they are not. Bibace and Walsh (1980) applied Piaget's concepts to children's concepts of illness and a body of research in this area has followed (e.g. Lin et al 2008, Olson et al 2007).

Piaget's ideas might lead one to only explain health to children depending on their cognitive stage, or to not try to get children to talk about health in more and more sophisticated ways. From a Vygotskian perspective, for children to learn and extend their skills they rely on social scaffolding from others around them: siblings, parents, carers and teachers. Instead of assuming a child is at a certain stage and cannot go beyond it, Vygotsky's theories remind us that there is a range of skills the child is learning, from easy skills they can do themselves at the lower limit of their ZPD, to skills they can do but only with direct guidance from others.

This suggests that it is worth pursuing conversations about health with children in both simple and more complex ways and that this will be what stretches the child's abilities and development. One should not expect children's reasoning and causal thinking to be sophisticated, but one can certainly encourage and guide more skills. Consider children with chronic illnesses such as cancer who, over repeatedly engaging in the treatment process, develop a complex understanding of their illness way beyond what might be expected in Piaget's theory.

different ages. These conflicts can result in good outcomes or poor outcomes depending upon the environment and the previous history of the individual. He proposed eight stages from infancy through to late adulthood (60 years old and beyond). Only the first five that are relevant to childhood development are discussed in this chapter; however, all of the stages are included in Table 2.2 because they will be considered in Chapter 3.

Notice that this sequence includes development relevant to family social relationships, cognitive development and friendship. This was shown through the ideas of Vygotsky and others, where being able to function successfully in social relationships is a prerequisite for any 'cognitive' or 'mind' development. Therefore, working in normal relations will facilitate the ZPD and lead to improvement in all theories that have been discussed in this chapter.

During infancy, according to Erikson, the main hurdle is to develop a basic sense of trust in people and the world, rather than to develop a general mistrust. He proposed that an optimal social environment or context would result in a person who will generally trust that their needs will be met and have confidence in themselves

Table 2.2	
ERIKSON'S DEVELOPMENTAL STAGES	
Erikson's stages	**Developmental stage (age)**
Trust versus mistrust	Infancy (first year)
Autonomy versus shame and doubt	Late infancy (years 1–3)
Initiative versus guilt	Early childhood (years 3–5)
Industry versus inferiority	Middle and late childhood (years 6 to puberty)
Identity versus identity confusion	Adolescence (years 10–20)
Intimacy versus isolation	Early adulthood (20s, 30s)
Generativity versus stagnation	Middle adulthood (40s, 50s)
Integrity versus despair	Late adulthood (60s onwards)

and the world they are in. In a social environment where an infant's needs are not met, then Erikson believed this child would develop to generally mistrust the world and the people around them and therefore not be willing to risk events with other people. This would mean that opportunities would be lost. It is not so much mistrusting that is the problem but the opportunities for further development that get restricted if a basic trust in people and the world is not present.

Later in infancy and toddlerhood, the task is for the child to begin acting independently and to be less reliant upon parents and others. This was characterised as a conflict between autonomy and shame or doubt, but the same thing can apply without those latter terms. A child who is too dependent might not develop self-doubt or shame, especially considering they are aged under three years at this point, but they still have not managed an important skill in the context of their future development; shame and doubt could develop as a consequence.

Similar comments apply to the stage in early childhood. The basic idea is that the child needs to have a context in which they can show initiative and start events by themselves. They need to get up in the morning, sometimes get food without asking or being told to, and need to initiate games and peer interaction. If this does not occur for the child, once again, numerous cognitive and social opportunities for further skill development will be missed. Though, as mentioned, we do not necessarily have to agree that the lack of initiative necessarily leads to guilt. A child might not even be aware or be able to verbalise what is going on if this contextual skill development is missed. But the basic process is still important and necessary for further development.

Erikson's fourth life task is the development of 'industry', meaning that things get done. The child is able to execute tasks. This includes all the cognitive, logical, social and other skills discussed in this chapter. Inability to do this is characterised as inferiority but, once again, we might temper this and say that children might grow up with different ideas of what they can and cannot do. Certainly in some circumstances this would lead to what is called a sense of inferiority but not in all cases. Some might accept (unwittingly) that this is just how things are and others might feel 'safer' not attempting everything.

Finally, adolescence is said to be characterised by the development of a sense of identity or a sense of identity confusion. This can have a couple of meanings. First, it can refer to the ways we learn to talk about ourselves to ourselves and others and what talk we can get away with. Are others agreeable with how we talk about who we think we are and what we can do? Second, it can mean a sense of taking on more adult-like roles and responsibilities and whether we do a good job – what special and unique things can I do and take responsibility for? Basically, how we talk about ourselves is related to whether we are good at doing these jobs and taking on responsibility.

SUMMARY OF DEVELOPMENTAL THEORIES

Key theorists have all spent extensive time observing behaviour or interacting with people; their theories were attempts to describe systematically the changes in development that they had observed, however biased or selective we might now view these to be. Some theorists emphasised that changes resulted from environmental changes, some from internal cognitive changes or biology and others tried to meld these two perspectives together. Perhaps the most useful approaches consider social influences as the key in understanding developmental changes because these are things that are observable or can change.

Major influences on developmental changes

In this section, we focus on some of the main influences on child development. There are obvious key events and people that influence children as they grow older. Most children in developed countries are given a long and complex education of some sort or another and this must impact on how they change. Children are exposed to family, friends and communities, and this exposure also impacts on how children change. There is also a huge array of media events that impact on children from television to computers, and from MP3 players to mobile phones.

PARENTS, FAMILY AND COMMUNITY

It is often assumed that parents comprise a major determinant of children's development. Freud, Skinner and ecological approaches would all suggest that parents are a major influence in the child's environment and surely influence development. However, there are two limitations to the view that parents are a major determinant of children's development. First, parent-centred life for children is not universal around the world or even within countries. For many children, parents are busy working and children spend more time with an extended family or with others in their wider community. The image in Western, English-speaking communities is that families comprise one or two parents and their children in a house (i.e. the 'nuclear' family) who make visits to other houses that contain relatives and family friends. However, many children spend a lot of time – or even live with – their grandparents or uncles and aunts, or even with strangers. In China, in fact, children as young as two from affluent families may board in childcare centres and only see their parents on the weekends (Brassard & Chen 2005). Most research, though, has focused on families in Western societies and the influence of parents. Whatever the findings, parents may have different impacts in the hugely diverse range of family and community settings.

Second, researchers are not unanimous in declaring parents a major influence (Collins et al 2000, Harris 1995). Research of this nature is very difficult to arrange so that clear answers are produced. We have to decide whether the evidence is that parents are not greatly influential over children or whether the research has not been done properly because of the difficulties in setting up such research. Showing whether a behaviour is primarily due to genetics or to the environment is not a simple dichotomous question and no methodology is straightforward. Let us outline both sides of the story.

Harris (1995) considered several lines of research to explore the case for parents having little or no influence on their children. For example, while twin studies show that twins reared apart are more different than those raised together (suggesting that the environmental factors such as parents are highly influential) it was pointed out that even identical twins reared together in the same home with the same parents are very different in many ways. News stories have focused on a few examples of twins amazingly liking or doing similar things that are unusual despite being reared apart, such as both wearing rubber bands on their wrists or reading magazines from back to front (Dowling 2004), but these cases are not common over the whole population. This suggests that environmental factors other than the parents are playing a major role in development. Harris argued that adolescent groups and friendships play a greater role in developmental changes, rather than the home environment of the parents.

Collins et al (2000) examined the quality of the research being cited. They suggested a greater role for parents than Harris (1995) but also argued that many of the research methods were flawed or had limitations. They worked within the types of ecological or biopsychosocial theories described earlier and identified roles for genetics, parents and peers.

Collins et al (2000) also pointed out that even if you show influences from peers, it takes a special research methodology to determine whether that peer influence was moderated by the parents in the first place. It could be that a child is influenced by peers at school but that the context for being influenced in such a way was produced by the parents (Hayes et al 2004). Similarly, Bamberg et al (2001) suggest that parents influence this selection of peers because adolescents who have parents who frequently smoke or drink alcohol are more likely to choose to associate with peers who display these behaviours. This is saying that there can still be a parental influence on children even if the children seem to be influenced by their friends, since the parents might facilitate or inhibit the children's receptivity to peer influence, or at least to certain types of peers. A child could be influenced by a peer at school, but the parental influence on friend selection might have encouraged their child to make friends with just that sort of peer. For example, a parent may tell a child, 'Only play with the nice boys when you get to school. Okay, Vincent?', or they may influence friend selection through their own networks such as by only inviting children of parents that they know over to play. This is shown more in the following sections.

In summary, children's development is influenced by parents, families, peers and communities but there is no single model for how much these play a role in all instances. As mentioned, communities and families are highly diverse, with some built on the nuclear family model and others with extended families and communities. Also, the many pathways through which parents, families and peers influence development are not clear and different contexts will produce different mixes of these. A single model of parental influence on children should perhaps not be expected.

Box 2.3 So, what makes good parenting?

This is a vexing question that does not have one answer. Different groups of people, communities and societies have different expectations of children that shape how they are raised. In Western countries such as Australia, New Zealand, the United Kingdom, the United States and Canada, independence from others and a strong education are the overriding concerns, whereas elsewhere, community spirit and cooperation are more valued.

One Western version suggests four dimensions to parenting (Baumrind 1991), of which one is clearly the one of choice for researchers in this context. *Indulgent* or *permissive* parenting both accepts what a child does and doesn't try to control the child. *Neglectful* or *uninvolved* parenting is unaccepting or unresponsive to the child and also does not try to control them. *Authoritarian* parenting is rejecting or being unresponsive while at the same time attempting to control the child and what they do. Finally, *authoritative* parenting is accepting and responsive while trying to control the child and protect them from mistakes. The latter approach is the one of choice for researchers in this context, but this must be kept in a context of the goals of people in Western societies (Darling & Steinberg 1993). If the child and parents live in a very harsh and risky environment then such indulgence might not be beneficial to children.

Some research has looked at these differences in parenting more openly when researching refugee or migrant groups that move into a Western society (Lin & Fu 1990). What we see is a range of parenting techniques that might have been appropriate for the homeland or for the refugee situation (which requires controlling the children strictly) but is no longer considered appropriate in the new country. Parents often need counselling about how they raise their children, but with a lifetime of advice from elders and experience of difficult situations, and current difficulties resulting from the migration experience and social exclusion, changing parenting strategies is difficult at best.

Another example of this is seen in research on slave families in the former United States colonies. Cultural practices are usually interpreted as 'internal' characteristics of those who were formerly colonised or oppressed, but they can also be seen as only having arisen in the first place because of that oppression. Of great relevance to those practising psychology, for example, is a misunderstanding as to why slaves raised their children with lots of punishment:

Cont... ▶

> *... at some point early affection had to give way to stern and perhaps arbitrary discipline – a cuffing without explanation – to turn the child towards automatic obedience and towards staying out of trouble with the white man.*
>
> (Wyatt-Brown 1988 p 1250)
>
> This is not something about the person or their race or ethnicity but relates to the deplorable situation they found themselves in as slaves.

Classroom activity

As a health professional, you will most likely find that you will interact with clients from a diverse range of cultural and linguistic backgrounds. Knowing some keywords, such as those for mother, father, family, children, boy and girl, from the languages of your clients can go a long way in either understanding what your clients are saying, or in showing your sensitivity.

In bilingual New Zealand, Māori words are often used interchangeably with English words. Consider words such as *whanau* (family) or *tamariki* (children).

Fill in the table below for your own situation and language.

Word	Your preferred language	English	Another language in your local area or that is common among people you might work with	Another language
Family				
Mother				
Father				
Children				
Boy/male				
Girl/female				

INFLUENCE FROM FRIENDS AND PEERS

In relation to peer influence, research methods can be limited in their ability to provide clear answers to what seem easy questions such as, how do peers influence children? As suggested earlier, peers are a strong force, though not as influential as some have argued, and it is often difficult to tease out parental influence on choosing peers in the first place (Collins et al 2000, Harris 1995, Hayes et al 2004).

But how might peer influence actually function in reality? A common view is that 'peer pressure' forces teenagers belonging to a group to do everything done by that

Research focus

Azize, P.M., Humphreys, A., Cattani, A., 2011. The impact of language on the expression and assessment of pain in children. Intensive and Critical Care Nursing 27, 235–243.

SUMMARY

This paper focuses on the importance of language in the expression of pain. How children describe their pain (i.e. how they encode) will influence how nurses or other health professionals will assess (or decode) the children's experience of pain. Variation in definitions of pain is presented (you may like to see Ch 12 on pain later in this textbook), together with a review of the evidence examining the impact language may have on the way pain is expressed linguistically. The implications for conducting research with children who speak different languages are explored. Strategies such as using non-linguistic methods of communication, additional time required for conducting interviews and the inclusion of research team members from the same ethnic or linguistic background are presented.

The authors present a table of research relating to children and their experience and communication of pain. For example, they refer to Goodenough et al (1999) and their research that found that children aged under eight could not distinguish between severities of pain, and that children aged over eight could determine the source of their pain. Also, Kortesluoma et al (2008) found that understanding of pain changes with age, but Piaget (1992) suggested that younger children are more intuitive about pain perception than older children.

The authors also provide a review of research that has shown poor pain assessment and under-treatment when clients are culturally or linguistically different from the healthcare provider. They suggest that it is critically important for health professionals to consider the ethnic, cultural and linguistic background, especially of children, to ensure pain is treated appropriately. Using interpreters or matching the cultural or linguistic abilities of health professionals with clients is one way to reduce under-reporting and under-treating pain.

Critical thinking

- What has been your experience in assessing pain in children?
- What experiences have you had of assessing pain in children who were linguistically or culturally different from you? How did that influence your practice? After reading this summary or the full article, would you do things differently? If yes, then how?
- What are some ways that culture and language influence children's experience of pain and therefore their description of pain? How would that then influence a health professional's assessment and treatment of pain? Why is this important?

Cont... ▶

> ■ What resources are available to nurses and other health professionals to facilitate working with culturally and linguistically different clients? (See Ch 8 for discussion on cultural safety.)

group. People commonly say that teenagers all dress the same and do the same things because of peer pressure (a causal theory). A child gets into a group and then that group pressures them to do the same things such as wear the same clothes, listen to the same music, or imbibe the same alcohol, drugs and tobacco. However, this view may be too simplistic.

As discussed earlier the way people view the influences from family, friends and communities is changing and new ways of thinking about these issues are emerging. Bauman and Ennett have explored the role of adolescent groups on smoking, drinking and drug use (Bauman & Ennett 1994, Chuang et al 2009, Ennett & Bauman 1993, 1994, Ennett et al 1994, Fisher & Bauman 1988) and others have shown similar results with other behaviours (Billy & Udry 1985, Kandel 1978). These challenge the common view that groups of peers pressure children into behaviours they would not do otherwise, but, more importantly, they expand our notions and see 'peer pressure' as one social strategy among others. Peer influence is bi-directional (i.e. peers influence each other) and these influences can be both positive and negative (Sumter et al 2009). Additionally, as adolescents get older, resistance to negative peer influence increases and girls have been found to be more resistant to peer influence than boys (Sumter et al 2009).

Research focus

Ennett, S.T., Bauman, K.E., 1993. Peer group structure and adolescent cigarette smoking: a social network analysis. Journal of Health and Social Behavior 34, 226–236.

SUMMARY

As an example, Ennett and Bauman (1993; for a more recent follow-up to this classic, see De Vries et al 2003) surveyed 1092 adolescent ninth-graders across five schools in a defined area. Seventy-five to 85% of those students completed a questionnaire in which they were asked for names of their three best friends. By using coded identification numbers, students from any of the five schools could be named as best friend and traced to their own data. While these friends could be anyone in the school system, 95% of network links were between children in the same school.

Ennett and Bauman used a computer program to categorise the children into three categories: cliques, liaisons and isolates. Cliques were tightly run groups in which most people referenced each other as their best friends. Liaisons were people who had friends in cliques but were not an integral part of any one clique. Last, isolates were those who did not have liking ratings that put them into a group of any sort. This does not mean

Cont... ▶

that they were loners, just that their friends might be elsewhere or they had a few friends who did not know each other all that well (enough to rate as one of three best friends anyway). They also measured the children's smoking behaviours.

The results were surprising. The common assumption is that smokers hang out in cliques that pressure members to smoke, but across the five schools the percentage of smokers on average were 26.9%, 10.3% and 10.2% for the isolates, liaisons and cliques respectively. That is, most of the smokers were isolates and there were fewer smokers in the cliques and liaison categories. So how do we explain these results? Ennett and Bauman (1993 p 233) came up with four possible explanations.

First, they suggested that being isolated might cause one to smoke or that being isolated means fewer social constraints. Second, it could be that cigarette smoking causes social isolation. Ennett and Bauman found that most cliques were comprised entirely of non-smokers and they might expel people from their group if they took up smoking. Let's come back to this 'exclusion' explanation in a moment. Third, both smoking and isolation could be caused through a third variable and have nothing to do with one another (a *mediational* theory). For example, adolescents who are depressed might become isolated and also take up smoking, even if these last two events are not otherwise related. Or, adolescents who had a job at night spent less time with school peers and also took up smoking, but these are otherwise unrelated. Finally, isolates could be in cliques outside of the school system. However, as mentioned earlier, 95% of the links were within the school system (Ennett and Bauman did not allow siblings to be named as the most liked friends). It could be that the isolates hung around with older siblings who smoked and there is actually some evidence for this (East & Rook 1992).

The evidence, then, is that peer pressure does not operate quite as thought (Ungar 2000). Bauman and Ennett's research (1994) suggests that *selection into and out of groups* is just as important as what goes on within those groups. If someone is a non-smoker then they are more likely to make friends with a non-smoker than a smoker and be selected into a non-smoking group – it is not that they just somehow get into groups and are then pressured to stop smoking. The sex, drugs and rock and roll behaviours are developed *to get into* those groups rather than *because of being in* those groups.

As suggested earlier when discussing parental influence, it is not that children become involved in groups that then pressure them in various ways but, rather, for a multitude of reasons (including parental influence) children *participate* in certain groups, get *expelled* from certain groups or are *selected* into groups. Participation in groups is very complex and requires further research, but it is also important not to oversimplify this complexity. Billy and Udry (1985) found a similar thing for sexual behaviours. People who were non-virgins tended to hang out with people who were also non-virgins and virgins tended to hang out with virgins, but their data showed that this does not mean that there is peer pressure to do what others in the group are doing (or not abstaining from). Rather, their longitudinal study found that when someone had sex for the first time they tended to join new groups of non-virgins. Therefore, it is once again the selection into and out of groups that make groups similar or homogeneous rather than pressure within a group for all the members to be similar.

There are four other points to consider in relation to this research. The first is that peer pressure is not necessarily negative. Ennett and Bauman (1993) found that most of their cliques tended to consist entirely of non-smokers. So, in this case, there is good argument that if there is peer pressure, it is beneficial in potentially reducing the number of smokers rather than acting to increase smoking. Second, research suggests that people overestimate the similarity among group members, especially groups other than their own. This is clearly part of the illusion that it is peer pressure that contributes to the behaviour of adolescents. Peers within groups are quite aware of small differences within their group, and outsiders (e.g. parents) may not be able to identify those differences. Third, it is in parents' best interests to portray their own children as innocent victims of peer pressure, rather than believe that their children actually self-select into groups. The final consideration is that far from adolescent smokers being compliant in a group of peers that pressure them to smoke, other research found that girls who smoked were more self-confident and socially skilled than non-smoking peers (Michell & Amos 1997) and therefore unlikely to be easily peer pressured into smoking.

From these strands of research you may find that the links between parents, peers and influences on a child's development are very convoluted and complex and simple generalisations are not useful.

Critical thinking

- To what extent is peer pressure the reason why children engage in behaviours they otherwise may not have engaged in?
- Describe the main influences on children's development.
- What sorts of contexts or situations may lead to different influences having a greater or lesser impact? For example, when might parents have a greater influence than school?

EDUCATION AND SCHOOLING

In this section, we consider the influence of education on children's development. First, we have seen that peers at school are one major influence on development, whatever the causal pathways. When children do not go to school then there might be less influence of non-related peers. Schooling in Western societies creates many opportunities for peer social influence and pressure that do not exist in other groups around the world.

Second, education is not the same as schooling and in many communities children are sometimes educated out of school more than in school. For example, families educate their children explicitly (even if informally) in and around the home and social environment. This might be in activities that are useful for the community and ritual activities, as well as reading, writing and arithmetic. Some families do not attempt to educate children except in a moral sense; they leave education to the schools. And in some cases, even moral education is left to the schools (as in religious or other private schools that may teach 'values'). Some parents, however, explicitly teach children, sometimes formally, as in home schooling.

The third point is that researchers who have studied children's cognitive or thinking development outside of the school setting may not show the full impact of the explicit education of children in how to think, count, etc. Many children, by the age of three or four years, are engaged in an education program aimed at facilitating or developing their abilities. Clearly, what is taught in kindergartens and schools will be a major influence on children. Discovering how children develop requires a perusal of formal schooling, as well as any peer or informal family education.

Stages, ages and milestones of development

Developmental milestones are a useful guide to parents, caregivers, educators and health professionals to gauge a child's development. Milestones can indicate whether a child is developing within a 'normal' range, although it is also important to acknowledge that deviations from these milestones do not necessarily mean there is anything wrong. Take, for example, talking. While talking among toddlers varies greatly, it would be important to explore why a toddler might not be talking by 24 months and to rule out physical causes such as hearing difficulties. For example, a toddler in a large family may not be talking because others in the family do all the talking, or they might be able to talk but do not do this out loud because they normally do not have a chance. There are many well-developed milestone charts that are used by parents and health professionals to help understand children's development. Some websites of developmental milestones are presented at the end of this chapter. You may find different charts or ways of presenting milestones more useful than others. It is worthwhile to explore different milestone charts and approaches to see their differences and to determine which ones work for you or the parents who you might be working with.

Conclusion

In this chapter several theories of human development have been explored, with an emphasis on understanding the key features of these theories. Theorists have attempted to explain the behaviours they observed in children and adolescents that were inexplicable or interesting.

Some of the main influences on development have been discussed and the relative weights of those influences were critically examined. Critical thinking has been encouraged about influences that are often taken for granted such as the influence of peers or parents on children's development. We also discussed the diversity of parenting practices and the complexities of schooling and education.

REMEMBER

- Theories of human development are influenced by the life contexts of the people developing the theories.
- Family, friends and school all influence child development.
- Parenting styles are diverse and can be influenced by context and history.
- Healthcare practice can benefit from knowledge and understanding of the influences and issues of childhood and adolescence.
- While developmental theories provide useful models for understanding human development they are not universally applicable.

Further resources

Christensen, P., Mikkelsen, M.R., 2008. Jumping off and being careful: children's strategies of risk management in everyday life. Sociology of Health & Illness 30, 112–130.

Coyne, I., Gallagher, P., 2011. Participation in communication and decision-making: children and young people's experiences in a hospital setting. Journal of Clinical Nursing 20 (15–16), 2334–2343.

Hawthorne, K., Bennert, K., Lowes, L., et al., 2011. The experiences of children and their parents in paediatric diabetes services should inform the development of communication skills for healthcare staff (the DEPICTED Study). Diabetic Medicine 28 (9), 1103–1108.

Morrow, A.M., Hayen, A., Quine, S., et al. (2011). A comparison of doctors', parents' and children's reports of health states and health-related quality of life in children with chronic conditions. Child: Care, Health and Development 38 (2), 186–195.

Wagmiller, R.L., Lennon, M., Kuang, L., 2008. Parental health and children's economic well-being. Journal of Health and Social Behavior 49, 37–55.

Weblinks

There are a number of useful sources of information regarding childhood developmental milestones. Below is a list of just a few of these. Remember, milestone charts are useful as an indicator of development, but many factors contribute to when these milestones are met. If a child has not reached a milestone this should be seen as an opportunity to rule out possible problems while also keeping in mind that variation in development is normal.

Dunedin Multidisciplinary Health and Development Research Unit at the University of Otago

dunedinstudy.otago.ac.nz

This site provides information conducted in the Dunedin Multidisciplinary Health and Development Research Unit including one of the largest ever longitudinal studies on human development, which has been going for nearly 40 years.

HealthInsite

www.healthinsite.gov.au

The Health Insite website from the Australian Government is a useful website for accessing information about a wide range of health issues. Search for 'developmental milestones' to access topic pages relevant to baby and child development.

Ministry of Health (New Zealand) Child Health section

www.health.govt.nz/our-work/life-stages/child-health

The child health section of the New Zealand Ministry of Health website provides useful information on a range of services offered in New Zealand relevant to child health as well as a link to publications.

Raising Children Network

www.raisingchildren.net.au

The Raising Children Network is a web resource for parents that is supported by the Australian Government and provides a wide range of useful materials and information about raising children and links to services and support.

The Community Child Health Service for Queensland Health

www.health.qld.gov.au/cchs/growth_approp.asp

This website provides a number of useful milestone guides in various languages.

US Department of Health and Human Services Centers for Disease Control and Prevention

www.cdc.gov/ncbddd/actearly/milestones

The US Department of Health and Human Services Centers for Disease Control and Prevention website includes an interactive milestones chart for parents as well as other developmental information for a range of age groups from the National Center on Birth Defects and Developmental Disabilities.

References

Andresen, J.T., 1990. Skinner and Chomsky thirty years later. Historiographia Linguistica 17, 145–165.

Aries, P., 1962. Centuries of childhood. Vintage Books, New York.

Azize, P.M., Humphreys, A., Cattani, A., 2011. The impact of language on the expression and assessment of pain in children. Intensive and Critical Care Nursing 27, 235–243.

Bamberg, J., Toumbourou, J.W., Blyth, A., et al., 2001. Change for the best: family changes for parents coping with youth substance abuse. Australian and New Zealand Journal of Family Therapy 22 (4), 189–198.

Bauman, K.E., Ennett, S.T., 1994. Peer influence on adolescent drug use. American Psychologist 49, 820–822.

Baumrind, D., 1991. The influence of parenting style on adolescent competence and substance use. Journal of Early Adolescence 11 (1), 56–95.

Bibace, R., Walsh, M.E., 1980. Development of children's concepts of illness. Pediatrics 66, 912–917.

Billy J.O.G., Udry, J.R., 1985. Patterns of adolescent friendship and effects on sexual behavior. Social Psychology Quarterly 48, 27–41.

Brassard, M.R., Chen, S., 2005. The boarding of upper middle class toddlers in China. Psychology in the Schools 42 (3), 297–304.

Bruner, J.S., 1973. Beyond the information given: studies in the psychology of knowing. Norton, New York.

Catania, A.C., 1997. An orderly arrangement of well-known facts: retrospective review of B F Skinner's verbal behavior. Contemporary Psychology 42, 967–970.

Chomsky, N., 1959. A review of B F Skinner's verbal behavior. Language 35, 26–58.

Chuang, YC., Ennett, S.T., Bauman, K.E., et al., 2009. Relationships of adolescents' perceptions of parental and peer behaviors with cigarette and alcohol use in different neighborhood contexts. Journal of Youth and Adolescence 38, 1388–1398.

Collins, W.A., Maccoby, E.E., Steinberg, L., et al., 2000. Contemporary research on parenting: the case for nature and nurture. American Psychologist 55, 218–232.

Darling, N., Steinberg, L., 1993. Parenting style as context: an integrative model. Psychological Bulletin 113 (3), 487–496.

De Vries, H., Engels, R., Kremers, S., et al., 2003. Parents' and friends' smoking status as predictors of smoking onset: findings from six European countries. Health Education and Research 18 (5), 627–636.

Dowling, J.E., 2004. The great brain debate. Joseph Henry Place, Washington DC.

East, P.L., Rook, K.S., 1992. Compensatory patterns of support among children's peer relationships: a test using school friends, nonschool friends and siblings. Developmental Psychology 28, 163–172.

Ennett, S.T., Bauman, K.E., 1993. Peer group structure and adolescent cigarette smoking: a social network analysis. Journal of Health and Social Behavior 34, 226–236.

Ennett, S.T., Bauman, K.E., 1994. The contribution of influence and selection to adolescent peer group homogeneity: the case of adolescent cigarette smoking. Journal of Personality and Social Psychology 67, 653–663.

Ennett, S.T., Bauman, K.E., Koch, G.G., 1994. Variability in cigarette smoking within and between adolescent friendship cliques. Addictive Behaviors 19, 295–305.

Erikson, E.H., 1959. Identity and the lifecycle – selected papers 1959. International University Press, New York.

Erikson, E.H., 1963. Childhood and society. Norton, New York.

Fisher, L.A., Bauman, K.E., 1988. Influence and selection in the friend-adolescent relationship: findings from studies of adolescent smoking and drinking. Journal of Applied Social Psychology 18, 289–314.

Freud, S., 1917. A general introduction to psychoanalysis. Washington Square Press, New York.

Goodenough, B., Thomas, W., Champion, G.D., et al., 1999. Unravelling age effects and sex differences in needle pain: ratings of sensory intensity and unpleasantness of venipuncture pain by children and their parents. Pain 80 (1–2), 179–190.

Gottesman, I.I., Hanson, D.R., 2005. Human development: biological and genetic processes. Annual Review of Psychology 56, 263–286.

Guerin, B., 2001. Individuals as social relationships: 18 ways that acting alone can be thought of as social behavior. Review of General Psychology 5, 406–428.

Guerin, B., 2004. Handbook for analyzing the social strategies of everyday life. Context Press, Reno.

Harms, L., 2005. Understanding human development: a multidimensional approach. Oxford University Press, Melbourne.

Harris, J.R., 1995. Where is the child's environment? A group socialization theory of development. Psychological Review 102, 458–489.

Hayes, L., Smart, D., Toumbourou, J.W., et al., 2004. Parenting influences on adolescent alcohol use, Research report No. 10. Australian Institute of Family Studies, Canberra.

Hayes, S.C., Hayes, L.J., Sato, M., et al, (Eds.), 1994. Behavior analysis of language and cognition. Context Press, Reno.

Kandel, D.B., 1978. Homophily, selection and socialization in adolescent friendships. American Journal of Sociology 84, 427–436.

Kortesluoma, R.L., Punamaki, R.L., Nikkonen, M., 2008. Hospitalized children drawing their pain: the contents and cognitive and emotional. Journal of Child Health Care 12, 284–300.

Lin, C.Y.C., Fu, V.R., 1990. A comparison of child-rearing practices among Chinese, immigrant Chinese and Caucasian-American parents. Child Development 61, 429–433.

Lin, H.P., Mu, P.F., Lee, Y.J., 2008. Mothers' experience supporting life adjustment in children with T1DM. Western Journal of Nursing Research 30, 96–110.

Michell, L., Amos, A., 1997. Girls, pecking order and smoking. Social Science and Medicine 44, 1861–1869.

Nelson, E.E., Guyer, A.E., 2011. The development of the ventral prefrontal cortex and social flexibility. Developmental Cognitive Neuroscience 1, 233–245.

Olson, L.M., Radecki, L., Frintner, M.P., et al., 2007. At what age can children report dependably on their asthma health status? Pediatrics 119 (1), e93–e102.

Peterson, C., 2009. Looking forward through the lifespan, fifth ed. Pearson Education, Frenchs Forest.

Piaget, J., 1952. The origins of intelligence in children (M. Cook, Translation). International Universities Press, New York.

Piaget, J., 1954. The construction of reality in the child. Basic Books, New York.

Piaget, J., 1962. Play, dreams and imitation. WW Norton, New York.

Piaget, J., 1992. The child's conception of the world. Routledge, New York.

Santrock, J.W., 2008. Lifespan development, eleventh ed. McGraw-Hill, New York.

Skinner, B.F., 1938. The behavior of organisms. Appleton-Century-Crofts, New York.

Skinner, B.F., 1957. Verbal behavior. Appleton-Century-Crofts, New York.

Skinner, B.F., 1969. Contingencies of reinforcement: a theoretical analysis. Prentice Hall, Englewood Cliffs.

Stiles, J., 2011. Brain development and the nature versus nurture debate. Progress in Brain Research 189, 3–22.

Sumter, S.R., Bokhorst, C.L., Steinberg, L., Westenberg, P.M., 2009. The developmental pattern of resistance to peer influence in adolescence: Will the teenager ever be able to resist? Journal of Adolescence 32, 1009–1021.

Ungar, M.T., 2000. The myth of peer pressure. Adolescence 35, 167–180.

Vygotsky, L.S., 1978. Mind in society: the development of higher psychological functions. Harvard University Press, Cambridge.

Wyatt-Brown, B., 1988. The mask of obedience: male slave psychology in the old South. American Historical Review 93, 1228–1252.

Chapter 3
Lifespan: Middle and later years (adulthood to ageing)

PAULINE GUERIN & BERNARD GUERIN

Learning objectives

The material in this chapter will help you to:

- describe the major developmental theories relevant from early to late adulthood
- discuss the diversity of partner selection, marriage and family structures
- discuss the complexities of employment, career and lifestyle during adulthood and the implications of these for health.

Key terms

- Lifespan development – middle and later years
- Developmental theories
- Milestones of adulthood
- Family and partnerships
- Parenting and caregiving
- Employment, career and lifestyle
- Chronic and other health issues
- Death, dying and bereavement

Introduction

In this chapter we examine theories of adulthood and ageing in the context of health psychology. The period from emerging adulthood to end-of-life spans a huge part of human experience, with a wide range of events taking place. While it is not possible to review all the health psychology material relevant to adulthood in one chapter, a range of issues relevant to adulthood will be covered and this will, perhaps, inspire you to seek out more information on related topics. The purpose is to give you a developmental perspective when confronting issues in your healthcare practice.

A common practice among researchers and theorists is to partition adulthood into stages or milestones, even though these might not apply universally. The broad stages of early, middle and late adulthood show major differences in physical, social, emotional and cognitive abilities, as well as circumstances. Theorists have observed quantum changes in how people behave across these periods. Additionally, theorists have more recently been discussing the transition from adolescence to adulthood, referring to this stage as *emerging adulthood* (Arnett 2000, Arnett et al 2011, Arnett & Tanner 2006). However, a drastic change in, for example, economic circumstances in contemporary society, can result in changes to adult circumstances. For example, young adults may find they live at home with their parents longer than they have in the past when economic circumstances were more favourable.

In this chapter, we will focus on adulthood as the time in a person's life in which they have taken on greater responsibility, whether through employment, marriage or partnership, having children or living away from primary caregivers. The times at which these events occur varies substantially in different people's lives and it is therefore essential to have an understanding of the various conceptions of age, such as chronological, psychological, social and biological.

Chronological age, or the number of years since someone was born, becomes important during emerging adulthood for a number of legal issues, such as being able to drive, vote or have certain jobs, or to get access to healthcare benefits. Chronological age, however, does not necessarily correlate with *psychological age*, which relates to an individual's ability to adapt to various circumstances compared with others who might be the same chronological age. Psychological age also differs from *social age*, or the social roles and expectations relative to chronological age. While someone might be functioning at an advanced social age (relative to their chronological age), this does not necessarily imply that they are also advanced psychologically, although these tend to be related.

Biological age, or the age in terms of physical health and development, is yet another conception of age. For example, while a 14-year-old female may biologically be capable of motherhood, the social role of motherhood is often considered more appropriate for women in their 20s or 30s in Western societies (social age). Similarly, at the other end of the spectrum are the wide differences between older people of various chronological ages and biological ages. For example, a 60-year-old may participate in competitive athletics and be healthier than many 40-year-olds, but both these differ from a 60-year-old who has been diagnosed with dementia and has had double knee replacements.

Chronological age is the concept that is almost exclusively used in healthcare practice, but it has many limitations and health professionals need to be careful about basing health judgments on this alone. Because of the extreme variability in the health of older people, some have argued that healthcare should not be related to chronological age but, instead, should be relevant to need, health conditions or biological age. For example, because policies are related to healthcare provision relevant to specific chronological ages (e.g. various cancer screening programs are only available for certain age groups), those who do not 'fit' in this conception (e.g. residents from refugee backgrounds or Aboriginal and Torres Strait Islander Australians with chronic conditions) can miss out on important healthcare (see, for example, the case study: Jane on page 67).

Theories

The theories of human development usually outline various stages of life pinned to chronological ages. However, others have argued that imposing chronological age on human development is imprecise at best (Hendry & Kloep 2002, Kloep et al 2009) and can be demeaning, or even damaging at worst. We will consider some of the stage theories while also bringing in other views of what occurs during human development. In this section, we will first review Erikson's theory, and will then explore Bronfenbrenner's ecological theory, Kohlberg's theory of moral judgment, and Hendry and Kloep's lifespan model of developmental challenge.

ERIKSON'S THEORY

Erik Erikson is probably the most well known developmental psychologist whose lifespan theory extends into adulthood. Other theorists, such as Freud and Piaget, only extended their theories to puberty (Freud's 'genital stage') and around age 11 (Piaget's 'stage of formal operations'. See Chs 1 and 2 for more information on these.). Perhaps the complexities with adulthood and the lack of well-defined, discrete, developmental stages directly related to age have challenged theorising in this area.

The three main stages of Erikson's theory relevant to adulthood are the stages of intimacy versus isolation, generativity versus stagnation and integrity versus despair (Erikson 1950, 1982, Erikson & Erikson 1997) (see Ch 2, Table 2.2). The stage of *intimacy versus isolation* is characterised by either the seeking of companionship and intimate love with another person or becoming emotionally isolated and fearing rejection or disappointment. This stage is usually said to occur during early adulthood and is often associated with the chronological ages of 18–24 years. In terms of healthcare practice, health professionals who recognise that people at this stage may be struggling to come to terms with intimacy issues and those multiple factors that contribute to isolation can serve a very useful role in assisting clients to successfully resolve this stage. For example, linking clients with support services, community organisations or self-help programs and groups can go a long way in preventing issues that could become more serious if left unrecognised and reinforce their isolation. This is supported by considering the relationship between social isolation and mental disorders such as schizophrenia (e.g. Cantor-Graae 2007) and that three in four mental disorders occur before age 24 (Kessler et al 2005).

Middle adulthood, according to Erikson, is characterised by a contribution to the next generation, usually through work or employment or having a family (i.e. *generativity*) or by becoming socially inactive (i.e. *stagnation*). One of the limitations of the application of Erikson's theory is that it can be interpreted as an either/or dichotomy; whereas, in reality, adults may find that in some aspects of their lives they have been generative but in other aspects have a sense of stagnation. Take, for example, a woman who is highly successful in her career but who never had children. While she may have a strong sense of generativity in her career, she may have regrets for not having had children (being stagnant in that area), although we must not assume that someone who has not had children would have regrets. However, it is also usually not this simple. For example, many families also contribute to their siblings' families rather than have their own families (see section on adoption later in this chapter) and this could be considered either generativity or stagnation, depending upon how the person sees it. It is therefore important to consider diversity in the development and understanding of these concepts and the importance of considering assumptions that might be made around these concepts. Always check with clients about their own understanding of where they are at in life.

Finally, in Erikson's theory, older adults make sense of their lives either as having *integrity* (i.e. being meaningful) or they may *despair* about the things that they did not achieve or accomplish in life. Erikson's theory is usually considered in the context of an individual and his or her resolution of these stages. However, the wider social context has much to contribute to these stages of development. For example, health professionals, again, can serve an important role in assisting clients to develop a sense of integrity rather than despair when working with people who are chronically ill or those nearing the end of life.

KOHLBERG'S THEORY

Kohlberg's theory of moral reasoning (1976) included three levels and six stages, roughly from age four to adulthood (see Table 3.1). Level I, or preconventional morality, includes stages 1 (orientation towards punishment and obedience) and 2 (individualism and exchange). Level II, or conventional morality, generally relates to children aged 10–13 and includes stages 3 (maintaining mutual relations and approval of others) and 4 (social concern and conscience or maintaining the social order). Level III, or postconventional morality, includes stages 5 (social contract or individual rights and democratically accepted law) and 6 (morality of universal ethical principles). Stages 5 and 6 are most relevant to adulthood and healthcare, although Kohlberg postulated that some people never enter these stages. In stage 5, people are rational and can be thoughtful and critical of laws and legal issues but inevitably will conform to laws and human rights as morally ideal. In stage 6, however, universal ethical principles will outweigh legal concerns in a moral dilemma. Kohlberg also later included a stage 7 (the cosmic stage) in which people would be able to see the impact of their action on the greater world, rather than only their immediate world (Kohlberg & Ryncarz 1990).

Table 3.1	
KOHLBERG'S THEORY OF MORAL REASONING	
Level I: preconventional	
Stage 1	Punishment and obedience
Stage 2	Individualism and exchange
Level II: conventional	
Stage 3	Maintaining mutual relations and approval of others
Stage 4	Social concern and conscience or maintaining the social order
Level III: postconventional	
Stage 5	Social contract or individual rights and democratically accepted law
Stage 6	Morality of universal ethical principles
Stage 7	The cosmic stage: able to see impact of actions on the greater world

In terms of healthcare, the relevance of Kohlberg's theory is obvious. There are many moral and ethical dilemmas that health professionals contend with on a regular basis and the resolution of these dilemmas will partly depend on where a person is at in terms of these stages and how the dilemmas are resolved. But it is perhaps too restrictive to view these as internal stages of moral development. Dealing with moral dilemmas regularly and the social and structural systems in place to facilitate this, such as the quality of debates with coworkers or the policies in place surrounding moral dilemmas, will influence the resolutions of these dilemmas. Take, for example, the issue of euthanasia or, for a less contentious issue, the use of a medication that has serious side effects. Kohlberg's theory would suggest that how you think about these issues can differ with a more or less developed sense of moral reasoning. Therefore, health professionals need to consider all forms of reasoning and not just believe there is only one right or wrong answer to euthanasia or medication.

Health professionals will not only benefit from understanding Kohlberg's theorising in their own practice, but consideration of Kohlberg's stages in respect of clients will help in treating clients. For example, issues of violence, drug abuse and even parenting can be understood better by considering these stages of moral development. Health professionals might consider that some clients will be thinking about these issues very differently and this may influence how health professionals will interact with and understand their clients.

Carol Gilligan is a theorist who argued that human development theories (especially Kohlberg's) do not adequately account for development as it relates to girls and women (Gilligan 1982). In her research with pregnant women contemplating abortion, she found that conflicts with responsibility to self and to others related to moral development for women that is not adequately addressed in Kohlberg's theory. Overall, Gilligan found that morality for women relates to an ethic of care and suggested that differences between men and women should not be minimised (Gilligan & Farnsworth 1995). Although some research (e.g. Jaffee & Hyde 2000) has shown that Gilligan's critiques of Kohlberg's theory were unjustified, her theorising drew attention to the often male-dominated theorising in human development.

OTHERS' THEORIES

Limitations to these classic theories have resulted in the need for theories that are more contextual and not so limited to Western notions of individuality and chronological age (Qin & Comstock 2005). These more recent theories include the ecological approach of Urie Bronfenbrenner (1979, 2004), Paul Baltes' lifespan perspective (Baltes 2000, Baltes & Baltes 1990, Baltes et al 2006) and the lifespan model of developmental challenge (Hendry & Kloep 2002, Kloep et al 2009).

Bronfenbrenner's (1979, 2004) theory considers individual development in a wider social context that includes micro (e.g. family and work), meso (the interactions between the individual's social connections e.g. your mother interacting with your partner), exo (the social connections that the individual's social connections have e.g. your partner's work colleagues) and macro systems (e.g. religion and politics). Bronfenbrenner's system, also called a 'bioecological' system, is multidirectional in that it is not only the social systems that impact on the individual but that the individual also impacts on those systems (Fig 3.1). 'Development is not something that just "happens" to the individual person but an interactive, dynamic process that involves all the system levels of a society' (Hendry & Kloep 2002 p 12).

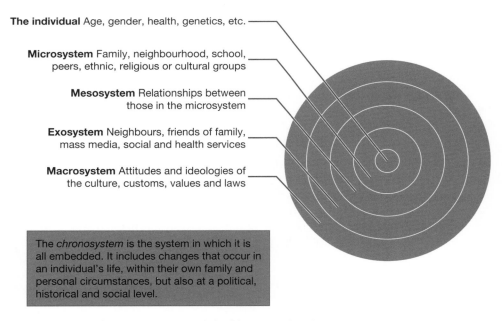

The individual Age, gender, health, genetics, etc.

Microsystem Family, neighbourhood, school, peers, ethnic, religious or cultural groups

Mesosystem Relationships between those in the microsystem

Exosystem Neighbours, friends of family, mass media, social and health services

Macrosystem Attitudes and ideologies of the culture, customs, values and laws

The *chronosystem* is the system in which it is all embedded. It includes changes that occur in an individual's life, within their own family and personal circumstances, but also at a political, historical and social level.

Figure 3.1 Bronfenbrenner's model of human development

Based on Urie Bronfenbrenner's 1979 model

CASE STUDY

You are a nurse doing a late shift in the emergency department of a major metropolitan hospital. A mother and father come in with their 18-month-old daughter, who has had severe diarrhoea and vomiting for the past four days. You find out that the mother and daughter are new arrivals and have just flown in from a small African country four days ago. The vomiting and diarrhoea started during the flight. The father is a postgraduate student at the local university and it is unclear who is responsible for the cost of the healthcare. Despite that, the baby is rushed in to see the paediatrician. The baby is severely dehydrated and the staff attempt to insert a line for a drip, but the dehydration combined with the baby's dark skin is making it difficult to find a vein. You notice that even though the baby is crying, the mother keeps going to the back of the room to sit in a chair with her head in her hands. You ask if the couple have other children and the father tells you no. After some time, you ask if the baby has been this sick before and the mother tells you that they had another baby who died at one year from diarrhoea, just before they fell pregnant with this baby.

Critical thinking

- Consider Bronfenbrenner's model of human development and identify socioeconomic issues that you would need to consider as a health professional in this situation.
- What might you need to know about Africa (broadly) to care for this family?
- What social, developmental and psychological issues might you need to consider during your further treatment of the baby and family?

Lifespan perspectives, or lifespan theories, of human development consider development across the full lifespan and suggest that to fully understand someone's development, one needs to consider how life events influence development. The lifespan perspective also considers important social and political factors that impact on development such as policies impacting on Aboriginal Australians (like the 'stolen generations') or economic conditions (such as the global financial crisis). Marion Kloep and Leo Hendry, proposed such a lifespan model of developmental challenge (Hendry & Kloep 2002, Kloep et al 2009). In their model, the concepts of challenges, resources, stagnation and decay feature prominently (2002). Basically, in this model, people have 'potential resources', and these resources influence how an individual will respond to various challenges ('potential tasks') that will occur throughout life. Resources include an individual's biology, social resources, skills, self-efficacy and structural resources. An interesting feature of this model is the relationship between task demands (whether there are many or few) and the availability of resources and how they relate to feelings of anxiety or security, and whether the task is then a risk, a challenge or routine. If tasks are often routine and the resources exceed the task, then stagnation can result. Also, if there are not enough resources and the tasks are risky, then decay can result.

Take, for example, a person who is overworked with high family demands but on a low income. Over time, the resource pool will deplete and the person's development risks 'decay'. Success, in this model, is 'development' and development can contribute more resources to the pool. However, people can be in a state of 'dynamic security' in which their resource pool is full and there are not many challenges. This is not necessarily an ideal situation because boredom can ensue. It is in this way that the model is also interesting, in that individuals are active players through their seeking or not seeking challenges to continue their development. If people do not seek out a challenge they may then be in a state of 'contented stagnation'. On the contrary, 'unhappy stagnation' occurs when there are no challenges but the individual does not have the resources to seek them out.

Kloep and Hendry's lifespan model of developmental challenge (Fig 3.2) is useful for health professionals because it reflects the complex realities of people's lives that we observe in real situations. Health professionals are in a position where they may see people experiencing a challenge (e.g. a health condition or an accident) and can determine whether people and their families have the resources to successfully develop through the challenge. From the client's perspective, a health professional who assists in identifying these factors will contribute to improved outcomes, both from the healthcare situation and more holistically for the client.

Hendry and Kloep's lifespan model of developmental challenge. Depiction of the relationship between potential resources, potential tasks and the context.

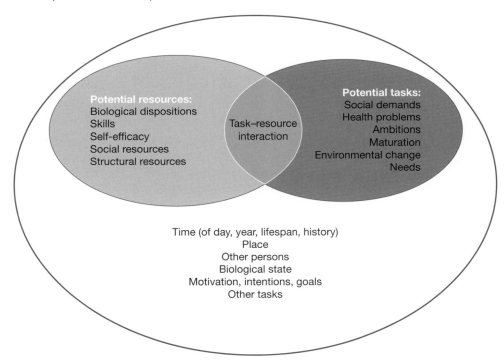

Figure 3.2 Hendry and Kloep's lifespan model of developmental challenge

From Lifespan development: resources, challenges and risks by Hendry L B, Kloep M 2002, Thomson, Australia, page 24. Reproduced by permission of Cengage Learning EMEA Ltd.

Milestones of adulthood

So far in this chapter we have examined theories of lifespan development in adulthood that delineate *stages*. We will now look at adulthood from the perspective of the main milestones of adulthood and the complexities associated with these. As key examples of milestones of adult development, we will discuss: marriage, partnership and family; parenting, mothering and caregiving; employment and career development; lifestyle, leisure, spirituality and wellbeing; retirement and the development of chronic or other illness during adulthood; and dying, death and bereavement.

MARRIAGE, PARTNERSHIP AND FAMILY

Being in a close relationship with another person, either through marriage, a civil union or co-habitation, is perhaps one of the most significant milestones of human life. With around 50% of the adult population currently married, and certainly many more in other forms of close and lasting relationships, and a variety of health and legal implications for those who are married or not, it is certainly an important topic for health professionals. Marriage and civil unions are also currently a highly politically charged topic worldwide. Although some countries now have legalised civil unions (i.e. a legally recognised relationship between people of either the same or opposite sex), same-sex relationships are not nationally legally recognised in many countries including Australia (although civil unions are recognised in some states, Australian Marriage Equality 2012). In New Zealand, the *Civil Union Act 2004* came into effect in 2005 (Department of Internal Affairs 2011). Even so, in Australia, in 2009–10, there were 23,000 documented same-sex couple families (Australian Bureau of Statistics (ABS) 2011).

With the huge religious and cultural diversity of Australia, mate selection, marriage, partnership and family are correspondingly diverse (de Vaus 2004, Hartley 1995). We might think that differences in marriage fall into distinct categories of 'love marriages' or 'arranged marriages' or we may have our own ideas about what it is that makes up a family. These ideas are strongly influenced by our own family, the media and other social influences.

A family, according to the ABS, is two or more people, one of whom is at least 15 years of age, who are related by blood, marriage (registered or de facto), adoption, step or fostering, and who are usually resident in the same household (ABS n.d.). This definition is a very Western conception and revolves around the concept of the 'nuclear' family. In that definition, for example, 'family' who do not live in the same household are not considered to be part of that family unit. The ABS also identifies couple families with and without children, one-parent families, step families and blended families but these, too, are basically variations on 'nuclear' family conceptions. However, how families are conceptualised can differ quite drastically in different cultural groups. For example, for some, the 'family' would not exclude those who 'are not usually resident in the same household' and the relevance of the 'household' may have different meanings for different people and groups. For some people, companion animals are very much considered to be part of the 'family', though they would not be included in official records or documentation.

Marriage is generally considered to be a permanent and legally recognised arrangement between two people that includes both a sexual and an economic relationship with mutual rights and obligations. An *endogamous* marriage is one where the bride and groom are from the same group (like Italians marrying other Italians or Jewish people marrying other Jewish people) and an *exogamous* marriage is one in which the partners are from differing groups (like a Catholic marrying a Muslim or someone from Iraq marrying someone from France). For example, for some Australian Aboriginal groups it is important to marry outside of one's 'skin group' and to marry someone from certain other skin groups only.

While only *monogamous* marriages are legal in Australia and New Zealand (i.e. only have one husband or wife), it is perhaps useful to know that this is not the case in all countries around the world, and with increasing migration from non-Western countries, health professionals should be aware of other types of marriage arrangements. For example, *polygamy*, or marriage to multiple spouses, is desirable in many Islamic countries and communities, where it is acceptable and even expected for men to have up to four wives (also called *polygyny*), but this arrangement is illegal in Australia. Less common are *polyandrous* marriages where a woman has more than one husband at the same time. Perhaps more common in Australia and New Zealand is *serial monogamy*, or successive marriages that may be short or long term.

There are also various notions of relatives that are important for health professionals to recognise. For example, *consanguineal kin* are people who are related by blood, ancestry or descent and *affinal kin* are people who are related by marriage. In-laws and their relatives are therefore affinal kin. *Adopted kin* are family created through adoption and *fictive kin* are those who you might consider to be related to you, like calling your best friend your sister or a family friend your 'aunt'.

Figures 3.3 and 3.4 illustrate only two of the many ways that relationships in a family can be construed. Figure 3.3 shows the *Euro kinship* pattern while Figure 3.4 illustrates the *Dravidian kinship* pattern. The Euro kinship pattern is common in Western groups, while the Dravidian system is found in South India and in some Aboriginal and Oceanic groups. These are only two kinship patterns and there are a number of other ways in which relationships between blood and marriage can be understood. However, in Australia and New Zealand, perhaps the Dravidian and the Euro patterns are most common.

In Euro kinship, siblings are called brothers and sisters and offspring from the brothers and sisters of one's mother and father are called cousins. The brothers and sisters of one's mother and father are not distinguished and are referred to as aunts or uncles, based on gender. Similarly, the parents of one's parents are referred to as grandmother or grandfather, again, depending on gender.

In Dravidian kinship, on the other hand, a person can have multiple mothers and fathers and sisters and brothers who are outside the immediate family unit. For example, the sister of one's mother is also called mother and the daughter or son of that mother is called a brother or sister. In terms of parenting (discussed next), this kinship pattern can be very useful. For example, if a teenage boy, whose biological

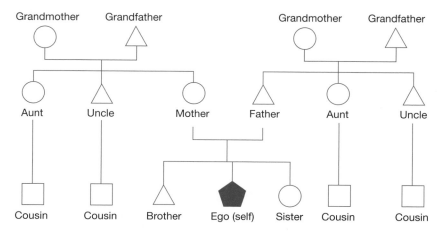

Figure 3.3 Euro kinship

DOUSSET, Laurent 2011. Australian Aboriginal Kinship: An introductory handbook with particular emphasis on the Western Desert. Marseille: pacific-credo Publications.

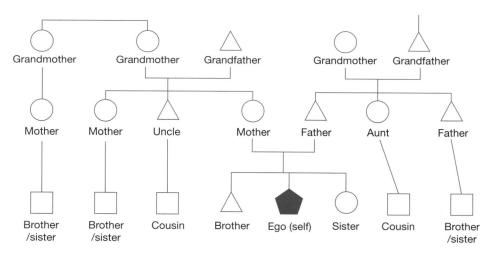

Figure 3.4 Dravidian or Australian Aboriginal kinship

DOUSSET, Laurent 2011. Australian Aboriginal Kinship: An introductory handbook with particular emphasis on the Western Desert. Marseille: pacific-credo Publications.

father is not available, is getting into trouble, then another 'father' may be called upon to offer guidance. In terms of healthcare, a mother's sister may take children to healthcare appointments in her role as another mother. Another characteristic in Aboriginal kinship systems is 'avoidance relationships', which is the avoidance of, or not interacting with, certain relatives out of respect. For example, a man and his mother-in-law constitutes an avoidance relationship.

Critical thinking

- Is development in adulthood related to chronological age or to life experiences? Or is it related to both? Take, as your examples, a 60-year-old with small children and a 40-year-old with teenagers.
- How can an understanding of different kinship patterns influence healthcare practice?

Overall, the number of marriages per year, and the marriage rate, has decreased over time (Hayes et al 2011, Statistics New Zealand 2012). Age at marriage has been steadily increasing, and living together before getting married (i.e. cohabitating) is now a very common practice (Hayes et al 2011, Statistics New Zealand 2012).

Marriage is an important consideration of health professionals because of the research showing various relationships between marriage (or being single) and health (Jaffe et al 2007). For example, people who are married have a longer life expectancy: 'Marriage reduces the risk of an earlier death as a person is less likely to participate in risky behaviour and more likely to nurture or "guardian" each other's health through promoting good diet and physical care' (Elliot 2008 p 1). A large study in the United States by the Centers for Disease Control and Prevention (CDC) (Schoenborn 2004) found that married people were overall (except in bodyweight) healthier than people who were not married. This research also showed that marriage benefits the health of men more so than women. This better health includes being less likely to suffer various conditions such as headaches or back pain, as well as healthier lifestyle factors such as not smoking, not drinking alcohol or not being physically inactive. Married men, however, were more likely to be overweight, which might lend some credibility to the old saying that the best way to a man's heart is through his stomach! Interestingly, the patterns did not hold for people who were living together but not married. Their health was similar to the poorer health reported by divorced or separated adults (Schoenborn 2004).

DIVORCE AND FAMILY BREAKDOWN

Like marriage, partnership and having a family, divorce and family breakdown are major milestones in adult development when they occur, and can have both positive and negative consequences. These effects depend on the social contexts and consequences of the divorce or family breakdown. For example, divorce with children involved can be very complicated, but the outcomes largely depend on how these complications are managed (Amato 2010). While there is a large body of research showing negative health consequences of divorce (Amato 2010, Schoenborn 2004), staying in violent marriages or in highly dysfunctional relationships may be more harmful (Amato 2010, Emery 2009). Whether those involved marry again is another consideration in the interpretation of the health consequences of divorce. When working in healthcare with people who have divorced or separated from long-term partners, or children of parents who have divorced, it is important to get a full contextual picture of the family situation before making assumptions about the health and social effects.

Classroom activity

PARTNER SELECTION AND MARRIAGE

In small groups, discuss your knowledge and experience with marriage, partnership or civil unions, and divorce.

1. How did you or your parents get married?
   - Think about how you or they met or were introduced to each other. What sort of ceremonies and social events took place related to the engagement and marriage?
2. What are the dating or partner selection experiences in your family or culture?
3. Discuss similarities and differences with others in the group.

PARENTING, CAREGIVING AND RE-CONCEPTUALISING CHILDREN

Data indicate that the average Australian family includes roughly 1.7 children who are, on average, 18 months different in age (Hayes et al 2010). The mother would have been about 30 years old when she had her first child and chances are the couple will have divorced after 12 years of marriage. While this can contribute to a static and narrow view of families in Australia and New Zealand, the reality is that family composition, parenting and divorce are highly diverse and change drastically over time (Cribb 2009, de Vaus 2004, Hayes et al 2010). Take, for example, sole-parent households, blended families, teenage parents, same-sex parents, fostering, adoption and grandparents taking responsibility for bringing up their grandchildren. Becoming a parent or the caregiver of children is a major milestone of adulthood, challenging identity and social roles. In fact, being a parent or carer of children changes almost everything a person does and can do.

As discussed in Chapter 2, parenting is an important contributor to children's development, but it is highly complex and diverse. One of the complexities of parenting relates to the different ways of parenting or interacting with children. Most research has been conducted in Western countries, with corresponding biases in terms of what is considered to be 'good parenting', as well as how parenting styles are represented.

For example, as discussed in Chapter 2 (see Box 2.3) one popular version of parenting includes four dimensions: authoritative, indulgent, neglectful and authoritarian (Baumrind 1991, Baumrind et al 2010). Although authoritative parenting is generally considered a preferable parenting style in the Western context, there are communities and contexts in which this parenting style would be considered inappropriate. Consider a context in which the environment is socially or physically dangerous, such as a socially and economically depressed locale with high rates of violence. In this context, authoritative parenting might not be beneficial and authoritarian parenting might have better health and social outcomes for children. Similarly, in a context in which being educated is the most important and useful goal and the environment is less risky, then authoritative or even indulgent parenting may be preferable.

Another issue related to parenting style is the way a society or parents view children. In some contexts children are viewed as an economic resource for parents because they can gain employment and bring money into the household, or they can work around the house and thereby relieve the parents for employment purposes, or they will marry into another family and attract wealth. In some contexts, babies may be considered dispensable in poverty conditions or other problematic conditions (Omokhodion & Uchendu 2010, Scheper-Hughes 1985). In contexts with greater social and economic stability, such as in the West, children may be viewed more idealistically and seen as people in themselves rather than as resources for the family.

Dharmalingam (1996) studied family size preferences in a small village in southern India where there were two major industries: a brickwork and a beedi factory (beedis are a type of cigarette). Children could begin employment at the age of five years. Dharmalingam found several interesting things. First, villagers who were more economically disadvantaged reported wanting more children than those who were better off. About 50% of those who wanted more children reported wanting as many as possible or as many as God gave them. From a Western perspective this seems irrational because those with less money and fewer resources should want fewer children. However, the social logic is quite clear when children are considered as resources: those who are economically more disadvantaged have greater benefits with more children because they attract more resources than what they use. However, when Dharmalingam asked the villagers about their reasons for having boys or girls, direct economic reasons were usually ranked third. But the major reasons for having boys were so that they could inherit the property, provide security against risks and provide for the parents in their old age. All of these are to do with economic resources.

Importantly, when children are considered as a resource, parenting patterns will be very different from when children are not seen in that way (Scheper-Hughes 1985). Advising people in different social and economic contexts to reduce the number of children they have because of the problems associated with the increasing world population, while good-intentioned, may inadvertently result in compromising their standard of living and social and economic resources. The values that are derived in one social and economic context can be harmful when applied in a different context.

In greater socially and economically advantaged contexts, having fewer children has greater advantages and benefits, especially in relation to education and the cost of education, particularly in many Western contexts. Having fewer children provides for a greater share of the resources because of the way that resources are allocated or structured in Western societies. Therefore, having fewer children and educating them better has the same social logic spelt out by Dharmalingam's participants but built upon the particular social and economic context.

Health professionals are often in the position to observe family dynamics and interactions between caregivers and children and it is important to recognise and not be critical of dynamics that may seem unusual or different from one's own way of doing things. Family relationships and how children are viewed within the family depends heavily on the context, milieu or culture in which people have been raised and it is these factors that may not be easily accessible to health professionals.

CASE STUDY: JANE

Jane is a community health worker who conducts education sessions for a group of elderly refugee women from East Africa. Before starting the education sessions Jane found out that life expectancy for the countries where the women are from is less than 50 years and that, roughly, there is only one health professional for every 100,000 people. Jane also knows that all of the women are Muslim and that she may need to be sensitive to issues of modesty. Jane organises a session about breast and cervical cancer screening. On the night of the session, when Jane introduces the speaker and the topic, many of the women say they do not get cancer in Africa and that it is a Western disease.

Classroom activity

In small groups discuss:

1. Considering what Jane knows about healthcare and life expectancy in East Africa, how might she approach discussing the issue of cancer screening with the women?
2. How might an understanding of human development be influenced by differences in life expectancy for different population groups or for migrants or refugees from countries with very different life expectancies from the new country of residence?

PARENTING AND ATTACHMENT THEORY

With an increasing diversity of family composition and parenting roles, particularly in developed Western countries, there has been greater attention to the role of 'mothering' in society and in families. Early theorists such as John Bowlby emphasised that mothers are of crucial importance to children and developed his original attachment theory primarily based on clinical observations and monkeys raised without their mothers. He believed, and the ethos at the time agreed wholeheartedly, that mothers are of special importance to raising healthy and happy children as the primary caregiver, and described this bond as of 'lasting psychological connectedness between human beings' (Bowlby 1969 p 194).

While the early attachment of children to parents and others is not disputed and has had a revival of late (Holmes 2011), attachment no longer refers solely to mothers and their children. Depending on how mothering is defined, it may or may not involve only women as mothers. Consider, for example, Arendell's (2000) definition of a mother as someone who does the relational and logistical work of child rearing. This work can be done by men or women. For example, currently, in Sweden, men can be considered to be 'mothering' under some conditions of work practice and have time off work. However, others have argued that the role of motherhood is unique for women and that men cannot fully be 'mothers' (Doucet 2006). Riggs and Due (2010) discuss the complexities in relation to gay male parents and surrogacy in India, arguing for greater recognition of issues of gender as well as power and privilege and how that intersects with roles of mothering and caretaking.

In terms of considerations for health professionals, again, the diversity of parenting roles and relationships cannot be underestimated. How health professionals manage diversity in practice can significantly impact on healthcare and health outcomes.

Adoption or fostering

Adoption or fostering of children provides another interesting example of the diversity of family dynamics and the role of children within families. Often, in Western countries, a child may be homed through adoption or fostering because the mother or parents cannot look after her or him. This may be because of poverty, drug habits, violence, neglect, death or illness, and so a child may be taken as a ward of the state or country. In many circumstances an opportunity is first provided to other family members, such as grandparents, aunts or uncles, to look after the child. In many cases this is not possible so people who are completely unrelated (biologically) may adopt or foster and raise the child. These adoptive parents are also becoming increasingly diverse in their circumstances. For example, consider that with greater recognition of same-sex partnerships, that these couples may opt for fostering or adoption as a way to raise children. While there are some lay views that these 'non-traditional' parenting arrangements are problematic, a recent study on adoptions by gay or lesbian couples found very few differences to heterosexual couples who raised adopted children (Farr et al 2010).

However, in many non-Western countries, and in many communities within Western countries, forms of adoption and fostering are and have always been a common event. Children may be raised by kin (with full knowledge of their origin) with no problematic situations and within very healthy contexts. This is common, for example, in both traditional and contemporary Māori social relations. For example, a woman might ask her sister if she would raise one of her children and this can be arranged even before the child is born. This arrangement can be viewed as an ultimate gift from sister to sister. These arrangements can be made for a wide range of reasons. For example, it may be that the adopting sister has had problems conceiving and therefore would like a child. In other cases the adopting sister might already have a family but still be asked to raise a child, maybe because of her parenting skills. This sort of adoption process can be seen as another way of facilitating and maintaining bonds and relationships between people in kin-based communities.

It is important to emphasise that, in some circumstances, when this kind of fostering or adoption occurs, it does not necessarily indicate that any of the people involved are having problems such as the baby being in danger of neglect or that the family are not fully able to raise the child. Sometimes grandparents might raise children and the grandparents might not be much older than the parents. It is unlikely, as would be the case for many Western families, that a 70-year-old grandmother would raise a newborn baby for her daughter. But a 40-year old grandparent might easily raise a grandchild.

One important element in this fostering scenario is that the context involves a kin-based community in which everyone spends time together and is close (even if conflict occurs regularly). This means that the child would know his or her 'biological' parents and see them regularly, which is unlike how adoption was conducted until very recently in most Western systems – where the child was made anonymous and the 'biological' parents' names were kept secret. There are numerous examples of this sort of kin-adoption or fostering and reports of this from all corners of the world, mainly where extended or kin-based families remain intact. This practice is still common among Māori in New Zealand, for example (e.g. Cameron 1966, Hegar 1999, Hegar & Scannapieco 1999, McRae & Nikora 2006, Shirley et al 1997).

Overall, the stage of adult life involving parenting and child rearing is common and important. This is not just for the children involved but also for the parents. Nevertheless, while disagreement exists between some researchers and theorists regarding exactly how this developmental phase operates in adult life, there is agreement that what is considered 'normal' adult behaviour at this stage is now diverse and changing. These early life contexts also contribute significantly to health outcomes, the development of health and health issues, and influence the effectiveness of healthcare interventions. Healthcare services will be much more effective when health professionals are informed with even a basic understanding of these contexts and complexities of their clients.

EMPLOYMENT, CAREER AND LIFESTYLE

Employment and careers are obviously important to our life stages, but research shows that the nature of career development has changed over time. While parents or grandparents may have been employed in the same place for their entire adult life, many people today make substantial career changes throughout their working life. Again, while the majority of Australians and New Zealanders will finish high school and then go on to either trades training or university before moving into a career, there is a substantial minority who will not navigate such a clear path to employment opportunities and career options.

In Australia Census data show that the percentage of families with children with both parents employed has gradually increased to 63% in 2009–10, while the percentage of families with children where neither parent is employed has gradually decreased from 7% in 1996 to 5.4% in 2006 and 5% in 2009–10 (ABS 2011). The employment status of parents is related to the age of dependent children in the household (ABS 2011). For example, as children get older, there is a higher proportion of parents employed. Overall, the 2009–10 data show an increase in the employment of mothers, with 66% of mothers employed in couple families with dependent children (compared with only 59% in 1997) (ABS 2011). Additionally, in lone mother families with dependent children, in 2009–10, 60% were employed, but in 1997 only 46% were employed. Although there are a number of economic benefits for families when the caregivers are employed, this also means that there are many children in homes where the only parent is working. There are many social and health effects of these arrangements and they are not necessarily all positive.

'Being employed' is a major aim and milestone of adulthood and has a number of health benefits. Equally, being unemployed can negatively impact on health, as can being employed in the wrong job or in poor working conditions (Bambra et al 2010, Benach et al 2010). *Underemployment* is when someone is employed at a level lower than their qualifications or skills. *Overemployment*, in contrast, is the employment of someone in a position that requires greater skills or knowledge than what the person has. Both of these conditions can be stressful and adversely impact on health. Additionally, poor work environments and high-risk jobs can make employment more problematic than beneficial.

Lifestyle patterns largely develop during early adulthood with the development of social circles, employment and education and family (married or not, having children or not). Lifestyle patterns that develop during early adulthood – such as smoking, alcohol or other drug consumption; religious or spiritual activity; physical activity; and dietary habits – reveal their impacts in middle adulthood. Lifestyle, in health psychology, has largely been a concept relevant to individuals and research, and intervention in this area has largely focused on individual behaviour change. However, lifestyle is inextricably linked with social conditions, economic circumstances such as employment, place of residence and the larger community.

Classroom activity

1. Before coming to class, have a discussion with either a parent, aunt, uncle, grandparent or an 'elder' who you are close to about their lifetime lifestyle experiences. Consider the following questions in your discussion. Bring these responses to discuss in a small group.
   - What sorts of things do you do to relax?
   - Do you do anything for exercise, physical activity or leisure (sports, walking, gardening, housework, etc.)?
   - What sorts of things did you do for exercise, physical activity or leisure when you were in your 20s? 30s? 40s? 50s? (as appropriate)
   - Would you say that your lifestyle/leisure activities have changed much in your life? If so, what would you say contributed to those changes? If not, what things do you think contributed to maintaining your lifestyle behaviours or what things might have been barriers to changing or doing things differently?
2. In small groups discuss the following:
   - Did your discussion with your interviewee change your ideas about how you think about lifestyle and what is 'good' and 'bad' (such as what is exercise or physical activity and how your interviewee changed in their life with respect to these activities) especially for older people.
   - Did you learn anything in your interview that you didn't know about before? What did you learn and how has that impacted on you? If you didn't learn anything new, was there anything interesting or noteworthy about your conversation with this person?

SPIRITUALITY AND WELLBEING

The massive growth in literature and research relating to spirituality and religion and their relevance to wellbeing and health is testament to the importance of these topics for contemporary health professionals. During adulthood, religious or spiritual development can change dramatically depending on many factors such as social groups that one is involved with, employment situations and major life events (especially traumatic ones). Additionally, beliefs and practices may change more than once. This is known as 'religious mobility' or 'religious switching'. For example, someone may become involved in a new church through the invitation of someone at work, but then, perhaps after moving to a new town, may find that their church attendance ceases, but they commence other activities, such as joining a social running group.

Overall, research generally finds that religiosity or spirituality contribute to improved wellbeing and can contribute to health improvements and healing from illnesses (Koenig et al 2012), although these benefits can change with religious switching (Scheitle & Adamczyk 2010). Spirituality, while once (and still often) synonymous and used interchangeably with 'religion' and organised religious practices (e.g. Catholicism, Islamism and Buddhism), has become a field of study on its own, encompassing both secular and religious practices. In this sense, the definition proposed by Gomez and Fisher (2003) is apt: '... spiritual well-being can be defined in terms of a state of being reflecting positive feelings, behaviours, and cognitions of relationships with oneself, others, the transcendent and nature, that in turn provide the individual with a sense of identity, wholeness, satisfaction, joy, contentment, beauty, love, respect, positive attitudes, inner peace and harmony, and purpose and direction in life' (Gomez & Fisher 2003 p 1976).

La Cour and Hvidt (2010) described the three domains of secular, spiritual and existential orientations in terms of meaning-making in relation to health and illness. They consider the three domains in relation to knowing (cognition), doing (practice) and being (importance), providing a useful tool to extract some of the complexities of these important topics. For example, using this framework, researchers can tease out some of the relationships between religion and health such as the social supports often associated with some religious practices (e.g. going to church) or the influence of meditation or prayer activities on health.

Given the importance of links between religion or spirituality and health, health professionals may find it very beneficial for clients to have their religious or spiritual needs considered, particularly in acute care or end-of-life contexts. For example, a recovering alcoholic undergoing inpatient cancer treatment may find it helpful for healthcare staff to assist with locating a local 12-step recovery meeting. Twelve-step recovery groups are based on spiritual principles and belief in a 'higher power' to relieve one of their addictions. Health professionals may also recommend, when appropriate, that clients explore religion or spirituality as part of their healing processes.

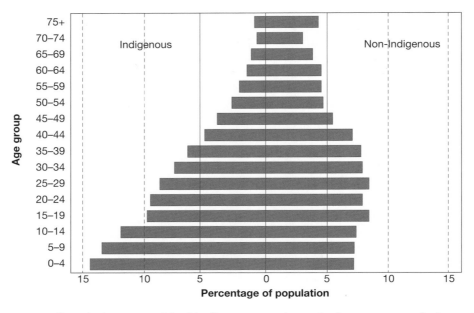

Figure 3.5 Population pyramid of Indigenous and non-Indigenous populations of Australia, 2011

Source: HealthInfoNet 2011

DEMOGRAPHY

In order to appreciate the importance of age and ageing in healthcare practice, a look at the statistics or the demography of the population is essential. For example, different population groups have different age structures. This is shown in 'population pyramids' such as depicted in Figure 3.5.

Figure 3.5 illustrates the percentage of the population in five-year age groups for the Indigenous and non-Indigenous population of Australia. We can deduce from this figure that the social issues for human development might vary considerably for Indigenous and non-Indigenous Australians. For example, while non-Indigenous Australians have a greater proportion of people in the middle-age groups, Indigenous Australians have a greater proportion of the population represented in the younger age groups. The social impact of that is the greater demand on older Indigenous Australians for child care (compared with non-Indigenous Australians) but greater demands on non-Indigenous Australians for elderly care. These data illustrate the importance of a wide range of factors (in this case, population structure) when considering human development.

Other demographic factors that are important to consider in healthcare include, for example, the populations living in urban, rural or remote areas and access to health services. It is also important to consider gender and place of birth and languages spoken as important considerations in healthcare. With an understanding of the demographics of the places where we live and work, we can potentially anticipate and prepare for ensuring that the health services we provide are appropriate and meeting the needs of the clients we see.

Research focus

Smith, K., LoGiudice, D., Dwyer, A., et al., 2007. Ngana minyarti? What is this? Development of cognitive questions for the Kimberley Indigenous Cognitive Assessment. Australasian Journal on Ageing 26 (3), 115–119.

ABSTRACT

Objectives

To describe the processes used to develop an instrument to assess cognition in the older Indigenous community of the Kimberley region of Western Australia, given the diverse history and culture of the region.

Methods

Cognition questions were discussed with Indigenous organisations, councils, linguists, interpreters and health professionals. Existing assessment tools were reviewed. The cognition questions and the way in which they were approached were trialled with older Indigenous participants.

Results

Questions to assess cognition were developed and incorporated into the Kimberley Indigenous Cognitive Assessment (KICA) instrument, which has since been demonstrated to be a valid and reliable assessment of cognition in older Indigenous Australians in the Kimberley.

Conclusion

The KICA questions in the survey tool provide the first specific instrument for assessing cognitive decline in older Indigenous Australians. This instrument, or a modification of this instrument, is likely to have broader applicability across Indigenous communities in northern Australia.

Key points

In any study of Indigenous people, it is important to consult with a range of community members and specialists to gain support and advice on how to develop appropriate questions for research instruments.

Community studies of older Indigenous people require awareness of historical, cultural and linguistic factors.

Indigenous people are heterogeneous and there is a need to trial tools with people from different areas, language groups, ages and levels of cognitive impairment.

In this article, the authors report that Indigenous Australians are often not diagnosed with dementia until the dementia has progressed to late stages. While this may be due to complex factors such as language barriers, developing a dementia screening tool would assist in identifying dementia in early stages. The researchers included a consultation process as a part of their project and the project itself provided a useful tool for the people involved.

Critical thinking

- Will the KICA tool be useful for other Aboriginal groups in Australia?
- Why or why not?
- What history of the Aboriginal people in the Kimberley may be relevant to understanding cognitive assessment with this group?

CHRONIC ILLNESS AND OTHER HEALTH ISSUES

Chronic illness, disability and other health issues increasingly become a part of reality as people age. Health psychology has also gained an increasing role in chronic and other illnesses because of the growing recognition of behavioural and social factors contributing to these conditions. For example, in 2010, ischaemic heart disease, cerebrovascular disease and dementia and Alzheimer's disease were the top three underlying leading causes of death in Australia (ABS 2012). With the 'ageing' population of Australia, it is perhaps not surprising that for the leading causes of death in Australia, dementia and Alzheimer's disease have gone from rank 8 in 1997 to rank 6 in 2001 to rank 4 in 2006 and in 2010, rank 3. Deaths from dementia and Alzheimer's disease have nearly doubled since 1997 (from 3294 in 1997 to 6542 in 2006) and are more likely to affect women than men (ABS 2008).

For health professionals, these statistics suggest that illnesses are more common partly because people are living longer. But, more importantly, as people age and certain illnesses become more prevalent, people will increasingly need care and specialised processes and equipment. For example, there has been an increase in the need for dialysis machines for kidney disease stemming from diabetes. Therefore, not only are there a greater number of people with various illnesses, but also people are required to travel to access specialised equipment and care and their final years may be involved with hospitals rather than living close to families.

DEATH, DYING AND BEREAVEMENT

The topics of death, dying and bereavement are often addressed in the context of older people but obviously they can affect people of all ages. They are discussed here because death, dying and bereavement become more likely as people grow older and therefore are a major part of human development for adults. Death, dying and bereavement may affect people differently depending on many factors such as the contexts of the death (e.g. whether by an accident or after a long illness), the family and support situation available (to both the person who dies and those who love or have cared for them), and economic circumstances.

Bereavement has been defined as the 'objective situation of a person who has suffered the loss of someone significant' (Boerner & Wortman 2001 p 1151) and grieving relates to the emotional experience of a bereavement. Perhaps the most well known theory of stages of bereavement is Elizabeth Kubler-Ross' model, which suggests that people go through stages of denial, anger, bargaining, depression and acceptance. While the model has been useful in helping people understand their emotional experiences during a time of bereavement, it has been argued that this theory has been taken too literally, is too simplistic and has not necessarily been supported in the literature (Boerner & Wortman 2001). The idea of staged bereavement can also contribute to professionals placing too much emphasis on the stages and then pathologising people who do not go through the stages in the way a model, such as Kubler-Ross', predicts (Boerner & Wortman 2001). Some research has looked at applying ideas from stress and coping to understand grieving (Stroebe & Schut 2001).

A review by Stroebe et al (2007) of the health outcomes of bereavement suggested that there are a number of risk factors that increase vulnerability to problems with bereavement. Death of a spouse, in terms of stressfulness of life events, ranks as the most stressful experience that people have (Holmes & Rahe 1967). Grieving after someone dies is normal and, indeed, not grieving, especially if the death was of a close family member or friend, would be seen as problematic. Reactions to bereavement are generally classified according to affective (emotional), cognitive (thought-based), behavioural, physiologic-somatic and immunological and endocrine changes. Overall, bereavement increases physical ill health and physical health complaints, as well as the incidence of seeking healthcare. *Complicated grief*, however, is when the psychological and social aspects of grieving exceed what might be considered 'normal' (Ray & Prigerson 2007).

As with research on other topics relevant to health psychology (e.g. trauma and stress), it should not be surprising that research in bereavement is also exploring the positive aspects of grief and challenging previously held notions. For example, Schaefer and Moos (2001) looked at positive growth (see also literature on *posttraumatic growth*) following bereavement and Heilman (2005) looked at the diversity of the grief experience, particularly the positive dimensions, following the 9/11 attacks on the World Trade Center in New York. Other research has explored the possibilities of creativity and art as therapy in bereavement (Bolton 2007). Chapter 11 also examines loss resulting from death, dying and bereavement.

Critical thinking

In Davis and Bartlett's article the authors discuss some of the health benefits of rural living, such as fresh air, peace and quiet, lower housing costs and less violence and crime. The authors also discuss some of the things that make it harder to live healthily in rural settings. Some of these include the higher costs of food, fuel and transportation and barriers to social activities and access to health services.

- How might knowledge of rural Australia contribute to your practice? Consider if you are working in an urban centre and have clients from rural or remote areas. What might you need to consider in your treatment?
- What issues might health professionals working in a rural or remote area need to consider? Consider access to equipment, specialists and options in emergency situations.

Research focus

Davis, S., Bartlett, H., 2008. Healthy ageing in rural Australia: issues and challenges. Australasian Journal on Ageing 27 (2), 56–60.

ABSTRACT

Approximately 36% of the rural Australian population is 65 years or older. In fact, many rural and remote communities have higher proportions of older people than metropolitan centres. The rate of growth, patterns of migration, higher levels of health risk factors and of social and economic disadvantage all impact on healthy ageing in rural communities. Older people in rural communities have become marginalised by longstanding misconceptions about rural life and urban-centric policies, much of which goes unchallenged because of a paucity of research in key areas and a lack of intrarural research. Understanding the complexities of rural healthy ageing is challenging and more research is required to develop a stronger empirical base. The aim of this review was to critique the literature related to rural ageing in Australia to identify the issues and challenges for rural healthy ageing and implications for policy and practice.

Key points

- Approximately 36% of the rural-dwelling population in Australia is aged 65 or older.
- Rural living presents a range of challenges for optimising healthy ageing.
- Perceptions about rural ageing are often inaccurate and do not reflect the diverse nature of the rural experience.
- More research into the differences between and within rural communities is needed to inform policy and practice to support healthy ageing in rural areas.

Conclusion

To summarise, this chapter explored various stage theories in adult developmental psychology, including Erikson, Kohlberg, Bronfenbrenner, and Hendry and Kloep. Developmental milestones, such as marriage and employment, were explored and the relevance of these to healthcare practice was discussed. All of these theories and ideas can be critiqued and exceptions made to the stages or theories. While stages and generalisations about adulthood and ageing can be made, it is important to consider different circumstances at different ages and how people of various ages in differing situations might be affected. It is not possible to determine exactly how people will behave at different times of their lives, but learning how to identify differences and to expect these differences will improve the appropriateness of healthcare practice.

For example, knowing that a client in your health clinic is 21 years old provides very different health expectations compared with knowing that a client is 50 or 80 years old. However, expectations and treatment would differ greatly for a single 21-year-old client who grew up in urban Australia compared with a 21-year-old client with three children and recently arrived from the Middle East. Theories about developmental stages of adulthood can provide a guide to understanding clients but cannot predict exactly the lived human experience.

Developing an understanding of developmental (st)ages is at least partly dependent on personal experience, in addition to experience with others to understand the diversity of people's lives. With so much diversity, asking your clients about their contexts, circumstances, milestones and stages of life will go far in ensuring that the healthcare provided is appropriate and relevant.

REMEMBER

- The lived experiences of adulthood are amazingly diverse in Australia and New Zealand, relative to socioeconomic status, ethnicities, disabilities, genders, geographic locations, and types of religions and spiritualities.
- Understanding the diversity of adult lives can improve healthcare practice and outcomes.
- While developmental theories provide useful models for understanding human development they are not always universally applicable.

Further resources

Breen, L.J., O'Connor, M., 2007. The fundamental paradox in the grief literature: a critical reflection. Omega 55, 199–218.

Hildon, Z., Smith, G., Netuveli, G., et al., 2008. Understanding adversity and resilience at older ages. Sociology of Health & Illness 3, 726–740.

Liu, H., Umberson, D.J., 2008. The times they are a changin': marital status and health differentials from 1972 to 2003. Journal of Health and Social Behavior 49, 239–253.

Slater, C.L., 2003. Generativity versus stagnation: an elaboration of Erikson's adult stage of human development. Journal of Adult Development 10, 53–65.

Teachman, J., 2008. Complex life course patterns and the risk of divorce in second marriages. Journal of Marriage and Family 70, 294–305.

Weblinks

Australian Indigenous Health*InfoNet*

www.healthinfonet.ecu.edu.au

The Australian Indigenous Health*InfoNet* is an innovative web resource that makes knowledge and information on Indigenous health easily accessible to inform practice and policy.

Australian Institute of Family Studies

www.aifs.gov.au

The Australian Institute of Family Studies provides bibliographies on a range of topics of interest to health psychology and lifespan development including:

- separation and divorce
- grandparents
- Indigenous families.

Australian Institute of Health and Welfare

www.aihw.gov.au

The AIHW website provides an extensive range of publications and information relevant to material covered in this chapter. See, for example, Australia's Health 2008 Chapter 6 'Health across the life stages'.

HealthInsite

http://www.healthinsite.gov.au/topics/Family_Breakdown

HealthInsite provides some useful resources relating to family breakdown and divorce.

Multicultural Mental Health Australia

www.mmha.org.au

MMHA provides national leadership in building greater awareness of mental health and suicide prevention among Australians from culturally and linguistically diverse (CALD) backgrounds. Through unique partnerships with Australian mental health specialists, services, advocacy groups and tertiary institutions, MMHA actively promotes the mental health and wellbeing of Australia's diverse communities through a series of campaigns, projects and information fact sheets. MMHA also produces a series of resources and training for specialist and mainstream mental health professionals.

References

Amato, P.A., 2010. Research on divorce: continuing trends and new developments. Journal of Marriage and Family 72 (3), 650–666.

Arendell, T., 2000. Conceiving and investigating motherhood: the decade's scholarship. Journal of Marriage and the Family 62, 1192–1207.

Arnett, J.J., 2000. Emerging adulthood: a theory of development from the late teens through the twenties. American Psychologist 55, 469–480.

Arnett, J.J., Kloep, M., Hendry, L.B., et al. (Eds.), 2011. Debating emerging adulthood: stage or process? Oxford, New York.

Arnett, J.J., Tanner, J.L. (Eds.), 2006. Emerging adulthood in America: coming of age in the 21st century. American Psychological Association, Washington DC.

Australian Bureau of Statistics (ABS), 2008. Causes of death, Australia 2006, 3303.0. Online. Available: http://www.abs.gov.au/ausstats/abs@.nsf/0/2093DA6935DB138FCA2568A9001393C9 11 Aug 2008.

Australian Bureau of Statistics (ABS), 2011. Family characteristics, Australia 2009–10, 4442.0. Online. Available: http://www.abs.gov.au/ausstats/abs@.nsf/Latestproducts/4442.0Main%20Features22009-10?opendocument&tabname=Summary&prodno=4442.0&issue=2009-10&num=&view= 11 Nov 2012.

Australian Bureau of Statistics (ABS). n.d. Family and community glossary. Online. Available: http://www.abs.gov.au/websitedbs/c311215.NSF /43b68f1dafb94862ca256eb0000221a5/dc61793ed26c330bca25715500193159! OpenDocument 11 Aug 2008.

Australian Bureau of Statistics (ABS), 2012. Causes of death, Australia 2010, 3303.0. Online. Available: http://www.abs.gov.au/ausstats/abs@.nsf/Products /6BAD463E482C6970CA2579C6000F6AF7?opendocument 11 Nov 2012.

Australian Marriage Equality, 2012. Civil unions in Australia, Online. Available: http:// www.australianmarriageequality.com/civilunions.htm.

Baltes, P.B., 2000. Life-span developmental theory. In: Kazdin, A. (Ed.), Encyclopedia of psychology. American Psychological Association & Oxford University Press, Washington DC & New York.

Baltes, P.B., Baltes, M.M., 1990. Psychological perspectives on successful aging: the model of selective optimization with compensation. In: Baltes, P.B., Baltes, M.M. (Eds.), Successful aging: perspectives from the behavioural sciences. Cambridge University Press, New York.

Baltes, P.B., Lindenberger, U., Staudinger, U.M., 2006. Lifespan theory in developmental psychology. In: Damon, W., Lerner, R.M. (Eds.), Handbook of child psychology: Vol 1, Theoretical models of human development, sixth ed. Wiley, New York, pp. 569–664.

Bambra, C., Gibson, M., Sowden, A., et al., 2010. Tackling the wider social determinants of health and health inequalities: evidence from systematic reviews. Journal of Epidemiology and Community Health 64, 284–291.

Baumrind, D., 1991. The influence of parenting style on adolescent competence and substance use. Journal of Early Adolescence 11 (1), 56–95.

Baumrind, D., Larzelere, R.E., Owens, E.B., 2010. Effects of preschool parents' power assertive patterns and practices on adolescent development. Parenting: Science and Practice 10, 157–201.

Benach, J., Muntaner, C., Chung, H., et al., 2010. The importance of government policies in reducing employment related health inequalities. British Medical Journal 340, c2154.

Boerner, K., Wortman, C.B., 2001. Bereavement: international encyclopedia for the social and behavioral sciences. Elsevier, pp. 1151–1155.

Bolton, G. (Ed.), 2007. Dying, bereavement and the healing arts. Jessica Kingsley, London.

Bowlby, J., 1969. Attachment and loss. Attachment, Vol. 1. Basic Books, New York.

Bronfenbrenner, U., 1979. The ecology of human development. Harvard University Press, Cambridge.

Bronfenbrenner, U. (Ed.), 2004. Making human beings human: bioecological perspectives on human development. Sage, Thousand Oaks.

Cameron, B.J., 1966. Adoption. In: McLintock, A.H. (Ed.), 2007 (originally published in 1966). An encyclopaedia of New Zealand. Online. Available: http:// www.teara.govt.nz/1966/A/Adoption/Adoption/en 26 Sep 2008.

Cantor-Graae, E., 2007. The contribution of social factors to the development of schizophrenia: a review of recent findings. Canadian Journal of Psychiatry 52, 277–286.

Cribb, J., 2009. Focus on families: New Zealand families of yesterday, today and tomorrow. Social Policy Journal of New Zealand 35, 4.

Davis, S., Bartlett, H., 2008. Healthy ageing in rural Australia: issues and challenges. Australasian Journal on Ageing 27 (2), 56–60.

de Vaus, D., 2004. Diversity and change in Australian families: a statistical profile. Australian Institute of Family Studies, Canberra.

Department of Internal Affairs Te Tari Taiwhenua, 2011. Civil unions. Online. Available: http://www.dia.govt.nz/diawebsite.nsf/wpg_URL/Services-Births-Deaths-and-Marriages-Civil-Union?OpenDocument 18 Apr 2012.

Dharmalingam, A., 1996. The social context of family size preferences and fertility behaviour in a South India village. Genus 52, 83–103.

Doucet, A., 2006. Do men mother? Fatherhood, care, and domestic responsibility. University of Toronto Press, Toronto.

Dousset, L., 2011. Australian Aboriginal Kinship: An introductory handbook with particular emphasis on the Western Desert. Marseille: Pacific-credo Publications.

Elliot, J., 2008. Marriage increases life expectancy. Minister for Ageing, Canberra. Online. Available: http://www.health.gov.au/internet/ministers/publishing.nsf/Content/mr-yr08-je-je135.htm 11 Aug 2008.

Emery, C.R., 2009. Stay for the children? Husband violence, marital stability and children's behavior problems. Journal of Marriage and Family 71 (4), 905–916.

Erikson, E.H., 1950. Childhood and society. WW Norton, New York.

Erikson, E.H., 1982. The life cycle completed. WW Norton, New York.

Erikson, E.H., Erikson, J.M., 1997. The life cycle completed. WW Norton, New York.

Farr, R.H., Forsell, S.L., Patterson, C.J., 2010. Parenting and child development in adoptive families: Does parental sexual orientation matter? Applied Developmental Science 14 (3), 164–178.

Gilligan, C., 1982. In a different voice: psychological theory and women's development. Harvard University Press, Cambridge.

Gilligan, C., Farnsworth, L., 1995. A new voice for psychology. In: Chester, P., Rothblum, E.D., Cold, E. (Eds.), Feminist foremothers in women's studies, psychology, mental health. Harrington Park Press, Binghamton.

Gomez, R., Fisher, J.W., 2003. Domains of spiritual well-being and development and validation of the spiritual well-being questionnaire. Personality and Individual Differences 35, 1975–1991.

Hartley, R., 1995. Families and cultural diversity in Australia. Allen and Unwin, Sydney.

Hayes, A., Weston, R., Qu, L., et al., 2010. Families then and now: 1980–2010. Australian Institute of Family Studies, Canberra.

Hayes, A., Qu, L., Weston, R., et al., 2011. Families in Australia 2011: sticking together in good and tough times Australian Institute of Family Studies. Online. Available: http://www.aifs.gov.au/institute/pubs/factssheets/2011/fw2011/index.html 11 Nov 2012.

HealthInfoNet, 2011. What details do we know about the Indigenous population? Online. Available: http://www.healthinfonet.ecu.edu.au/health-facts/health-faqs/aboriginal-population 18 Apr 2012.

Hegar, R.L., 1999. The cultural roots of kinship care. In: Hegar, R.L., Scannapieco, M. (Eds.), 1999. Kinship foster care: policy, practice and research. Oxford University Press, New York, pp. 17–27.

Hegar, R.L., Scannapieco, M. (Eds.), 1999. Kinship foster care: policy, practice and research. Oxford University Press, New York.

Heilman, S.C. (Ed.), 2005. Death, bereavement and mourning. Transaction, New Brunswick.

Hendry, L.B., Kloep, M., 2002. Lifespan development: resources, challenges and risks. Thomson, Australia.

Holmes, J., 2011. Attachment, autonomy, intimacy: some clinical implications of attachment theory. British Journal of Medical Psychology 70 (3), 231–248.

Holmes, T.H., Rahe, R.H., 1967. The social readjustment rating scale. Journal of Psychosomatic Research 11, 213–218.

Jaffe, D.H., Manor, O., Eisenbach, Z., et al., 2007. The protective effect of marriage on mortality in a dynamic society. Annals of Epidemiology 17 (7), 540–547.

Jaffee, S., Hyde, J.S., 2000. Gender differences in moral orientation: a meta-analysis. Psychological Bulletin 126 (5), 703–726.

Kessler, R.C., Berglund, P., Demler, O., et al., 2005. Lifetime prevalence and age-or-onset distributions of DSM-IV disorder in the National Comorbidity Survey replication. Archives of General Psychiatry 62, 593–602.

Kloep, M., Hendry, L., Saunders, D., 2009. A new perspective on human development. Conference of the International Journal of Arts and Sciences 1 (6), 332–343.

Koenig, H.G., King, D.E., Carson, V.B., 2012. Handbook of religion and health. Oxford, Auckland.

Kohlberg, L., 1976. Moral stages and moralization: the cognitive developmental approach. In: Lickona, T. (Ed.), Moral development and behaviour: theory, research and social issues. Holt, New York, pp. 33–35.

Kohlberg, L., Ryncarz, R.A., 1990. Beyond justice reasoning: Moral development and consideration of a seventh stage. In: Alexander, C.N., Langer, E.J. (Eds.), Higher stages of human development. Oxford University Press, New York, pp. 191–207.

La Cour, P., Hvidt, N.C., 2010. Research on meaning-making and health in secular society: secular, spiritual and religious existential orientations. Social Science and Medicine 71 (7), 1292–1299.

McRae, K.O., Nikora, L.W., 2006. Whangai: remembering, understanding and experiencing. MAI Review 1, 1–18.

Omokhodion, F.O., Uchendu, O.C., 2010. Perception and practice of child labour among parents of school-aged children in Ibadan, southwest Nigeria. Child Care and Health Development 36 (3), 304–308.

Qin, D., Comstock, D.L., 2005. Traditional models of development: appreciating context and relationship. In: Comstock, D.L. (Ed.), Diversity and development: critical contexts that shape our lives and relationships. Thomson, Australia.

Ray, A., Prigerson, H., 2007. Grieving. In: Fink, G. (Ed.), Encyclopaedia of stress, second ed, Vol. 2. Elsevier, Australia, pp. 238–242.

Riggs, D.W., Due, C., 2010. Gay men, race, privilege and surrogacy in India. Outskirts 22. Online. Available: http://www.outskirts.arts.uwa.edu.au/volumes/volume-22/riggs 1 May 2012.

Schaefer, J.A., Moos, R.H., 2001. Bereavement experiences and personal growth. In: Stroebe, M.S., Hansson, R.O., Stroebe, W. et al. (Eds.), Handbook of bereavement research: consequences, coping and care. American Psychological Association, Washington DC, pp. 145–167.

Scheitle, C.P., Adamczyk, A., 2010. High-cost religion, religious switching, and health. Journal of Health and Social Behavior 51 (3), 325–342.

Scheper-Hughes, N., 1985. Culture, scarcity and maternal thinking: Maternal detachment and infant survival in a Brazilian shantytown. Ethos 13, 291–317.

Schoenborn, C.A., 2004. Marital status and health: United States, 1999–2002. Advance data from vital and health statistics; no 351. National Center for Health Statistics, Hyattsville.

Shirley, I., Koopman-Boyden, P., Pool, I., et al., 1997. New Zealand. In: Kamerman, S.B., Kahn, A.J., 1997 Family change and family policies in Great Britain, Canada, New Zealand and the United States. Oxford University Press, New York, pp 207–304.

Smith, K., LoGiudice, D., Dwyer, A., et al., 2007. Ngana minyarti? What is this? Development of cognitive questions for the Kimberley Indigenous Cognitive Assessment. Australasian Journal on Ageing 26 (3), 115–119.

Statistics New Zealand, 2012. Marriages, civil unions, and divorces: year ended December 2011. Online. Available: http://www.stats.govt.nz/browse_for_stats/people_and_communities/marriages-civil-unions-and-divorces/MarriagesCivilUnionsandDivorces_HOTPYeDec11.aspx 11 Nov 2012.

Stroebe, M.S., Schut, H., 2001. Models of coping with bereavement: a review. In: Stroebe, M.S., Hansson, R.O., Stroebe, W. et al. (Eds.), Handbook of bereavement research: consequences, coping and care. American Psychological Association, Washington DC, pp. 375–404.

Stroebe, M.S., Schut, H., Stroebe, W., 2007. Health outcomes of bereavement. The Lancet 370, 1960–1973.

Chapter 4
Health and health psychology

PATRICIA BARKWAY

Learning objectives

The material in this chapter will help you to:

- understand the complex dynamics of the concept of health
- understand the role of health psychology in healthcare practice
- describe the biomedical model of health and illness
- describe the biopsychosocial model of health and illness
- explain the contribution of psychology and, in particular, health psychology to understandings of health, illness and health behaviours
- analyse and critique the interrelationship between biological, psychological and social factors in health and illness behaviours and in the delivery of healthcare services.

Key terms

- Health
- Psychology
- Health psychology
- Sociology
- Biomedical model
- Biopsychosocial model

Introduction

In this chapter health is presented as a dynamic concept that is constantly changing, is multidimensional and is influenced by factors that are both internal and external to the individual. The biomedical (also called bioscience) model of health and illness, which dominated healthcare delivery up until the middle of the 20th century and perpetuates the notion of a mind–body split, is examined and critiqued. Finally, it will be argued that the biopsychosocial model, which utilises research evidence, theory and clinical practices from a range of health disciplines including bioscience, psychology and sociology, offers a more comprehensive explanation for health behaviours and health outcomes than is provided by the biomedical model alone. In particular, health psychology (a branch of psychology) is examined for the contribution it makes to understandings of human behaviour in relation to health and illness and thereby to the clinical practice of not only psychologists but of all health professionals.

Psychological theories offer complementary and, at times, contradictory views of human behaviour that reflect different assumptions about the nature of individuals and how they should be studied. These varying theoretical perspectives include bioscience, psychoanalytic, behavioural (or learning), cognitive and humanistic theories. These explanations are described in detail in Chapter 1 and underpin the approaches used in health psychology. You will discover that each theoretical position offers a different perspective on human behaviour and each may provide useful explanations in specific situations. Nevertheless, none provide a universal explanation of behaviour that is applicable to all people in all situations.

What is health?

Health is a construct that can be defined in both broad and narrow terms. Narrow interpretations are provided by the biomedical model, which emphasises the presence or absence of disease, pathogens and/or symptoms. A broader interpretation is provided by the biopsychosocial approach that proposes that health is influenced by a complex interaction of biological, psychological and social factors. See Table 4.1 for sociological, psychological and biomedical factors that influence health.

Additionally, health can be examined both objectively and subjectively. Objective measures such as an x-ray or scan can indicate health or illness, while an individual's subjective interpretation will report whether he or she feels healthy or ill, but there may be no correlation between the two. For example, a person may report feeling healthy but have dangerously high blood pressure, or another person may report pain for which physical pathology cannot be identified. Therefore, given the range of criteria and the different perceptions that can influence a definition of health, it is not surprising that many interpretations exist and that debate surrounds an agreed definition of the concept (Australian Institute of Health and Welfare (AIHW) 2010, Jormfeldt et al 2007).

Table 4.1

MODELS OF HEALTH AND THEIR INFLUENCE

Models of health		
Biomedical	Psychological	Sociological
Pathogens	Thoughts	Social
Genetics	Feelings	Cultural
Biochemical	Behaviours	Ethnicity
Hormonal	Unconscious drives	Economics
Injury	Learning	Politics
Environment	Environment	Environment

Furthermore, health can have different meanings for the general public or laypeople than it does for health professionals. Three consistent themes arise in research into laypeople's understanding of the concept of health. They are: health is not being ill; health is a prerequisite for life's functions; and health involves both physical and mental wellbeing (Baum 2008 p 7). Baum suggests that these lay definitions have more in common with the World Health Organization's (WHO) definition of health (more than the absence of disease) than biomedical interpretations do.

BIOMEDICAL MODEL

Throughout history, explanations for illness have included somatic imbalance, demonology, witchcraft and environmental pathogens. In Western-industrialised countries up until the middle of the 20th century, health was generally viewed as the absence of disease, and illness was seen as a pathological state. With the emergence of the public health movement in the 19th century the biomedical approach (also called the medical model) rose to prominence and dominated Western medicine for more than 200 years. The biomedical model proposes organic, pathological theories to explain and treat illness. Essentially, this approach is an illness-based model with the underpinning assumption that illness and disease are caused by disequilibrium in the body that is brought about by one or more of the following:

- biological pathogens such as viral or bacterial infection
- trauma or injury such as acquired brain injury
- a biochemical imbalance in the body such as hypothyroidism or diabetes
- degenerative processes such as arthritis or dementia.

From the 19th century, public health strategies utilising a biomedical approach such as mass vaccinations and sanitation have achieved a worldwide reduction in many communicable diseases like polio, smallpox and pneumonia, and an increase in life expectancy (Brannon & Feist 2009, Frieden 2010). In the 20th century, the discovery of antibiotics, psychotropic medications and the development of sophisticated surgical techniques such as organ transplantation have enabled previously life-threatening diseases and conditions to be treated and, in many instances, cured.

However, by the latter half of the 20th century it became apparent that the *treatment* era of the previous decades did not live up to the expectations of the scientific or wider community. In Western countries, for example, diseases related to lifestyle, like diabetes and cardiovascular disease, now pose a greater threat to health than that of infectious diseases. Also, with regard to the treatment of infectious diseases, some bacterial strains have developed resistance to antibiotics (e.g. methicillin-resistant *Staphylococcus aureus*) and for many cancers neither a cure, nor preventive vaccination has been discovered. In the main, many cancer prevention and chronic illness management strategies are related to lifestyle and the environment, such as ceasing cigarette smoking, using sun protection, being physically active, eating a healthy diet and maintaining weight within the healthy range.

In the mental illness field the unwanted side effects of antipsychotic drugs are often problematic and can contribute to non-adherence to treatment, for example, the rapid and sustained weight gain and iatrogenic diabetes mellitus experienced by some patients taking atypical antipsychotic medication to treat schizophrenia (Hasnain et al 2009, Kim et al 2010). Such consequences of treatment present a challenge to both patients and health professionals with regard to the relative cost–benefit of the treatment. For patients, the unwanted social and health consequences may interfere with adherence to the recommended treatment. For health professionals, there is the ethical dilemma of encouraging adherence to a treatment for one health condition such as schizophrenia that carries a high risk that the patient will develop another serious health condition such as diabetes mellitus.

Challenges to an exclusive biomedical approach

Initially, the biomedical model held great promise to improve the health of individuals and communities. Scientific research in the 20th century led to the discovery of medications that could cure, or eliminate, many diseases. Sulphur drugs – developed in the 1930s – and other antibiotics revolutionised the treatment of infection. In the mental health field the first antipsychotic medication (chlorpromazine) was introduced in 1950. At the time it was lauded as a breakthrough in the treatment of schizophrenia because of its ability to reduce disruptive behaviour (Meadows et al 2012). Patients who would have been in straitjackets and lived out their lives in a mental institution could now be discharged and returned to live in the community.

However, by the middle of the 20th century concerns were mounting regarding the cost escalation of scientific, technological medicine; worldwide there was recognition of the need for sustainable environments. It was also evident, particularly in Western countries, that the diseases that threatened communities were no longer infectious and acute but were chronic and related to lifestyle. For example, the health conditions that now carry the greatest burden of disease are mental illness, cancer, cardiovascular disease, diabetes, substance abuse and interpersonal violence (AIHW 2010, Marmot & Wilkinson 2006).

Challenges to the biomedical model as the *exclusive* framework for understanding health and to structure the delivery of healthcare services began to emerge from the middle of the 20th century, the major criticism being that an exclusive biomedical approach fails to take into account the contribution of broader psychological, sociological, political, economic and environmental factors that influence health and illness. A further criticism of an exclusive biomedical approach is that health resources are directed to costly curative services rather than to health promotion or illness prevention. Baum argues that 'there needs to be more research on the ways in which social and economic factors affect health and what social, educational, housing and health interventions most improve health and health equity' (Baum 2008 p 145).

Questioning of the dominance of the biomedical model by policymakers, commentators and clinicians coincided with the United Nations establishing WHO in the 1940s. WHO was given the brief to work towards 'the attainment by all peoples of the highest possible level of health' and in 1946 the organisation released its then groundbreaking definition of health that stated:

Health is a state of complete physical, mental and social wellbeing and not merely the absence of disease or infirmity.

(WHO 1946)

This definition was developed in response to the changing healthcare needs of populations. The WHO explanation contested the efficacy of the prevailing biomedical view of health at the time by recognising the contribution of not only physical factors to health and illness but social and psychological factors as well. WHO's broadening of the definition of health signalled the introduction of what became known as the biopsychosocial approach in which the contribution of individual, lifestyle and social factors to health outcomes is acknowledged. It also laid the foundation for the emergence in the 1970s of the primary health care/new public health movement.

Nevertheless, while the WHO definition of health is a comprehensive one, it has its limitations. The use of the word 'complete' is problematic. Is it possible to be completely healthy in all areas identified (physical, mental and social) and at all times? And if this is not possible does it necessarily follow that an individual who has one health issue is unhealthy? Consider, for example, a person with a well-managed chronic illness (asthma) or a disability (vision impairment) who is otherwise in good health. If you asked either of these two individuals to rate their health do you think they would describe themselves as unhealthy? They probably would not. When asthma is managed by medication and vision impairment corrected by glasses the person does not experience limitations from the health issue. Therefore, in seeking a comprehensive definition of health other factors must be considered including the individual's sense of control of and satisfaction with his or her health and life.

Furthermore, there are demonstrated links between income and health outcomes, that is, that poor people have worse health outcomes regarding morbidity and mortality than people who are wealthy. This occurs both within and between countries (Babones 2008, WHO 2008). For example, in a Finnish study Tarkiainen et al (2011) found a gap in life expectancy of 5.1 years for men and 2.9 years for women between people in the lowest and highest income groups. And, while life expectancy in New Zealand is 79 years, it is only 39 years in Angola (NationMaster 2011). WHO recognises the importance of addressing income inequities to improve health and stated in the Closing the Gap report that 'higher levels of better coordinated aid and debt relief, applied to poverty reduction through a social determinants of health framework are a matter both of life and death and of global justice' (WHO 2008 p 130).

Increased longevity over the past two centuries, in Western countries, is attributed not only to advances in medical treatments, but also to public health initiatives and population-level interventions such as access to safe water and sanitation, programs to address global road safety, tobacco control and vaccination programs for preventable diseases (Centers for Disease Control and Prevention 2011). In fact, the biggest increase in life expectancy that occurred in the first half of the 20th century is attributed mainly to public health initiatives and population-focused interventions, not advances in medical science (Frieden 2010). Yet, in 2007–08 the Australian Government spent only 21.6% if its $100 billion health budget on public health activities for whole populations or population groups (AIHW 2010 p 442). This means that almost 80% of the government's health budget was allocated to treatment interventions and services for illness and injury, yet the evidence suggests that this is not the most effective allocation of financial resources to achieve the best health outcomes for individuals and populations (Kickbusch et al 2011, Marmot 2010).

In summary, the biomedical model holds the view that health outcomes are influenced by physiology, with health occurring when the body is in a state of equilibrium and illness being a consequence of physical pathology or disequilibrium. The approach is limited as a theory to explain and understand health and the provision of healthcare services because it is a one-dimensional model that fails to take into account the complex interplay of other factors, namely, psychological and social factors that interact with biological factors and affect health.

BIOPSYCHOSOCIAL MODEL

As discussed, the philosophy that underpins the biopsychosocial model is that health or illness results from a complex interplay between biological, psychological and social factors. The model emerged in the 1970s in response to realisations regarding the limitations of the biomedical model in a changing world.

The notion of an alternative to the biomedical model was first proposed by Engel (1977) and quickly gained momentum among health professionals and policymakers. The biopsychosocial model is holistic in approach and thereby avoids the mind–body split inherent in the biomedical model. A further outcome of this approach is the recognition of the contribution made by allied health professionals to healthcare and the emergence of the multidisciplinary team as a mechanism for providing health services.

Health priorities

Australia's National Health Priority Areas (AIHW 2011) are health issues identified by the federal Department of Health and Ageing for focused attention because they contribute significantly to the burden of illness and injury in Australia. The eight priority areas are: cancer control; injury prevention and control; cardiovascular health; diabetes mellitus; mental health; asthma; arthritis and musculoskeletal conditions; and obesity – all of which have complex aetiology including lifestyle, biological, psychological and social factors. In addressing these health problems the holistic nature of the biopsychosocial model offers greater opportunity to improve health outcomes than a biomedical approach alone because the biopsychosocial approach addresses more than just the symptoms of the condition.

Nevertheless, despite the intrinsic appeal of the biopsychosocial model some critics argue that, generally, social issues are not sufficiently addressed in practice (Lyons & Chamberlain 2006, Yamada & Brekke 2008). Utilising another approach – primary health care/new public health that operates from a biopsychosocial framework *and* has a strong emphasis on social and political issues that impact on health – is proposed as a way to overcome this shortcoming.

PRIMARY HEALTH CARE/NEW PUBLIC HEALTH

The emergence of the primary health care/new public health movement also in the 1970s coincided with the growing awareness that psychological and social influences as well as physical and biological factors influenced health outcomes for individuals and communities. It was formally endorsed as a mechanism to achieve *Health for all by the year 2000* at the 1978 WHO conference in the Declaration of Alma-Ata in the former Soviet Union. The declaration was the culmination of a WHO–UNICEF sponsored conference at which representatives from 134 nations endorsed the declaration with the philosophical principles of: social justice; equity; access; empowerment; self-determination; political action; health promotion and illness prevention; collaboration between consumers, practitioners, countries, governments and those responsible for health; and striving for world peace.

Worldwide policymakers, health professionals and communities were increasingly looking beyond the biomedical model for answers to health problems (Baum 2008, Karlsson et al 2010, Marmot 2008). In 1981 Lalonde, the then Canadian Minister of National Health and Welfare, described four general determinants of health that he called human biology, environment, lifestyle and healthcare organisation. Supporting a shift from a biomedical approach to a broader approach acknowledging biopsychosocial factors Lalonde stated:

There can be no doubt that the traditional view of equating the level of health in Canada with the availability of physicians and hospitals is inadequate. Marvellous though healthcare services are in Canada in comparison with many other countries, there is little doubt that future improvements in the level of health of Canadians lie mainly in improving the environment, moderating self imposed risks and adding to our knowledge of human biology.
(Lalonde 1981 p 18)

In 1986, eight years after the Alma-Ata declaration, the first WHO International Conference on Health Promotion was held in Ottawa, Canada. Conference participants developed an action framework of five strategies (the Ottawa Charter) to achieve *Health for All*. These five strategies have become the cornerstone of the primary health care/new public health movement and the Charter continues to be a robust, insightful and useful document in contemporary healthcare policy and practice (Baum & Sanders 2011). Nevertheless, some commentators argue that health policy alone is insufficient to achieve health equity and social justice, and that a 'health in all policies' (e.g. education, welfare, housing) approach is needed to redress health inequities (Baum & Sanders 2011, Kickbusch et al 2011).

Table 4.2

ACTIONS OF THE OTTAWA CHARTER FOR HEALTH PROMOTION

Ottawa Charter strategy	Action
Build healthy public policy	Direct policymakers to be aware of the health consequences of their decisions and to develop socially responsible policy
Create supportive environments	Generate living and working conditions that are safe, stimulating, satisfying and enjoyable
Strengthen community action	Empower communities and enable ownership and control of their own endeavours and destinies
Develop personal skills	Support personal and social development through providing information, education for health and enhancing life skills
Reorient health services	Share responsibility for health promotion in health services among individuals, community groups, health professionals, health service institutions and government

HEALTH OF AUSTRALIANS AND NEW ZEALANDERS

When compared with other countries in the world, the health of Australians and New Zealanders ranks highly. They are rated among the top 10 developed countries in the world across a range of significant indicators. Life expectancy is ranked among that of the top nations in the world. See Table 4.3 for life expectancies for selected countries.

In addition, Australians born in the 21st century can expect to live 20–25 years longer than their ancestors born at the commencement of the 20th century. That is, a male born in 1901 had a life expectancy of 55.2 years, whereas a male born in 2008 has a life expectancy of 79.2 years (see Table 4.4).

Classroom activity

1. Examine the international life expectancy statistics in Table 4.3.
   - What do these statistics tell us?
   - What are the implications of this?
2. Before coming to class, select three countries (each with a short, medium and long life expectancy) and research the health issues in these three countries.
   - Identify the health priorities or significant health issues of the three countries.
   - Discuss and critique these health issues and priorities in class.
   - Identify biomedical, psychological and sociological contributors to these health issues.

Table 4.3

LIFE EXPECTANCY IN SELECTED COUNTRIES

Selected countries	Life expectancy at birth
Japan	82.25
Hong Kong	82.14
Singapore	82.04
Australia	81.81
Indigenous Australians	70.0
Korea (South)	79.05
United Kingdom	80.05
New Zealand	79.0
Māori	70.4
United States	78.37
China	74.68
Indonesia	71.33
Papua New Guinea	66.24
India	66.8
Angola	38.76

Source: AIHW 2010, NationMaster 2011, NZ Ministry of Social Development 2010

Table 4.4

AUSTRALIAN LIFE EXPECTANCY (YEARS) AT DIFFERENT AGES, 1901–1910 AND 2006–2008

Age	Males			Females		
	1901–1910	2006–2008	Percent increase	1901–1910	2006–2008	Percent increase
Birth	55.2	79.2	43.5%	58.8	83.7	42.3%
30 years	66.5	80.3	20.8%	69.3	84.5	21.9%
65 years	76.3	83.6	9.6%	77.9	86.6	11.2%
85 years	87.7	90.9	3.6%	89.2	92.0	2.8%

Source: Australian Institute of Health and Welfare

Classroom activity

1. Compare the life expectancy statistics for Australia in 1901–1910 and 2006–2008 in Table 4.4.
   - What do these statistics tell us?
   - Identify factors that have contributed to increased life expectancy in Australia.
2. It is predicted that the current generation of young Australians will be the first to not outlive their parents.
   - Identify factors that have led commentators to make this claim.

TWENTY-FIRST CENTURY HEALTH CHALLENGES

Regardless of the gains made in longevity over the past one hundred years in Australia and New Zealand there are some disturbing trends in the health statistics of these two nations. Life expectancy for Indigenous Australians is 11.8 years lower than the national average. While this gap has reduced from 17.5 years in 2005–07 the AIHW cautions that the decrease is more likely to be as a consequence of a change in how the Australian Bureau of Statistics (ABS) collects statistics rather than an actual increase in Indigenous life expectancy (AIHW 2010 p 234). Also, while the discrepancy is not as great in New Zealand as it is in Australia, Māori life expectancy is 8.6 years less than the New Zealand average (NZ Ministry of Social Development 2010). Furthermore, Indigenous Australians not only die younger than the national average, they also experience significantly more ill health and disability than other Australians (AIHW 2010 p 229).

Also of concern is cardiovascular disease, which, in Australia, is the leading cause of death (36% of deaths) and one of the leading causes of disability (6.9% of the population). And while mortality figures for most health conditions, including coronary heart disease, stroke, colon cancer and infant mortality, have improved over the past 25 years in Australia, the mortality figures have worsened for some other illnesses, such as diabetes mellitus, chronic obstructive pulmonary disease and accidental falls (AIHW 2010 p 29). Finally, Australia has the unenviable 'honour' of being ranked in the 'worst' third of OECD countries for obesity levels, measured by a body mass index greater than 30 (AIHW 2010 p 31). That puts these Australians at increased risk for lifestyle health conditions such as high cholesterol, hypertension, heart disease and some cancers.

FRAMEWORK FOR HEALTH

In conclusion, finding a universally applicable definition of health is challenging because health is a dynamic concept influenced by a complex range of factors that interact with and influence each other. Therefore, rather than pursuing an all-encompassing definition of health, a more useful approach is to utilise a *framework* for understanding health, such as the one developed by the AIHW (2012) (see Fig 4.1) that identifies individual, societal and environmental influences on health and the interrelationship between these factors.

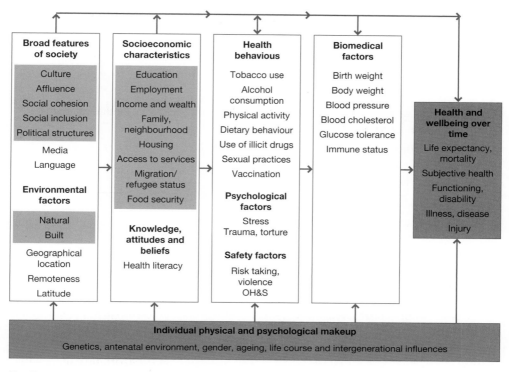

Note: Blue shading highlights selected social determinants of health.

Figure 4.1 Conceptual framework for the determinants of health

Source: Australian Institute of Health and Welfare

What is health psychology?

Health psychology emerged as a branch of psychology in the 1970s during the emergence of the biopsychosocial model and the primary health care/new public health movement. Influential in the development of health psychology was the changing health needs of populations, mounting dissatisfaction with the biomedical model and concerns regarding the escalating costs of a medically oriented healthcare system, alongside the growing realisation of the role psychological, social and lifestyle factors play in health and illness. Additionally, chronic illnesses were replacing acute illnesses as posing the greatest burden of disease to individuals, communities and healthcare resources. The prevailing view at this time was that individuals were primarily responsible for their own health and that health outcomes were a consequence of the individual's lifestyle choices (Marks 2002 p 9).

In 1980 Matarazzo provided a definition of health psychology that stated that health psychology was an:

[a]ggregate of the specific educational, scientific and professional contributions of the discipline of psychology to the promotion and maintenance of health, the prevention and treatment of illness, the identification of etiologic and diagnostic correlates of health, illness and related dysfunction and the improvement of the healthcare system and health policy formation.

(Matarazzo 1980 p 815)

This definition specified the scope of health psychology that was to:

- study the psychological aspects of how people engage in behaviours that maintain health and minimises health risks

- study how thoughts, feelings and personal qualities influence health behaviours and lifestyle choices

- study how thoughts, feelings and personal qualities influence responses to stress, pain, loss and chronic illness

- study how people recognise and respond to illness and how they decide to seek, start and complete treatment (or not)

- identify health promotion and illness prevention strategies and early intervention opportunities.

Contemporary critical health psychologists, however, question the moral and ethical stance of the psychological approaches to health that emerged in the 1970s and 1980s that blamed individuals for their health behaviours such as smoking or eating unhealthy food (Marks 2002 p 5). In the 21st century there is now abundant evidence that social determinants play a major role in health outcomes (Baum 2008, WHO 2008). Hence, contemporary critical health psychologists place increasing importance on the contexts in which individuals live their lives and advise that social, political and economic forces must be taken into consideration when exploring explanations of health behaviours (Brannon & Feist 2009, Marks 2002). As Murray (2012 p 38) observes, health psychology 'is not the steady accumulation of knowledge but rather a process of inquiry and action that is socially immersed.'

In summary, health psychology seeks understanding for human health behaviours within the psychosocial, economic and political contexts in which people live in order to: identify ways of maintaining positive health behaviours; identify strategies to assist people to avoid or modify negative health behaviours; and assist people to maintain new health behaviours. This not only enables individuals to achieve, maintain or improve health but it is important for wider society in that it can improve the health of its citizens and reduce the human and resource cost of illness.

HEALTH PSYCHOLOGY AS A CAREER

Health psychology is a specialised branch of psychology and has two career pathways: theoretical (research) or applied (clinical practice). Research psychologists develop and test theories and evaluate interventions, while clinical psychologists work in a range of healthcare settings as members of multidisciplinary teams. Entry to both of these career pathways requires a specialist postgraduate qualification in psychology. According to the Australian Psychological Society, health psychologists:

... specialise in understanding the relationships between psychological factors (such as behaviours, attitudes, beliefs) and health and illness. Health Psychologists practise in two main areas: health promotion (prevention of illness and promotion of healthy lifestyles) and clinical health (application of psychology to illness assessment, treatment and rehabilitation).

(Australian Psychological Society 2012)

Health psychology for health professionals

Moreover, health psychology makes a contribution to the education and practice of *all* health professionals. Theory and research from health psychology is a fundamental component in courses that prepare practitioners for all of the healthcare professions including, but not limited to, nursing, nutrition, medicine, occupational therapy, social work, speech pathology, paramedic practice and physiotherapy. Health professionals use knowledge and research findings from health psychology to understand the health behaviours of their patients and to plan treatment interventions, rehabilitation and recovery programs, illness prevention and health promotion programs.

Understanding health behaviours

Behaviours that promote health have long been known. For example, in 1983 Berkman and Breslow identified seven health practices that their research demonstrated could significantly reduce an individual's risk of dying at any age. They are:

- sleeping seven to eight hours per day
- eating breakfast
- rarely eating between meals
- being roughly appropriate weight for height
- not smoking
- drinking alcohol in moderation or not at all
- engaging in physical activity regularly (Berkman & Breslow 1983).

These practices continue to be relevant in the 21st century. In 2010 the AIHW cited tobacco smoking, physical inactivity, alcohol misuse, illicit drug use, poor nutrition and unsafe sex as behavioural determinants of health, which contribute significantly to disease burden in Australia (AIHW 2010).

Critical thinking

- Keep a diary for a week in which you record whether or not you observe the health behaviours identified by Berkman and Breslow.
- Identify your reasons for following or not following these identified health behaviours.

Influences on health behaviours

Psychological approaches to understanding health include: examinations of personality factors; perceptions and beliefs about personal control and individual; and environmental factors that reinforce behaviours. These will now be considered.

PERSONALITY

The psychological theories of personality that have particular relevance to the field of health psychology are the behavioural and cognitive models. Behavioural psychologists stress the role of learning, reinforcement and modelling in the initiation and maintenance of behaviours, while cognitivists argue that behaviours are influenced by the individual's beliefs and perceptions about themselves, events or circumstances. Additionally, personality traits and dispositions that are predictive of behaviour have been identified.

Personality types

The first description of a personality style that was purported to influence health was the type A personality type, which was described by two American cardiologists, who observed personality characteristics in their patients that they believed predisposed these patients to the risk of cardiovascular disease (Friedman & Rosenman 1959, 1974). Individuals with type A personality were considered to be competitive, impatient, time-conscious, hostile, unable to relax and had rapid, loud speech. Type B individuals were described as relaxed, quieter and less hurried than type A individuals.

While these categorisations have intuitive appeal it appears that the distinctions are not predictive of risk for coronary heart disease. For example, research conducted by Mitaishvili and Danelia examined the relationship between a range of psychological factors and coronary heart disease (CHD), and failed to find a significant relationship between CHD and personality. The researchers did find, however, that low socioeconomic status (SES) and jobs were associated with an increased risk of acute coronary events (Mitaishvili & Danelia 2006). This is similar to the finding of the landmark Whitehall study of the British civil service that found that workers in lower level positions with low job control experienced greater stress and had higher risk of CHD than higher level workers (Bosma et al 1997). See also Chapter 10.

Nevertheless, interest has been re-ignited recently in researching personality as a risk factor in the long-term prognosis of cardiac patients. With the introduction of the distressed personality type or type D, Denollet (2005) and Denollet and Pedersen (2009) described individuals who simultaneously experience high levels of negative affectivity or mood (NA) and high levels of social inhibition (SI). What this means is that when people with type D personality experience negative emotions they inhibit the expression of these emotions in social interactions. Chida and Steptoe (2009) undertook a meta-analysis review of 44 studies and concluded that anger and hostility were associated with CHD outcomes in both healthy populations and those with CHD, with the effect being greater in men than women. Denollet's research suggests it is not just the presence of negative emotions that may pose a risk factor for cardiac disease but also how that person copes with his or her negative emotions. This notion is further supported by research conducted by Williams et al (2008), as demonstrated in the following *Research focus*.

Research focus

Williams, L., O'Connor, R., Howard, S., et al., 2008. Type D personality mechanisms of effect: the role of health-related behavior and social support. Journal of Psychosomatic Research 64 (1), 63–69.

ABSTRACT

Objective

To (1) investigate the prevalence of type D personality (the conjoint effects of negative affectivity and social inhibition) in a healthy British and Irish population; (2) to test the influence of type D on health-related behaviour; and (3) to determine if these relationships are explained by neuroticism.

Methods

A cross-sectional design was employed, with 1012 healthy young adults (225 males, 787 females, mean age 20.5 years) from the United Kingdom and Ireland completing measures of type D personality, health behaviours, social support and neuroticism.

Results

The prevalence of type D was found to be 38.5%, significantly higher than that reported in other European countries. In addition, type D individuals reported performing significantly fewer health-related behaviours and lower levels of social support than non-type D individuals. These relationships remained significant after controlling for neuroticism.

Conclusion

These findings provide new evidence on type D and suggest a role for health-related behaviour in explaining the link between type D and poor clinical prognosis in cardiac patients.

Critical thinking

Williams et al (2008) state that the research findings 'suggest a role for health-related behaviour in explaining the link between type D and poor clinical prognosis in cardiac patients'.

■ What are the implications of their conclusion?

Resilience

Resilience is another personality trait that is linked to health outcomes. The word itself has a Latin derivation and means to spring or bounce back. In psychology resilience refers to a personality trait that is able to withstand and overcome adversity (American Psychological Association 2012).

Resilience was first described by Garmezy who, while researching risk factors for schizophrenia, observed that some children seemed to be thriving despite living in high-risk situations such as having a drug-addicted parent. Garmezy then shifted his research focus to examine what enabled such children to be successful, despite the adversity in which they lived. Subsequent research supports Garmezy's observation that resilient children are emotionally mature, that is they: possess high self-esteem and self-confidence; have the capacity to make and maintain friendships with peers; have the ability to gain the support of adults; are trusting; have a sense of purpose; possess a set of values and beliefs; and have an 'internal locus of control' (LOC) (Garmezy 1987).

Contemporary definitions of resilience include that it consists of individual and social components, that is, that resilience is a person's ability to adapt their emotions and to utilise social skills and resources when faced with adversity, which is mediated by culture and context (Howell 2011, Zraly 2010). Importantly, recognising the contribution of both the individual's personality traits and the role of wider society means that a person's ability to respond to negative events can be enhanced by intervening at the social level. By mobilising social resources the individual's ability to respond to and manage challenging experiences and events will be improved.

PERSONAL CONTROL

Beliefs about who or what is responsible for behaviours differ between individuals. There are many psychological concepts that attempt to explain these differences. Two of them are LOC and self-efficacy. Both will now be examined.

Locus of control

LOC is an attribution style that was identified by Rotter in his social learning theory (Rotter 1966). It refers to the individual's belief as to whether outcomes or events in their life are brought about by themselves (internal LOC), powerful others or are random (external LOC). The model predicts that a person with an 'internal' explanatory style will assume responsibility for whatever happens to him/herself, crediting their own efforts when they are successful and citing insufficient effort for failure.

Wallston et al (1978) applied Rotter's LOC theory to health and developed an instrument called the *multidimensional health locus of control scale* (health LOC). In the health LOC model the 'external' explanatory style of Rotter's LOC model is expanded to describe people whose explanatory style was either that health outcomes were the result of chance or were under the control of powerful others (doctors or other people). Wallston's three dimensions of control in relation to health are: internal health LOC; chance health LOC; and powerful others health LOC (Wallston 2005, 2007). The model predicts that if a person believes that they can control their health (internal attribution) then they will behave in ways that are health-enhancing. Alternatively if a person has an external attribution style (chance or powerful other) they will be less likely to take responsibility for managing their health.

Classroom activity

Jordan is a 35-year-old overweight man who has recently been diagnosed with type 2 (non-insulin-dependent) diabetes mellitus.

1. In pairs identify and discuss likely health behaviours in relation to the management of Jordan's diabetes for each of Wallston's multidimensional health LOC explanatory models.

Health LOC	Cognitions and beliefs	Predicted health behaviours
Internal	I will be able to control my diabetes if I am given sufficient information about the condition and its treatment.	
Powerful others	The doctor knows more about this condition than me. I will follow the medical advice.	
Chance	My father had diabetes so it is probably hereditary. Nothing I do can change that.	

2. Identify possible cognitions/beliefs and consequent health behaviours for 48-year-old Sandy who has smoked for 30 years and who has been advised to quit smoking following a bout of bronchitis.

Health LOC	Cognitions and beliefs	Predicted health behaviours
Internal		
Powerful others		
Chance		

Classroom activity

1. Complete the Multidimensional Health Locus of Control (Form A) (Wallston 2007) available at <www.vanderbilt.edu/nursing/kwallston/mhlcscales.htm> prior to attending your class.
2. Identify and reflect on your highest score.
   - What would be the implications of this if you had a health problem?
3. Bring your results to your class.
4. In small groups:
   - Compare and discuss your own perspective with the perspective of others.
   - Consider the implications of caring for a patient when his/her perspective is different from your own.

Self-efficacy

The concept of self-efficacy was first described by Bandura (1977) and refers to an individual's perceived ability to perform a certain task or achieve a specific goal in a given situation. Like health LOC, self-efficacy stresses the importance of the person's perceptions and beliefs about his or her personal control in a particular circumstance. However, self-efficacy also takes into account the expectation the person has about the consequences of action taken or not taken. For example, 'What will happen if I take no action?' (situation outcome expectancy); 'What will happen if I change my behaviour?' (action outcome expectancy); and 'Am I capable of changing my behaviour to achieve the goal?' (efficacy expectancy).

The theory speculates that an individual's level of confidence in his or her ability to succeed in a certain situation will influence whether the person engages in activities that will either facilitate success or failure. For example, when approaching an exam a student with a high level of self-efficacy who believes that he or she can pass the exam would engage in behaviours that lead to success such as managing their time to incorporate study, whereas a student who does not believe that they can pass the exam is likely to engage in behaviours that bring about failure such as procrastinating and avoiding preparing for the exam. Finally, while self-efficacy is considered a personality trait, it is amenable to modification through cognitive behavioural therapy (CBT) (Molaie et al 2010, Nash 2011).

Nevertheless, caution is advised in assuming that personality traits, resilience, internal LOC, high self-efficacy and an optimistic outlook are ideal in all circumstances. Consider the circumstance where the outcome cannot be controlled such as recurrence of cancer following a period of remission. The person who initially believed they could control their illness would have their belief seriously challenged by the recurrence and be vulnerable to depression according to Seligman's learned helplessness theory (Seligman 1994).

Research focus

Lee, L., Arthur, A., Avis, M., 2008. Using self-efficacy theory to develop interventions that help older people overcome psychological barriers to physical activity: a discussion paper. International Journal of Nursing Studies 45 (11), 1690–1699.

ABSTRACT

Background

Only a fifth of older people undertake a level of physical activity sufficient to lead to health benefit. Misconceptions about the ageing process and beliefs about the costs and benefits of exercise in late life may result in unnecessary, self-imposed activity restriction. Thus, adhering to a physical activity can be difficult, particularly when the benefits of exercise are often not immediate. Many of the barriers to engaging in physical activity among older people are attitudinal. It is therefore important to take account of the non-physical aspects of physical activity intervention programs, such as increasing confidence.

Cont... ▶

Self-efficacy is a widely applied theory used to understand health behaviour and facilitate behavioural modification, such as the increase of physical activity.

Aim

This paper aims to examine the ways in which self-efficacy theory might be used in intervention programs designed to overcome psychological barriers for increasing physical activity among older people.

Conclusion

A number of studies have demonstrated that exercise self-efficacy is strongly associated with the amount of physical activity undertaken. Evidence from some trials supports the view that incorporating the theory of self-efficacy into the design of a physical activity intervention is beneficial. Physical activity interventions aimed at improving the self-perception of exercise self-efficacy can have positive effects on confidence and the ability to initiate and maintain physical activity behaviour. There are a number of ways for nurses to facilitate older people to draw on the four information sources of self-efficacy: performance accomplishments; vicarious learning; verbal encouragement; and physiological and affective states. Research challenges that future studies need to address include the generalisability of exercise settings, the role of age as an effect modifier and the need for more explicit reporting of how self-efficacy is operationalised in interventions.

CASE STUDY: KARA

Kara is a 21-year-old third-year behavioural science student at a metropolitan university. She plans to pursue a career in sports psychology and work with elite athletes on completion of her studies. Health and fitness are priorities for Kara: she eats a healthy diet and trains three times a week at her local surf life saving club where she is a member of the current state champion surf boat team. Nevertheless, each weekend when she goes out with her friends Kara binge drinks to the point of not remembering what she did the night before. She brushes off her friends' concerns about her drinking and argues that the safe drinking limit for women is two standard drinks per day. Therefore she is only having her weekly quota if she has 14 drinks in one night.

Classroom activity

Read the case study above and revisit Chapter 1. Discuss in small groups:

1. What is your response to Kara's logic?
2. Reflect on how her engagement in healthy behaviours can be explained by:
   - classical conditioning (learning by association)
   - operant conditioning (learning reward or avoidance of an averse outcome)
   - modelling (observational/vicarious learning).
3. Reflect on how her engagement in unhealthy behaviours can be explained by:
   - classical conditioning
   - operant conditioning
   - modelling.

Social influences on health

Social influences on health are briefly identified here and are discussed in more detail in Chapter 5. Demographic data demonstrate health inequities for:

- *SES* – with lower income correlated with poorer health (Karlsson et al 2010, WHO 2008)

- *age* – the most pressing chronic health issue for young people is asthma, while it is arthritis for the elderly (AIHW 2010)

- *gender* – Australian and New Zealand women's life expectancy is almost five years greater than that of men's (AIHW 2010, Statistics New Zealand Tatauranga Aotearoa 2009)

- *ethnicity* – Higgins et al found that 'cultural and social factors … shape schizophrenia rehabilitation in China and India … including the use of traditional medicine and healers, emphasis on family involvement, stigma, gender inequality and lack of resources' (Higgins et al 2007).

Population groups considered at risk because of social inequities include: people from lower socioeconomic backgrounds; unemployed people; Indigenous peoples; people living in rural and remote areas; prisoners; refugees; and people with mental illness (AIHW 2010). Interestingly, in Australia, migrant populations and people in the defence forces experience better health than the overall population (AIHW 2010 p xi).

Critical thinking

- List reasons why you think that migrant populations and people in the defence forces experience better health than the wider population.

SOCIAL DETERMINANTS

WHO, in its publication *Social determinants of health: the solid facts* (Marmot & Wilkinson 2006), identified 10 key social and political factors that influence health. These different but interrelated social determinants of health are: the social gradient, stress, early life, social exclusion, work, unemployment, social support, addiction, food and transport. The authors stated that the publication of the *Social determinants of health* was intended to 'ensure that policy – at all levels in government, public and private institutions, workplaces and the community – takes proper account of the wider responsibility for creating opportunities for health' (Marmot & Wilkinson 2006 p 7).

Subsequently, WHO established the Commission on the Social Determinants of Health to examine and collate evidence on what could be done to bring about health equity and to foster a global movement to achieve it (WHO 2008). In the commission's report *Closing the gap in a generation: health equity through action on the social determinants of health* the commissioners called on governments worldwide to reduce health inequities through policy and programs that engage key sectors of the community, such as economic development, transport and education, and to include health in all policies because *health* policies and programs alone cannot achieve health equity or social justice (Irwin et al 2008, Kickbusch et al 2011, WHO 2008).

CROSS–CULTURAL INFLUENCES

Culture can be defined as the history, values, beliefs, language, practices, dress and customs that are shared by a group of people and that influences the behaviour of the members (Germov & Poole 2007). Commonly, culture is equated with ethnicity but this is a limited interpretation; other cultural groupings also exist based on shared understandings. For example, the phrase 'right hander' has different meaning for a surfer, a boxer or a schoolteacher. And, despite commonalities that define a culture, it cannot be assumed that all members of one culture necessarily share identical worldviews on any or all issues (McMurray 2010).

Different interpretations of health and explanations for illness exist between cultures that are *individualistic* (i.e. a society in which the smallest socioeconomic unit is the individual and independence is valued) and cultures that are *collectivist* (i.e. a society in which the smallest socioeconomic unit is the family and human interdependence is valued). Individualism is a cultural pattern mainly found in developed Western countries and is 'chiefly concerned with protecting the autonomy of individuals against obligation imposed by the state, family and community' (Kato & Sleeboom-Faulkener 2011 p 509). Individualist cultures attribute responsibility for health to the individual. Collectivist cultures, on the other hand, recognise the role of the extended family and community in all aspects of life. Members are 'usually characterized by a sense of emotional, moral, economic, social and political commitment to their collective' (Haj-Yahia 2011 p 333). For example, traditional Māori beliefs are that four domains influence health: family/community, physical, spiritual and emotional (Lyons & Chamberlain 2006 p 7).

Moreover, it is important to recognise that, in the main, psychological theories of behaviour were developed in Western Europe and the United States, which are individualistic cultures. Consequently, caution must be exercised when applying these psychological theories derived from research conducted in individualist societies to people from collectivist societies such as Australian Aboriginal and Torres Strait Islanders or New Zealand Māori, and the immigrant populations of the two countries (Lyons & Chamberlain 2006).

Conclusion

This chapter provides an overview of the many factors that influence health and health outcomes. In particular, the contribution that health psychology makes to understanding and managing health and illness is presented. While this branch of psychology generally focuses on understanding individual behaviour and the factors that influence health outcomes, the dynamic nature of health is acknowledged, particularly the social context in which individuals live. Health psychology, therefore, is located within the biopsychosocial framework – a model that recognises the interdependence and interrelationships between biological, psychological and social factors in understanding and managing health and illness.

REMEMBER

- Health and health outcomes are influenced by a complex interaction of biological, psychological and social factors.
- Health psychology proposes theories that attempt to explain why individuals engage in behaviours that maintain, enhance or threaten their health.
- An individual's thoughts, feelings and personal qualities can influence health behaviours and lifestyle choices.
- Understanding these influences enables health professionals to assist clients to engage in behaviours that maintain or enhance health and to cease behaviours that pose health risks.

Further resources

Australian Institute of Health and Welfare, 2012. Australia's health 2012. AIHW, Canberra.

Baum, F., 2008. The new public health, third ed. Oxford University Press, South Melbourne.

Lee, L., Arthur, A., Avis, M., 2008. Using self-efficacy theory to develop interventions that help older people overcome psychological barriers to physical activity: a discussion paper. International Journal of Nursing Studies 45 (11), 1690–1699.

McMurray, A., 2010. Community health and wellness: a socio-ecological approach, fourth ed. Elsevier, Sydney.

World Health Organization, 2008. Closing the gap in a generation: health equity through action on the social determinants of health. WHO Commission on Social Determinants of Health, Geneva.

Weblinks

American Psychological Association

www.apa.org/helpcenter/road-resilience.aspx

The APA provides general information about resilience and focuses on how the individual can develop and use a personal strategy to enhance resilience.

Australian Indigenous Health*InfoNet*

www.healthinfonet.ecu.edu.au

The Australian Indigenous Health*InfoNet* provides knowledge and information on many aspects of Indigenous health and support, 'yarning places' (electronic networks) that encourage information sharing and collaboration among people working in health and related sectors.

Australian Institute of Health and Welfare

www.aihw.gov.au

The AIHW is Australia's national agency for health and welfare statistics and information.

New Zealand Health Information Service/Te Paronga Hauora

www.nzhis.govt.nz

The New Zealand Health Information Service/Te Paronga Hauora contains health statistics and publications relevant to the health of New Zealanders.

The Social Report/Te Purongo Oranga Tangata

www.socialreport.msd.govt.nz/health

The Social Report/Te Purongo Oranga Tangata 2008 provides an overview of the current state of New Zealand's health and the likely trends in the future.

Hans Rosling's 200 countries, 200 years

http://www.youtube.com/watch?v=jbkSRLYSojo

This engaging presentation by Swedish Professor of Global Health Hans Rosling uses statistics to demonstrate the relationship between income, health and life expectancy changes throughout the world over the past 200 years.

References

American Psychological Association, 2012. The road to resilience. Online. Available: http://www.apa.org/helpcenter/road-resilience.aspx 12 Sep 2012.

Australian Institute of Health and Welfare (AIHW), 2010. Australia's health 2010. AIHW, Canberra.

Australian Institute of Health and Welfare (AIHW), 2011. Health Priority Areas. Online. Available: http://www.aihw.gov.au/health-priority-areas 12 Sep 2012.

Australian Institute of Health and Welfare (AIHW), 2012. Australia's health 2012: Australia's Health No. 12, AIHW cat. No. AUS122. AIHW, Canberra. Online. Available: www.aihw.gov.au 12 Sep 2012.

Australian Psychological Society, 2012. Specialist areas of Psychology. Online. Available: http://www.psychology.org.au/community/specialist 12 Sep 2012.

Babones, S.J., 2008. Income inequality and population health: Correlation and causality. Social Science and Medicine 66, 1614–1626.

Bandura, A., 1977. Self efficacy: towards a unifying theory of behaviour change. Psychological Review 84, 191–215.

Baum, F., 2008. The new public health, third ed. Oxford University Press, South Melbourne.

Baum, F., Sanders, 2011. Ottawa 25 years on: a more radical agenda for health equity is still required. Health Promotion International 27 (Supp 2), 253–257.

Berkman, L., Breslow, L., 1983. Health and ways of living: the Alameda County study. Oxford University Press, New York.

Bosma, H., Marmot, M., Hemingway, H., et al., 1997. Low job control and risk of coronary heart disease in Whitehall II (prospective cohort) study. British Medical Journal 314, 558–565.

Brannon, L., Feist, J., 2009. Health psychology: an introduction to behaviour and health, seventh ed. Wadsworth Cengage Learning, Belmont.

Centers for Disease Control and Prevention, 2011. Ten great public health achievements worldwide: 2001–2010 Morbidity and Mortality Weekly Report 24 June. Online. Available: http://www.cdc.gov/mmwr/preview/mmwrhtml/mm6024a4.htm 12 Sep 2012.

Chida, Y., Steptoe, A., 2009. The association of anger and hostility with future coronary heart disease: a meta-analytic review of prospective evidence. Journal of American College of Cardiology 53 (11), 936–946.

Denollet, J., Pedersen, S., 2009. Anger, depression and anxiety in cardiac patients. Journal of the American College of Cardiology 53 (11), 947–949.

Denollet, J., 2005. DS14: standard assessment of negative affectivity, social inhibition and type D personality. Psychosomatic Medicine (67), 89–97.

Engel, G., 1977. The need for a new medical model: a challenge for bio-medicine. Science 196, 129–135.

Frieden, T., 2010. A framework for public health: the health impact pyramid. American Journal of Public Health 100 (4), 590–595.

Friedman, M., Rosenman, R., 1959. Association of specific overt behavior pattern with blood and cardiovascular findings; blood cholesterol level, blood clotting time, incidence of arcus senilis, and clinical coronary artery disease. Journal of the American Medical Association 169 (12), 1286–1296.

Friedman, M., Rosenman, R., 1974. Type A behavior and your heart. Knopf, New York.

Garmezy, N., 1987. Stress, competence and development: continuities in the study of schizophrenic adults, children vulnerable to psychopathology and the search for stress-resistant children. American Journal of Orthopsychiatry 57 (2), 159–174.

Germov, J., Poole, M., 2007. Public sociology: an introduction to Australian society. Allen & Unwin, Sydney.

Haj-Yahia, M., 2011. Contextualising interventions with battered women in collectivist societies: issues and controversies. Aggression and Violent Behavior 16, 331–339.

Hasnain, M., Vieweg, W., Frederickson, S., et al., 2009. Clinical monitoring and management of the metabolic syndrome in patients receiving atypical antipsychotic medications. Primary Care Diabetes 3, 5–15.

Higgins, L., Dey-Ghatak, P., Davey, G., 2007. Mental health nurses' experiences of schizophrenia rehabilitation in China and India. International Journal of Mental Health Nursing 16 (1), 22–27.

Howell, K.H., 2011. Resilience and psychopathology in children exposed to family violence. Aggression and Violent Behavior 16, 562–569.

Irwin, A., Solar, O., Vega, J., 2008. The United Nations Commission of Social Determinants of Health. In: International Encyclopedia of Public Health. Elsevier, pp. 64–69.

Jormfeldt, H., Svedberg, P., Fridlund, B., et al., 2007. Perceptions of the concept of health among nurses working in mental health services. International Journal of Mental Health Nursing 16 (1), 50–56.

Karlsson, M., Nilsson, T., Lyttkens, C., et al., 2010. Income inequality and health: importance of a cross-country perspective. Social Science and Medicine 70, 875–885.

Kato, M., Sleeboom-Faulkener, M., 2011. Dichotomies of collectivism and individualism in bioethics: selective abortion debates and issues of self-determinism in Japan and 'the West'. Social Science & Medicine 73, 507–514.

Kickbusch, I., Hein, W., Silberschmidt, G., 2011. Addressing global health governance challenges through a new mechanism: the proposal for a Committee C of the World Health Assembly. Journal of Law, Medicine & Ethics Fall, 550–563.

Kim, S., Nikolics, L., Abbasi, F., et al., 2010. Relationship between body mass index and insulin resistance in patients treated with second generation antipsychotic agents. Journal of Psychiatric Research 44, 493–498.

Lalonde, M., 1981. A new perspective on the health of Canadians: a working document. Ministry of National Health and Welfare, Ottawa.

Lee, L., Arthur, A., Avis, M., 2008. Using self-efficacy theory to develop interventions that help older people overcome psychological barriers to physical activity: a discussion paper. International Journal of Nursing Studies 45 (11), 1690–1699.

Lyons, A., Chamberlain, K., 2006. Health psychology: a critical introduction. Cambridge University Press, Cambridge.

McMurray, A., 2010. Community health and wellness: a socio-ecological approach, fourth ed. Elsevier, Sydney.

Marks, D., 2002. Freedom, responsibility and power: contrasting approaches to health psychology. Journal of Health Psychology 7 (1), 5–19.

Marmot, M., 2010. Fair society, healthy lives: strategic review of health inequalities in England post 2010. The Marmot Review, London.

Marmot, M., 2008. Closing the gap in a generation: health equity through action on the social determinants of health. The Lancet 327 (8), 1661–1669.

Marmot, M., Wilkinson, R., 2006. Social determinants of health: the solid facts, third ed. World Health Organization, Geneva.

Matarazzo, J., 1980. Behavioral health and behavioral medicine: frontiers for a new health psychology. American Psychologist 35, 807–817.

Meadows, G., Farhall, J., Fossey, E., et al., 2012. Mental health in Australia: collaborative commnity practice, third ed. Oxford University Press, South Melbourne.

Mitaishvili, N., Danelia, M., 2006. Personality type and coronary heart disease. Georgian Medical News 134, 58–60.

Molaie, A., Shahidi, S., Vazifeh, S., et al., 2010. Comparing the effectiveness of cognitive behavioral therapy and movie therapy on improving abstinence self-efficacy in Iranian substance dependent adolescents. Procedia Social and Behavioral Sciences 5, 1180–1184.

Murray, M., 2012. Social history of health psychology: contexts and textbooks. Health Psychology Review. Online. Available: http://www.tandfonline.com/doi/full/10.1080/17437199.2012.701058 26 Sep 2012.

Nash, V., 2011. Cognitive behavioral therapy, self-efficacy and depression in persons with chronic pain. Pain Management Nursing 12 (2), e6.

NationMaster.com Health statistics: Life expectancy at birth. Online. Available: http://www.nationmaster.com/graph/hea_lif_exp_at_bir_tot_pop-life-expectancy-birth-total-population 12 Sep 2012.

New Zealand Ministry of Social Development, 2010. The social report – te pūrongo oranga tangata 2010. New Zealand Ministry of Social Development, Auckland.

Rotter, J.B., 1966. Generalized expectancies for internal versus external control of reinforcement. Psychological Monographs 80, 234–240.

Seligman, M., 1994. Learned optimism. Random House, Sydney.

Statistics New Zealand Tatauranga Aotearoa, 2009. New Zealand life tables 2005–2007. Online. Available: http://www.stats.govt.nz/browse_for_stats/health/life_expectancy.aspx 12 Sep 2012.

Tarkiainen, L., Martikainen, P., Laaksonen, M., et al., 2011. Trends in life expectancy by income from 1988 to 2007: decomposition by age and cause of death. Journal of Epidemiology and Community Health. Online. Available: http://jech.bmj.com/content/early/2011/03/04/jech.2010.123182.short 12 Sep 2012.

Wallston, K., Wallston, B., DeVellis, R., 1978. Development of multidimensional health locus of control (MHLOC) scales. Health Education Monographs 6, 160–170.

Wallston, K., 2005. The validity of the multidimensional health locus of control scales. Journal of Health Psychology 10 (5), 623–631.

Wallston, K., 2007. Multidimensional health locus of control (MHLC) scales. Online. Available: http://www.vanderbilt.edu/nursing/kwallston/mhlcscales.htm 26 Sep 2012.

Williams, L., O'Connor, R., Howard, S., et al., 2008. Type D personality mechanisms of effect: the role of health-related behavior and social support. Journal of Psychosomatic Research 64 (1), 63–69.

World Health Organization (WHO), 2008. Closing the gap in a generation: health equity through action on the social determinants of health. WHO, Geneva. Online. Available: http://www.who.int/social_determinants/thecommission/finalreport/en/index.html 12 Sep 2012.

World Health Organization (WHO), 1946. WHO constitution. WHO, New York.

Yamada, A., Brekke, J., 2008. Addressing mental health disparities through clinical competence not just cultural competence: the need for assessment of sociocultural issues in the delivery of evidence-based psychosocial rehabilitation services. Clinical Psychology Review 28, 1386–1399.

Zraly, M., 2010. Don't let the suffering make you fade away: an ethnographic study of resilience among survivors of genocide-rape in southern Rwanda. Social Science & Medicine 70, 1656–1664.

Chapter 5
The social context of behaviour

YVONNE PARRY & EILEEN WILLIS

Learning objectives

The material in this chapter will help you to:

- describe the social model and the social determinants of health
- understand the history and evidence leading to a social model of health as a counter to the biomedical model of health
- evaluate the social justice argument in support of a social model of health and the implications for government policy
- examine the relationship between the structural and the intermediary determinants of health as a way of understanding the relationship between the social determinants of health and psychological and behavioural explanations of health.

Key terms

- Social determinants of health
- Social model of health
- Biopsychosocial model
- Structural determinants
- Intermediary determinants
- Public policy

Introduction

In Chapter 4 it was argued that the biomedical model of health was inadequate in explaining the patterns of mortality and morbidity for populations and individuals. A biopsychosocial model of health was proposed and a brief outline of the social determinants of health presented. This chapter takes the 'social' aspects of the biopsychosocial model of health and examines the evidence, debates and theories that argue that illness and disease for individuals, populations and nations is not simply a matter of germs and viruses (biomedical) or individual psychology and behaviour (biopsychological) but a complex interaction between the social system of a given society and the individual (biopsychosocial) and their particular genetic inheritance (biomedical).

Traditionally there has been a stand-off between biomedical, biopsychological and social models of health. This stand-off is counterproductive and contrary to the evidence. Over the past three decades particular population groups within affluent nations have failed to make the promised biomedical and health promotion gains (Raphael et al 2005). Evidence of this has been obtained from long-term studies of health differences between sections of society in Western nations (Marmot & Wilkinson 2006, World Health Organization (WHO) 2008). Comparisons of health outcomes between individuals and nations have shown that although baseline improvements in life expectancy, infant mortality and death from childhood injury have occurred in countries such as the United Kingdom, Australia, New Zealand and the United States, there are marked differences in health status between individuals in these countries, as well as marked differences between countries (Marmot & Wilkinson 2006, WHO 2008).

These differences appear to be the result of life chances and the kind of social institutions and welfare policies a country has. For example, in the Scandinavian countries, while the gains in health have mirrored those in the United Kingdom, Australia, New Zealand and the United States, the population as a whole has made further health gains as the percentage of people on low incomes is lower than in English-speaking countries (Raphael 2006). This is best explained through the kinds of social policies in place in the Scandinavian countries.

The social model of health and the social determinants of health

THE SOCIAL MODEL OF HEALTH

There are two major components to a social model of health. First, health and illness are seen to be partly attributed to the social circumstances of individuals and populations. These social circumstances include their level of income in absolute terms and relative to other people in the population, their education, employment, gender, culture and status. Epidemiological evidence provides clear proof of differences in health status between individuals based on these factors. For instance, research on the social gradient (one of the social determinants of health) explains

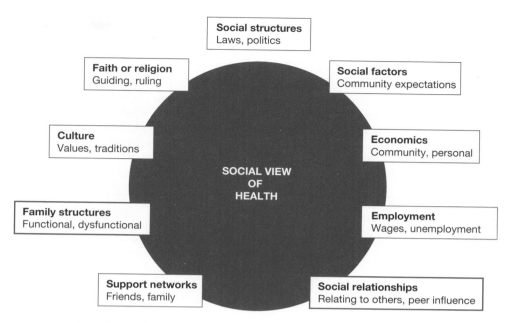

Figure 5.1 Social view of health

how the perception of one's social position can be a predeterminant of a chronic stress response that may create long-term physical and psychological illness (Marmot & Wilkinson 2006).

The second aspect of the social model of health suggests that the health of individuals and populations is influenced by the social, economic, political and welfare policies of a country. This includes policies covering: taxation; welfare payments and eligibility; public services such as health and education; and employment opportunities. A social model of health means that governments need to focus on policy at all levels, not just health policy. This is referred to as intersectorial collaboration across policy portfolios or a 'whole-of-government approach' to health.

Figure 5.1 illustrates the complex and multifaceted view of health portrayed by the social view of health. It incorporates the social, cultural, community, familial and economic circumstances that influence and determine health status.

THE IMPLICATIONS OF THE SOCIAL MODEL

The implications of taking a social model approach to health is that rather than focus solely on the individual's behaviour or their biological or genetic attributes, the focus shifts onto the attributes of society such as the level of wealth, differences in income, poverty and government policies dealing with these inequalities. This differs from the biomedical model that defines illness as a condition of the individual who may now have a disease or injury. It also differs from the biopsychological or behavioural model of health that suggests many illnesses result from the interaction between physical factors and the behaviour of individuals with the responsibility for treatment residing solely with the individual.

The difference can clearly be seen if we take the example of a student with the disability of cerebral palsy. In a biomedical analysis the individual has 'cerebral palsy', uses a wheelchair and therefore is not able to attend lectures due to the cerebral palsy. Conversely, the social model would assert that as the lecture theatre does not have wheelchair access, the person is discriminated against and denied access due to lecture theatre design. The social model acknowledges and describes aspects of life that are external to the individual that mediate how the individual can function and participate within a society. Clearly, in this example, the solution lies in government policy legislating equal access, building design and adequate funding. Illness and health are therefore tackled through social interventions.

A SOCIAL MODEL OF HEALTH IDENTIFIES THE SOCIAL DETERMINANTS OF HEALTH

The factors that make up the social model of health are known as the social determinants of health (SDH). These SDH explain the differences in health outcomes between individuals and populations. Each social determinant of health describes a set of circumstances that influences a particular health outcome. The SDH listed in Figure 5.2 were developed by Dahlgren and Whitehead (1991). In their model there are four layers of influence: individual lifestyle factors followed by three layers of social determinants. The first or outer layer includes the socioeconomic, cultural and environmental conditions; the second layer includes agriculture and food production, education, the work environment, unemployment, sanitation and water supplies, healthcare services and housing. Dahlgren and Whitehead add a third layer that

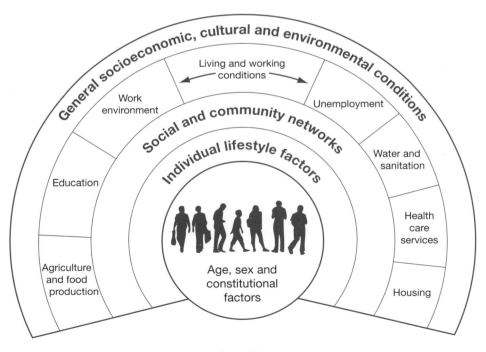

Figure 5.2 The social determinants of health

suggests that social networks also impact on health outcomes. It is not until the fourth layer that the individual and their behaviour are listed. This diagram is not simply a listing of features in a society. The authors are suggesting that the outer layers are features of a society that determine the health of its members and that each layer shapes the next inner layer.

Other theorists have suggested alternative social determinants. These include childhood poverty, differences in social class between groups, stress (Marmot 2001), social exclusion, unemployment (Marmot & Wilkinson 2006), type of work (Bartley et al 2006), lack of social support (Stansfeld 2006), social patterns of addiction (Jarvis & Wardle 2006), quality and quantity of food supplies (Robertson et al 2006) and transport (McCarthy 2006).

Figure 5.2 and the brief outline above have highlighted how complex and interdependent the SDH are. The SDH also provide a means of addressing inequalities in health outcomes in a manner that the biomedical model of health cannot. For example, by providing affordable, reliable, public transport to outer suburbs, a number of the social determinants could be addressed, such as access to health services. This is because transport contributes to a reduction in social isolation, increases the chance of people entering a city for employment and increases the opportunities to access health services. Thus, one government policy action can have a flow-on effect.

Classroom activity

AUSTRALIAN STUDENTS

Prior to your class:

1. Access the social health atlas for your state or territory (see <www.publichealth.gov.au/publications>).
2. Click on the fact sheet and read one of the identified areas, such as children, youth or women.
3. Examine this fact sheet and be prepared to bring information to class for your tutorial for discussion.
   - Select facts that highlight the social determinants of health.
   - Discuss in small groups.

NEW ZEALAND STUDENTS

Prior to your class:

- Go to the Social Report and click on 'Health Report' at <www.socialreport.msd.govt.nz/health>.
- Be prepared to come to class with information on the relationship between health, ethnicity and age.
- You could explore such relationships in terms of life expectancy, suicide and obesity.
- Discuss in small groups.

The history and the formation of the social determinants of health

The acknowledgment of the importance of the social model of health was demonstrated with the formation of WHO in 1948. The WHO constitution clearly outlines the need for a whole-of-government approach to health. Unfortunately, in the following 30 years governments around the world pursued a technologically driven model of health that only addressed the downstream, curative approach of health (Solar & Irwin 2007), thus failing to direct health policy towards the upstream, structural determinants of health. The term structural is used here to make the point that the problem lies in the organisation of a society or group, not in individual behaviour.

The 1978 *Alma Ata Declaration on Primary Health Care* and the *Health for All* movement attempted to revive action on the SDH through promoting a social model of health. While many governments in principle embraced the *Health for All* concepts and acknowledged the importance of incorporating a broader view of health that addressed aspects such as housing, education and employment on health (Solar & Irwin 2007), neo-liberal economic policies were gaining favour. The neo-liberal policies encouraged governments to reduce public spending on health, housing, employment and other welfare services, turning away from a social model.

However, work defining and refining the social model and the SDH has continued. The previously mentioned deficits in the biomedical model of health were highlighted by the seminal work of McKeown and Illich (Solar & Irwin 2007) and the *Black Report* in the United Kingdom (Turrell et al 1999). The works of McKeown, Illich and Black (and his colleagues) were instrumental in highlighting the gaps in health outcomes of population groups that were directly related to social conditions (Black et al 1980, Kelly et al 2006, Turrell et al 1999). The SDH have again risen to prominence in light of the mounting evidence that the efficiency models of the neo-liberal economic policies are exacerbating the health differences between the 'haves' and the 'have nots' such that, in Australia, there is now a 20-year mortality difference between those individuals in the highest socioeconomic group and those in the lowest (Royal Australasian College of Physicians (RACP) 2005). In 2003 WHO created the Commission on the Social Determinants of Health (Kelly et al 2006). The commission delivered its final report in 2008, which has placed the SDH and their ongoing refinement and definition firmly on the policy and research agenda (WHO 2008).

Why support a social model of health? The social justice argument and the implications for government policy

HEALTH AS A HUMAN RIGHT

As health professionals and as a society it is important to qualify our notions of health and the availability of health services. One way of achieving this is through defining and understanding health as a core value or human right. Values can be defined as:

... the beliefs of a person or group which contain some emotional investment or [are] held as sacrosanct; while core is the most essential or vital part of some idea.
(Morales & Gilner 2002)

The idea of health as a core value is espoused in the notion of health as a human right, as this places health as a central ideal and a 'right for all' (Lie 2004). If health is a right for all humans then it falls outside the individual to solely provide for it and becomes a joint responsibility of the individual and the government or society to provide. As a right for all, the provision of health becomes an entitlement and therefore falls on governments to ensure adequate provision (Baum et al 2009). By viewing health as a human right it enables governments to legislate to protect those rights and enables service providers to broaden the constructs of health to be inclusive of social conditions such as housing and education.

HEALTH AS A RIGHT ENSURES EQUITY

When governments incorporate health as a human right into their policy agenda the advancement of health equity is also ensured (Lie 2004). Where health is a human right, health services are provided regardless of people's socioeconomic position, gender, educational level, ethnicity or religion (Baum et al 2009, Solar & Irwin 2007). To charge people for health services is to charge them for something that is regarded as a right. Unfortunately, in many countries where healthcare is not free, factors such as socioeconomic position determine the level of health that can be enjoyed by an individual (Marmot & Wilkinson 2006).

Theoretical models for understanding the social determinants of health

If morbidity and mortality rates for a population are a result of social conditions it is important to identify what these SDH are and to introduce policy that will reduce the impact. One approach is to examine each SDH for how it impacts on health status and to make recommendations for the kind of social policy required to eliminate the negative effects (Raphael 2006). A number of social epidemiologists have taken this approach by identifying a range of social determinants they view as important in the higher rates of morbidity and mortality of some population groups.

Drawing on the work of these theorists the WHO Commission for the Social Determinants of Health has developed a model that integrates the social with the psychological model to form an explanatory psychosocial model. The psychosocial model acknowledges that there is a pathway or conduit between the social factors and the individual, their behaviour and mental states that influence health. This model is divided into three components: (1) the socioeconomic and political context, (2) the structural and (3) the intermediary social determinants of health.

THE SOCIOECONOMIC AND POLITICAL CONTEXT

The first factor impacting on the SDH is the socioeconomic and political context of a society. While this refers to the impact of the political and cultural system of a society on the health of the population, it is best understood in concrete terms as the impact of economic, social and public policy on the life chances of the population. Examples of economic policy include those governing industrial relations such as rates of pay and the casualisation of work for young people, including hours of work.

Social policies include those dealing with welfare issues such as access to housing, disability, old age and sickness benefits, while public policies cover issues such as access to education, the provision of healthcare and utilities such as power, water and communications. Policies that enable poor people to access resources such as power, water, education and healthcare, or protect workers from discrimination, or support workers during times of unemployment go some way towards achieving a reduction in inequality.

The kinds of policies a particular government puts in place will be very much influenced by its politics, values or beliefs. For example, where the political party in power believes health or education are human/citizen rights these services will be provided free by the government or at a cost that all can afford. Providing such services is referred to as the welfare state. Underpinning the welfare state is the idea that it is the responsibility of government to provide for its citizens' social insurance against hardship, poverty, illness or misfortune. The role of the welfare state is to redistribute the resources within a society from rich to poor, so that no one is destitute. This is usually done through taxation policies whereby everyone (rich and poor) subsidises those in need. The type and range of welfare provided by countries differs. A classic example is in healthcare. Some countries provide free, universal healthcare to all citizens; other countries have healthcare systems where patients must pay for the service, while elsewhere access to health services may be means tested or based on income.

The health impact of such policies is illustrated in the differences in mortality rates between the United Kingdom (free universal healthcare to all), the United States (private system with access to free healthcare means tested in its extension to the poor and elderly only) and Australia with a mixed public–private system. In 2007 the probability of a child under five years of age dying was 6/1000 in the United Kingdom and Australia and 8/1000 in the United States. These differences, while not stark, are explained partly as a result of healthcare policy where access to care is free in Australia and the United Kingdom, but not so in the United States (World Health Statistics 2007).

STRUCTURAL AND INTERMEDIARY DETERMINANTS

The SDH can be further categorised into those determinants that are 'structurally' produced and addressed through changes at a societal level via policy intervention and those determinants that act more directly on individuals and are 'intermediary' determinants that can be addressed through community health programs and individual health interventions and behaviour change (Solar & Irwin 2007). Dividing the SDH into these two categories makes health-promoting action clearer. The necessary policy for creating a healthy environment becomes evident whether this is through policy directed towards alleviating poverty (structural) or programs to help individuals change their behaviour (intermediary). The pathway between the structural and intermediary also goes some way to integrating the social and psychological.

STRUCTURAL DETERMINANTS OF HEALTH INEQUITIES

Structural determinants are those factors that generate or reinforce social divisions and power and status differences in a society, and as a result impact on people's life chances (Solar & Irwin 2007 p 26). The key to understanding the structural determinants lies in the concept of social stratification (Solar & Irwin 2007). Social stratification is the division created in a society between different groups. It can be based on income (class), gender, ethnicity, sexual preference, education or occupation. These factors describe one's social position in a society (Solar & Irwin 2007). Forms of social stratification differ between social and cultural groups but in all cases impact either positively or negatively on an individual's access to resources, education and employment and, ultimately, health.

The difficulty with using a measure such as social stratification is that it does not tell us how differences in status *impact* on health. Understanding the SDH requires more than identification – the pathway between each determinant and illness must also be understood or, if not completely understood, explored. A number of the social determinants described below can be broadly defined using the term socioeconomic position. This term has its origins in two theoretical positions: the first Marxist, the second Weberian. The first refers to social class. A person's social class tells us how much money they earn and have to use in their daily life. For example, they may own their own business, be a manager, boss or worker. A person who owns their own business has more control over their work than a person who works for an owner. In some cases their take-home money may be very similar but one gives the orders and the other performs the tasks. Influential studies by Michael Marmot (2001) have shown that even well-paid workers who must take orders from more senior managers have higher rates of illness. This would appear to be best explained by their lack of power in the workplace. This lack of power appears to impact on stress levels leading, for example, to higher rates of mental illness and heart disease (Marmot 2001). Marmot and his colleagues are continuing to work on understanding the pathway between the stress caused by lack of power and the consequent impact on morbidity and mortality levels for these populations.

Measuring socioeconomic position simply through one's class and power in the workplace is limited. There are other ways to access power besides money. These other variables include status (one's social power) and political affiliation. This theory was first described by Weber. An example of status power would be being a boy in a society that valued boys over girls, belonging to a religious or ethnic group that had access to all the best jobs or having a job with high prestige so one's opinion was more valued than lower status occupations. Political party power refers to one person's access to resources through affiliations with powerful groups or organisations. When sociologists combine class power (whether one is a worker or owner) with status power (social prestige) and political power (one's affiliations to powerful groups) they use the term socioeconomic position. The variables outlined below all contribute to one's socioeconomic position. The first is income.

Income

Income is the measure of the amount of money available to individuals and families to purchase the material assets necessary for life. These include food, healthcare, shelter (housing), employment and any other assets considered essential in that society. It is a commonly used indicator of socioeconomic position in society. Income has a direct positive relationship with health; as income improves, health improves. Correspondingly if income decreases, health decreases (Baum 2005). Income determines the amount of material wealth available to an individual or a family, as well as access to healthcare. It enables access to good food and determines the resources available to the children within the family. Adult health outcomes begin in childhood so that income and health have a cumulative effect over the lifespan (Blane 2006, McLaughlin et al 2011). The relationship between income and health status in Australia is evident across a variety of diseases. Poorer people have higher rates of arthritis (22% compared with 16%), higher rates of musculoskeletal problems (21% versus 17%) and higher rates of mental illness (16% come from disadvantaged areas and 9% from advantaged areas) (ABS 2006, 2009). Further, McLaughlin et al (2011) found that childhood socioeconomic status impacts on the onset, persistence and severity of mental illnesses.

Social class

Social class is closely related to income. One of the most intriguing findings related to social class has been the impact of the social gradient. This finding suggests that the steeper the income and social distance between people in a society, the wider the health gaps (Morrissey 2006). The impact of income differences is seen as one of the explanations for the poor health status of Aboriginal people in Australia. The income of Aboriginal people is higher than population groups in many underdeveloped countries, yet their mortality rates are higher. One explanation is that while Aboriginal people are not as poor as some population groups in Africa or Asia, the difference between Aboriginal people and non-Indigenous Australians is significant and a factor in explaining their poor health status (Morrissey 2006, Vos et al 2009). The link here may be one of comparison and it is through comparison that stress levels are affected and ill health results.

Education

Formal education is a reflection of both a child's and parents' circumstances. The kind of education an individual achieves is determined by their parents' social position, values and income. It is also determined by the social policies of the country. Where education is provided free, individuals have the opportunity to gain an education independent of parental income or values; where it is costly, their education will be determined by their parents' wealth or opinion about the value of education. Education as a variable of health status is a combination of both the baseline education (received during childhood and a result of the socioeconomic position of parents) and future education (one's own socioeconomic position) as an adult (Solar & Irwin 2007). It also influences occupational and employment outcomes, further impacting on access to healthcare and health resources as an adult. Education also enhances an individual's capacity to make healthy life choices because it exposes the adult to an array of health resources and services (Solar & Irwin 2007).

Occupation

Occupation is the type of work performed by an individual. It is an indicator of the amount of exposure to risk, social standing, income and level of education (Marmot et al 2006). Categorisation of individuals by occupation is a powerful predictor of inequalities in morbidity and mortality, especially workplace injury (Wadsworth & Butterworth 2006). Occupation also reflects one's social standing or value in a society and may result in access to privileges such as: better education, healthcare and nutrition; housing and community support; and facilities. Occupation may also provide the person with beneficial social networks and control and autonomy over their work. There is considerable research that suggests control over one's work reduces stress and impacts directly on health (Brunner & Marmot 2006, Marmot 2001).

Gender

All around the world women have less access to and control over resources such as health (female infanticide, genital mutilation, deliberate female underfeeding), income (economic dependency, lack of well-remunerated and secure employment or active discrimination in employment positions), education (nil or limited access to education) and housing (inability to inherit or secure housing without male support), and this has implications for the quality of life experience and health status (Solar & Irwin 2007). However, in Australia and New Zealand women have lower rates of mortality (they live longer) but higher rates of morbidity (they appear to be sicker) so the solutions are not clear cut. For example, in New Zealand the life expectancy for a male is 77.9 years but increases to 81.9 years for women (The Social Report 2007). Social stratification based on gender can only be addressed 'upstream' or structurally by governments through policy that legislates against gendered discrimination (Johnson et al 2006).

Critical thinking

- What factors might contribute to women having lower rates of mortality but higher rates of morbidity than men?

A caveat is worth noting at this point. Health inequities based on social stratification such as gender are unfair and unjust because they are socially produced, but they do not explain all variations in the health between men and women within a country. For example, differences in rates of prostate cancer between males and females are a consequence of being male rather than any inequity between men and women, since women do not have prostate glands (Braveman 2004). This is a difference based on one's sex. However, gender differences in health, such as the differing immunisation rates for boys over girls, is a clear form of social stratification causing health inequality (Braveman 2004).

Ethnicity

Similar to gender, ethnicity is a social construct (Solar & Irwin 2007). The active exclusion of particular groups due to their race/ethnicity has consequences for both psychological and physical health and is a result of discrimination (Nazroo & Williams 2006). Discrimination also impacts on access to income and stable employment (Nazroo & Williams 2006). Currently in Australia the life expectancy of Aboriginal and Torres Strait Islanders is almost 20 years behind non-Indigenous

Classroom activity

In small groups:

1. Make a list of occupations that might produce inequalities in morbidity and mortality.
2. What provision does the government make for workers and their families who are injured or die?
3. What provision does the government make for people with a disability that prevents them from working?
4. How is this paid for?

For information in addressing these questions visit the Australian Department of Families, Housing, Community Services and Indigenous Affairs website at <www.facs.gov.au> or the New Zealand Ministry of Social Development site at <www.msd.govt.nz>.

people (AIHW 2011, RACP 2005, Solar & Irwin 2007). For example, inequalities exist for Aboriginal people in South Australia across every variable of age and environment (Glover et al 2006). Further, Aboriginal people have the highest levels of disadvantage regarding life expectancy and this is reflected in that fact that an Aboriginal man has 18 years less life expectancy than the population average, while the most disadvantaged non-Indigenous male population groups have only 3.6 years less life expectancy than the population average (AIHW 2011). As discrimination is a structurally defined social and cultural concept, research and policy directives are hard to determine due to the intertwining nature with other aspects of stratification such as education, housing, health, employment and income. For example, the statistics noted above about gender differences in life expectancy need to be changed to accommodate ethnicity. In New Zealand life expectancy for Māori males is 69 years and 73.2 years for females (The Social Report 2007). In both cases there is up to an eight-year difference between Māori and non-Māori. It is the responsibility of governments to legislate against this active discrimination.

INTERMEDIARY DETERMINANTS OF HEALTH INEQUITIES

The intermediary determinants form the bridge between the structural determinants and the individual manifestations of the health inequalities (Solar & Irwin 2007). While social epidemiologists differ on what to include in the intermediary determinants of health, Solar and Irwin (2007) note the following: (1) material circumstances; (2) the social environment or psychosocial environment; (3) behavioural and biological factors; (4) the quality of the welfare-state aspects of the health system of the country; and (5) two cultural variables – social capital and social cohesion.

Material circumstances refer to aspects of the physical environment such as the quality of housing and access to transport, food and neighbourhood resources. Considerable research has been conducted to illustrate the impact of these factors on health. For example, people living in remote regions of Australia have higher rates of morbidity and mortality than people living in urban areas. There are many explanations as to why but at the intermediary level they have limited access to fresh foods and will often have to pay a higher price than people in cities. In cities supermarkets are often more numerous and better placed in high-income suburbs than in poorer neighbourhoods (Melchers et al 2009, Smith et al 2004), resulting in poorer people paying higher prices or having to travel further. The *Research focus* below provides an example of this.

Research focus

Pearce, M., Willis, E., McCarthy, C., et al., 2006. A response to the National Water Initiative from Nepabunna community, Report for the Aboriginal Affairs and Reconciliation Division of the Department of the Premier and Cabinet, South Australia, the Commonwealth Department of Family, Community Services and Indigenous Affairs, CRC for Aboriginal Health, Desert Knowledge CRC and United Water

ABSTRACT

The Anangu Pitjantjatjara (APY) Service Resource Management Project 'Cost of Living Study' (Tregenza & Tregenza 1998) was prepared in response to a proposal from the South Australian Government to charge Aboriginal people the full cost of electricity on their lands. In order to convince the government that this policy would have a detrimental impact on the health of the community, John and Elizabeth Tregenza constructed a hypothetical Aboriginal family of two adults employed through the 'work for the dole' program (officially called the Community Development Employment Program or 'CDEP'), one pensioner and three children (two of whom were under 15) to determine a typical weekly wage.

Using data derived from a range of communities across the APY Lands, they determined that the maximum (not average) wage for a family employed through CDEP was $600 per week once community-based deductions for rent, funerals and other items were taken into account. While not all families cleared $600 per week, this amount was used to determine the impact of a move to user-pays for electricity across the APY Lands. Indeed, in some instances families earning less than the hypothetical $600 per week figure went without food in the days prior to pension or CDEP payments.

The $600 was used to explore the ability of the hypothetical family to purchase food and household items linked to five of the nine Healthy Living Practices (Nganampa Health Council, South Australian Health Commission and the Aboriginal Health Organisation of SA 1987). These five practices are the capacity to:

- wash children and adults
- wash clothes and bedding
- buy, store and prepare healthy food
- control dust
- control temperature.

Cont... ▶

Family weekly costs included adequate food determined in consultation with a nutritionist, cleaning agents linked to health hardware such as brooms, mops, buckets, blankets, clothes and cooking utensils as well as health consumables such as cleaning agents and some medicines purchased monthly, quarterly or yearly. In total the items cost 23% more at community stores on APY Lands than the cost of the same items in Alice Springs (the closest capital city). The food basket comprised 85% or $500 of the family's income. The authors noted that few if any families on the APY Lands could afford to purchase whitegoods such as refrigerators or energy-efficient appliances, both essential prerequisites for maintaining the health hardware of the house. Personal income for sufficient food, health, hardware, adequate storage and energy-efficient appliances was seen as an essential building block to enable people to make healthy choices. Therefore, increasing the cost of living through user-pays for essential water and energy services would decrease the wellbeing of individuals, especially children.

The study formed the basis for the Mai Wiru Regional Stores Policy, which argued for increased subsidies on the APY Lands. In 2008 the South Australian Government provided subsidies to the APY community stores through a reduction in electricity costs. This was done to enable the stores to sell food at a cheaper rate and represents an example of healthy public policy.

Social, environmental or psychological factors include the stress of debt linked to poverty, uncertainty about employment and the impact of income differentials across a society discussed earlier. Material circumstances leading to overcrowding may also generate increased domestic violence or crime in the area, further impacting on the psychological health and wellbeing of the population. Behavioural and biological factors include the prevalence of smoking, alcohol consumption and eating patterns. Research demonstrates differences in these lifestyle factors based on socioeconomic status. The exact causal link between behaviour and illness is complex and not clearly understood. While there does appear to be a cultural factor, whereby poorer people are more likely to smoke, be physically inactive or have a poor diet, it would appear that there is also a stress factor associated with other aspects of their living conditions. For example, smoking may be a response to stress, and a diet high in saturated fats may lead to higher rates of heart disease. It is also possible, however, that stress linked to a social issue such as unemployment may activate the hormonal system, leading to high blood pressure (Brunner & Marmot 2006).

The resources and structure of the health system itself are intermediary factors (Solar & Irwin 2007) already explored. Countries with free universal health services usually have lower mortality and morbidity rates than those that rely on a market-based healthcare system where the consumer must pay for all services. The impact of the healthcare system goes beyond providing free access to acute medical services. It includes public health measures such as free immunisation and adequate financial support for those with chronic illness, those with a disability or those in need of rehabilitation.

The final intermediary determinant refers to social capital and social cohesion. Briefly, it is argued that population groups that have access to social networks,

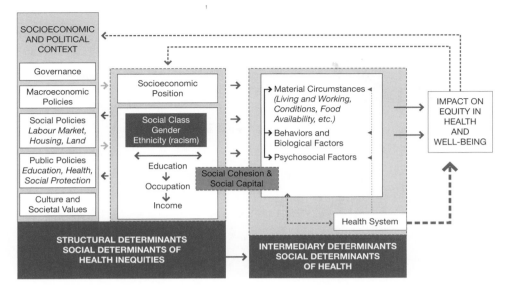

Figure 5.3 Framework for the social determinants of health

Solar O, Irwin A. A conceptual framework for action on the social determinants of health. Social Determinants of Health Discussion Paper 2 (Policy and Practice), ISBN 978 92 4 150085 2, © World Health Organization 2010

friends, neighbours and relatives who can assist them to improve their economic conditions have better health outcomes. Communities where there is a strong sense of collaboration and trust are also likely to enjoy better health. Importantly, these cultural factors cannot substitute for sound policy and structural reform.

The intermediary determinants create a causal chain of influence over the lifespan (Solar & Irwin 2007). The intermediary determinants provide the means of direct intervention (Solar & Irwin 2007). Interventions can be through direct policy or through health promotion initiatives that assist individuals and communities to change their behaviour. Clearly health promotion activities need to take account of the structural factors. Blaming poor people for their health status denies the causal factors found in their material circumstances and its subsequent stress. Figure 5.3 consists of all the SDH that interact to determine health outcomes for individuals. This overriding final framework devised by Solar and Irwin for the Commission on the Social Determinants of Health explains and visually represents the determinants that are currently used to inform WHO's research and policy recommendations (Solar & Irwin 2007).

Social determinants of health and psychology

While there is irrefutable evidence that socioeconomic position impacts on health, the exact biopsychosocial pathway from the structural and intermediary determinants to the presence of physical illness, mental illness or disease within an individual's body or in an entire population is only just beginning to be investigated. Understanding how it is that low income or discrimination based on gender or ethnicity means higher mortality or morbidity is difficult to explain. A number of

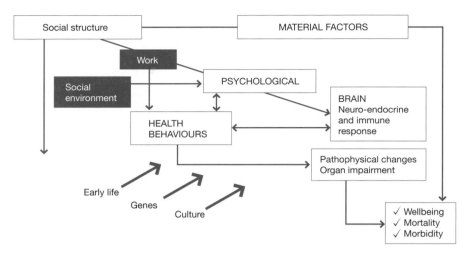

Figure 5.4 Connections between life factors and their psychosocial outcomes

Brunner E, Marmot M 2006 Social organization, stress and health. In: Marmot M, Wilkinson R (eds) Social determinants of health. Oxford University Press, Oxford

theories are proposed. These include explorations of the impact of the human *fight or flight* response on hormonal levels, metabolic rates or endocrine transmitters. The argument suggests that people in low socioeconomic groups are overloaded with psychological fight or flight demands (Brunner & Marmot 2006). This is covered in more detail in Chapter 10. Brunner and Marmot also suggest high levels of stress may make poorer people more susceptible to infection as a result of immune compromise. It is not our intention to describe the range of possible pathways as it is beyond the remit of this chapter. However, Figure 5.4 illustrates the connections between different factors in life and the psychosocial outcomes for individuals.

Further, mental illness correlates with social patterns. Poorer people are likely to have higher rates of mental illness; this has been highlighted by several studies (Draine et al 2002, Heneghan et al 2006, McLaughlin et al 2011, Petrilla et al 2005). Biopsychological illnesses follow distinct social boundaries, with those in the lowest income quintile having a much higher incidence of mental and physical illness. For example, 34% of the population with mental illnesses are people living in one-parent households, while only 55% of people with a severe disorder are employed (Australian Government 2010 p 35). Draine et al's (2002) research highlights the improvements in mental illness outcomes following the implementation of a program that addressed social disadvantage. Draine et al (2002) assert that programs that do not address the social causes and the sociopolitical context of psychological illness perpetuate and maintain these illnesses.

Conclusion

This chapter first clarified the aspects of health external to the individual and individual health behaviours that determine health outcomes. The social model of health broadens the view of health beyond both the biomedical model and the biopsychological model to examine the influences on health that are determined by social circumstances. The social aspects of health have formed the basis of the SDH.

The chapter argued that the social model of health suggests that health is a human right and responsibility for providing the determinants of health resides with governments as well as individuals.

In the second section of the chapter the SDH, such as education, income, gender, ethnicity and social class, were outlined. Those SDH that are described as structural are directly influenced by the social and political environments and institutions within society, and can be addressed by changes to policy in the areas of health, education, housing and so on. The SDH that are intermediary in nature are downstream and closer to the individual, and are addressed through community and individual health interventions. Both the structural and the intermediary SDH have short- and long-term effects on the physical and psychological outcomes of citizens within a society and mediate the level of health that can be attained. Importantly, the social determinants present health professionals with a dilemma. Having diagnosed, treated and cured the illness or disease, health professionals know that in many instances they discharge the patients back into the same illness-producing social system. Consequently, health professionals need to be social reformers!

REMEMBER

- The physical health of individuals is often thought to be the result of physical and psychological factors, however, mortality and morbidity rates appear to also be caused by social factors.
- These social factors are referred to as the 'social determinants of health'.
- Social epidemiologists and social theorists attempt to explain how the social determinants of health translate to health or illness and disease for individuals and populations.
- While the evidence is clear that mortality and morbidity rates are influenced by social factors, there is considerable debate on how these social determinants impact on the psychological health or behaviour of individuals or cause physical illness.

Classroom activity

In small groups:

1. Make a list of the social determinants of health that impact on people in your city, town or region.
2. There is a clear relationship between poverty, gender, ethnicity and morbidity and mortality rates.
   - Could it be argued that there are cultural practices that contribute to poorer health outcomes and cultural practices that are responses to these factors? Discuss.
   - If so, identify illness-producing behaviours and identify whether they arise from the culture or structure of a society.

Cont... ▶

3. In this chapter we have suggested that structural determinants rather than individual behaviours explain many differences in mortality and morbidity rates for population groups.

   ■ How does a structural explanation differ from a cultural explanation?

4. If you were Minister for Health how might you go about reducing mortality and morbidity rates for people living in rural and remote regions?

   ■ In giving an answer consider the situation for a specific population group such as men, youth, families, Māori or Aboriginal people.

Further resources

Australian Bureau of Statistics (ABS), 2009. National health survey: summary of results, Australia 2004–05 Cat. No. 4364.0. ABS, Canberra.

Brunner, E., Marmot, M., 2006. Social organization, stress, and health. In: Marmot, M., Wilkinson, R. (Eds.), 2006. Social determinants of health. Oxford University Press, Oxford.

Jarvis, M.J., Wardle, J., 2006. The life course, the social gradient and health. In: Marmot, M., Wilkinson, R. (Eds.)., Social determinants of health. Oxford University Press, Oxford.

Marmot, M., Siegrist, J., Theorell, T., 2006. Health and the psychosocial environment at work. In: Marmot, M., Wilkinson, R. (Eds.), 2006. Social determinants of health. Oxford University Press, Oxford.

Nganampa Health Council, South Australian Health Commission and the Aboriginal Health Organisation of SA, 1987. Uwankara Palyanyku Kanyintjaku report: an environmental and public health review within the Anangu Pitjantjatjara lands. UKP Report, Adelaide.

World Health Organization (WHO), 2008. Closing the gap in a generation: health equity through action on the social determinants of health. Final report of the Commission on Social Determinants of Health. WHO, Geneva.

Weblinks

All students

World Health Organization report into health inequities

http://whqlibdoc.who.int/publications/2008/9789241563703_eng.pdf

The final report from the WHO Commission on the Social Determinants of Health discussing the disparities between population groups and the action required to address these health inequities.

World Health Organization report into the social determinants of health

http://whqlibdoc.who.int/publications/2007/interim_statement_eng.pdf

This report outlines the social determinants of health and discusses their sociopolitical context, offering various theoretical explanations for the occurrence of the SDH. It also includes suggestions for researching the SDH and the policy actions required to address the SDH.

World Health Organization statistics

www.who.int/healthinfo/statistics/en

This report presents the statistics from 193 states on healthcare within nations covering material wealth, preventable diseases, mortality rates and health trends.

Australian students

The Social Atlas

http://www.publichealth.gov.au/publications/a-social-health-atlas-of-australia-[second-edition]—volume-1:-australia.html

This report describes the social aspects of Australia and provides information collected over several years outlining the disparities between population groups within Australia.

New Zealand students

The Social Report

www.socialreport.msd.govt.nz/health

This webpage features the health section of *The Social Report*, outlining the disparities and deprivation that occurs between people within New Zealand. It includes information such as avoidable deaths, levels of education and other factors that determine an individual's wellbeing and health.

References

Australian Bureau of Statistics (ABS), 2006. Musculoskeletal conditions in Australia: a snapshot 2004–05. ABS, Canberra.

Australian Bureau of Statistics (ABS), 2009. National health survey: summary of results, Australia 2004–05. Cat. No. 4364.0, ABS, Canberra.

Australian Government, 2010. The changes to Medicare primary care items. Department of Health and Ageing, Canberra. Online. Available: www.health.gov.au/internet/mbsonline 10 Mar 2011.

Australian Institute of Health and Welfare (AIHW), 2011. Comparing life expectancy of indigenous people in Australia, New Zealand, Canada and the United States: conceptual, methodological and data issues. Cat. no. IHW 47. AIHW, Canberra. Online. Available: http://www.aihw.gov.au/publication-detail/?id=10737420537 25 Sep 2012.

Bartley, M., Ferrie, J., Montgomery, S.M., 2006. Health and labour market disadvantage: unemployment, non-employment and job insecurity. In: Marmot, M., Wilkinson, R. (Eds.), Social determinants of health. Oxford University Press, Oxford.

Baum, F., 2005. Who cares about health for all in the 21st century? Journal of Epidemiology and Community Health 59, 714–715.

Baum, F., Begin, M., Houweling, T., et al., 2009. Changes not for the faint hearted: reorienting healthcare systems towards health equity through action on the social determinants of health. American Journal of Public Health 99 (11), 1967–1974.

Black, D., Morris, J.N., Smith, C., et al., 1980. Report of the working group on inequalities in health. Stationery Office, Department of Health and Social Security, London.

Blane, D., 2006. The life course, the social gradient and health. In: Marmot, M., Wilkinson, R. (Eds.), Social determinants of health. Oxford University Press, Oxford.

Braveman, P., 2004. Defining equity in health. Health Policy and Development 2 (3), 180–185.

Brunner, E., Marmot, M., 2006. Social organization, stress and health. In: Marmot, M., Wilkinson, R. (Eds.), Social determinants of health. Oxford University Press, Oxford.

Dahlgren, G., Whitehead, M., 1991. Policies and strategies to promote social equity in health. Institute for Future Studies, Stockholm.

Draine, J., Salzer, M., Culbane, D., et al., 2002. Role of social disadvantage in crime, joblessness and homelessness among persons with serious mental illness. Psychiatric Services 53 (5), 565–573.

Glover, J., Hetzel, D., Glover, L., et al., 2006. A social health atlas of South Australia, third ed. The University of Adelaide, Adelaide.

Heneghan, C.J., Glasziou, P., Perera, R., 2006. Reminder packaging for improving adherence to self-administration of long-term medications. Cochrane Database System Review 1:CD005025.

Jarvis, M.J., Wardle, J., 2006. The life course, the social gradient and health. In: Marmot, M., Wilkinson, R. (Eds.), Social determinants of health. Oxford University Press, Oxford.

Johnson, M., Mercer, C.H., Cassell, J.A., 2006. Social determinants, sexual behaviour and sexual health. In: Marmot, M., Wilkinson, R. (Eds.), Social determinants of health. Oxford University Press, Oxford.

Kelly, M.P., Bonnefoy, J., Morgan, A., et al., 2006. The development of the evidence base about the social determinants of health. World Health Organization Commission of Social Determinants of Health Measurement and Evidence Knowledge Network. WHO, Geneva.

Lie, R.K., 2004. Health, human rights and mobilization of resources for health. BMC International Health and Human Rights Journal 4, 4–12.

Marmot, M., 2001. Aetiology of coronary heart disease: foetal and infant growth and socioeconomic factors in adult life may act together. British Medical Journal 323, 1261–1262.

Marmot, M., Siegrist, J., Theorell, T., 2006. Health and the psychosocial environment at work. In: Marmot, M., Wilkinson, R. (Eds.), 2006. Social determinants of health. Oxford University Press, Oxford.

Marmot, M., Wilkinson, R. (Eds.), 2006. Social determinants of health. Oxford University Press, Oxford.

McCarthy, M., 2006. Transport and health. In: Marmot, M., Wilkinson, R. (Eds.), 2006. Social determinants of health. Oxford University Press, Oxford.

McLaughlin, K.A., Breslau, J., Green, J.G., et al., 2011. Childhood socio-economic status and the onset, persistence and severity of DSM-IV mental disorders in a US national sample. Social Science & Medicine 73 (7), 1088–1096.

Melchers, K.G., Klehe, U.-C., Richter, G.M., et al., 2009. I know what you want to know: the impact of interviewees' ability to identify criteria on interview performance and construct-related validity. Human Performance 22, 355–374. doi:10.1080/08959280903120295.

Morales, F., Gilner, L., 2002. Sage English dictionary 2002. Computer program. Sage, London.

Morrissey, M., 2006. The Australian state and Indigenous peoples 1990–2006. Journal of Sociology 24 (4), 347–354.

Nazroo, J.Y., Williams, D.R., 2006. The social determination of ethnic/racial inequalities in health. In: Marmot, M., Wilkinson, R. (Eds.), Social determinants of health. Oxford University Press, Oxford.

Nganampa Health Council, South Australian Health Commission and the Aboriginal Health Organisation of SA, 1987. Uwankara Palyanyku Kanyintjaku report: an environmental and public health review within the Anangu Pitjantjatjara Lands. UKP Report, Adelaide.

Pearce, M., Willis, E., McCarthy, C., et al., 2006. A response to the National Water Initiative from Nepabunna community, Report for the Aboriginal Affairs and Reconciliation Division of the Department of the Premier and Cabinet, South Australia, the Commonwealth Department of Family, Community Services and Indigenous Affairs, CRC for Aboriginal Health, Desert Knowledge CRC and United Water.

Petrilla, A.A., Benner, J.S., Battleman, D.S., et al., 2005. Evidence-based interventions to improve patient compliance with antihypertensive and lipid-lowering medications. International Journal of Clinical Practice 59 (12), 1411–1451.

Raphael, D., 2006. Social determinants of health: Present status, unanswered questions and future directions. International Journal of Health Services 36 (4), 651–677.

Raphael, D., Macdonald, J., Colman, R., et al., 2005. Researching income and income distribution as determinants of health in Canada: gaps between theoretical knowledge research practice and policy implication. Health Policy 72, 217–232.

Robertson, A., Brunner, E., Sheiham, A., 2006. The life course, the social gradient and health. In: Marmot, M., Wilkinson, R. (Eds.), Social determinants of health. Oxford University Press, Oxford.

Royal Australasian College of Physicians (RACP), 2005. Inequity and health: a call to action. Addressing health and socioeconomic inequality in Australia. Policy statement RACP.

Smith, A., Coveney, J., Carter, P., et al., 2004. The Eat Well SA Project: an evaluation-based case study in building capacity for promoting healthy eating. Health Promotion Journal 19 (3), 327–334.

Social Health Atlas of Australia, 2011. Online. Available: http://www.publichealth.gov.au/publications/a-social-health-atlas-of-australia-[second-edition]-volume-1:-australia.html 5 Mar 2011.

Solar, O., Irwin, A., 2007. A conceptual framework for action on the social determinants of health. Discussion paper for the Commission of Social Determinants of Health. Draft. April. WHO, Geneva.

Stansfeld, S., 2006. Social support and social cohesion. In: Marmot, M., Wilkinson, R. (Eds.), Social determinants of health. Oxford University Press, Oxford.

The Social Report New Zealand, 2007. Online. Available: http://www.socialreport.msd.govt.nz/health/index.html 5 Mar 2008.

Tregenza, J., Tregenza, E., 1998. Cost of living on the Anangu Pitjantjatjara Lands, Survey report. AP Services.

Turrell, G., Oldenburg, B., McGuffog, I., et al., 1999. Socioeconomic determinants of health: towards a national research program and a policy and intervention agenda. Queensland University of Technology, School of Public Health, AusInfo, Canberra.

Vos, T., Barker, B., Begg, S., et al., 2009. Burden of disease and injury in Aboriginal and Torres Strait Islander peoples: the Indigenous health gap. International Journal of Epidemiology 38, 470–477.

Wadsworth, M., Butterworth, S., 2006. Early life. In: Marmot, M., Wilkinson, R. (Eds.), Social determinants of health. Oxford University Press, Oxford.

World Health Organization (WHO), 2008. Closing the gap in a generation: health equity through action on the social determinants of health, WHO commission on Social Determinants of Health. Online. Available: http://www.who.int/social_determinants/final_report/en/index.html 5 Sep 2008.

World Health Statistics, 2007. Health data and statistics. Online. Available: www.who.int/healthinfo/statistics/en 13 Mar 2008.

Chapter 6
Research for health professionals

PATRICIA BARKWAY

Learning objectives

The material in this chapter will help you to:

- distinguish and describe various research paradigms used in psychological and health research
- describe how research shapes healthcare practice
- describe the role of health professionals as research consumers
- critically appraise research reports and draw conclusions appropriate for practice
- describe the ethics of research participation and in particular the advocacy role played by health professionals.

Key terms

- Qualitative research
- Quantitative research
- Evidence-based practice
- Research consumer
- Research ethics

Introduction

This chapter examines how psychological and health research findings influence healthcare practice and provides an overview of research paradigms, methodologies and methods. It is not within the scope of this chapter to provide a detailed account of *how* to conduct research as this is covered in more detail and depth elsewhere in your course and in specific research textbooks. Rather, this chapter focuses on how research findings influence healthcare practice and how health professionals can use research in their day-to-day clinical practice and, thereby, be competent *consumers* of research (Schneider et al 2013). Being a competent consumer of research involves knowing how to access, critique and utilise research findings to inform your everyday clinical practice. Finally, the role of the health professional in the ethical conduct of research is addressed.

Healthcare research: an overview

Research is a process of inquiry that seeks to develop new knowledge or to expand existing knowledge. In the health arena research findings are used to: identify the health needs of populations; test and choose appropriate interventions and treatments for illness and health problems; plan and implement intervention strategies for illness prevention and health promotion; evaluate programs and interventions; and assist with resource allocation.

Research can be either basic or applied. *Basic* research aims to develop new theory and/or knowledge, while *applied* research examines the application of knowledge in certain circumstances. A study of the factors that influence an individual's decision to follow or disregard a recommended health treatment, for example, is basic research; and a randomised control trial (RCT) testing a new drug to treat cancer is an example of applied research.

A further important distinction between research studies is whether they are experimental, observational, interpretive or critical. Experimental studies utilise quantitative methods and are a powerful research method because people (subjects/participants) can be allocated to receive an exposure of interest, such as a new treatment or healthcare practice, or an intervention, such as allergen avoidance or dietary advice. In such studies, independent variables that distort the association between another independent variable and the problem (confounding factors) can be controlled and, therefore, the level of evidence obtained is high.

Observational research, also called descriptive studies, utilises either quantitative (e.g. census) or qualitative (e.g. ethnography) methods. They are less powerful for measuring associations; nevertheless, they are a valuable method for: measuring the effects of non-modifiable risk factors such as age or gender; measuring the effects of exposures to which people cannot be ethically randomised, such as breastfeeding or environmental tobacco smoke; or understanding human experience and social issues.

Interpretive and critical approaches are located within the qualitative research paradigm and aim to describe, explore and seek understanding of human and social phenomena. Interpretative research is focused on understanding or creating meaning, while critical research has the additional goal of bringing about social and political change.

Research paradigms

Various methods can be utilised to conduct research and the choice of method is driven by the methodology (or the philosophical and theoretical tradition that underpins the inquiry). Methodologies, also referred to as paradigms, are the theoretical and philosophical positions that underpin the research approach. They are a broad framework of perception, understanding and beliefs within which theory and practice operate.

There are two main research paradigms: quantitative and qualitative. The *quantitative* research paradigm is scientific and positivist and seeks objective answers to the research question. It assumes that an objective answer to the question exists. The *qualitative* research paradigm is interpretative and critical and seeks greater meaning and understanding of the issue under investigation. It acknowledges the subjective nature of human experience.

QUANTITATIVE RESEARCH

Quantitative research is steeped in the conventional scientific tradition. It involves collecting data that are quantifiable and measurable and, therefore, can be analysed and interpreted numerically. It takes a positivist philosophical position and is underpinned by the view that reality is objective, measurable and separate from the researcher. In this way quantitative research follows a scientific tradition of objective observation, prediction and testing of causal or correlational relationships (Bragge 2010, Swanwick 2010).

Quantitative research generally involves extensive data collection and, thereby, seeks a *broad* understanding to enable explanations and predictions to be made. Hypotheses can either be supported or rejected by applying statistical tests of significance to the data. The data collected in quantitative research can be: *nominal*, when the data distinguish categories (like male/female); *ordinal*, when the data distinguish degree like never, sometimes, always; or *numerical*, when the data measures numbers like how many cigarettes smoked per day. Examples of quantitative methods include experiments (e.g. RCTs, questionnaires and surveys), structured interviews and census collection.

Quantitative research designs include: *experimental*, which attempt to show that one thing causes another; *quasi experimental*, which is an experimental design but does not have random allocation to the control group or an experimental group; *descriptive*, which summarises and describes a set of measurements; and *correlational*, which explores the relationship between two variables.

Focus on quantitative research: randomised control trials (RCTs)

In RCTs with human subjects, participants agree to enrol following informed consent and are then randomly allocated to the experimental (receive the intervention) or control (don't receive the intervention) group. Depending on the type of study, the control group may receive a placebo intervention or may receive current best practice. Placebo interventions are usually only used when a new treatment method is being assessed and, for this reason, placebo-controlled trials usually have a small sample size because they are seen as an intermediary step in the process of showing the efficacy of a new treatment.

RCTs provide the highest level of evidence because the random allocation of participants to study groups minimises the influences of selection bias, of known and unknown confounders and of prognostic factors such as participant characteristics on the study results. Blinding (not informing the participants and/or the research team about which participants are in which group) can also reduce the effects of other biases.

The inclusion criteria are an important issue in RCTs. In trials to measure the effectiveness of a treatment or intervention, participants who have an identified health problem are enrolled. However, in interventions designed to prevent an illness or condition from developing, participants who are 'at risk' are enrolled before the illness or condition has developed. Although RCTs provide the most scientifically rigorous research method available, they are often difficult to conduct and low response rates may reduce the generalisability of the results. Table 6.1 summarises the strengths and weaknesses of RCTs.

Table 6.1	
STRENGTHS AND WEAKNESSES OF RCTs	
Strengths	**Weaknesses**
Provide a high level of evidence	Selection bias may be an issue if potential participants have treatment preferences
Confounders, prognostic factors and exposures are balanced between groups	Follow-up bias may be influential if control group participants selectively drop out because they are receiving a placebo or existing treatment
Allocation, reporting and observer bias can be controlled by blinding	Low participation rates may reduce the generalisability of the results
Willingness to participate does not influence group allocation	Long-term outcomes may not be measured

Critical thinking

- Is Barlow et al's research basic or applied?
- What is the rationale for your decision?
- The authors recommend further research. What further research can be undertaken to identify the support needs of parents?

Research focus

Barlow, J., Powell, L., Gilchrist, M., et al., 2008. The effectiveness of the Training and Support Program for parents of children with disabilities: a randomized controlled trial. Journal of Psychosomatic Research 64, 55–62.

ABSTRACT

Objective

The Training and Support Program (TSP) was designed to equip parents of children with disabilities with a simple massage skill for use with their children in the home environment. The effectiveness of the TSP was examined in an RCT with a wait-list control group.

Methods

Parents were trained in massage by suitably qualified therapists in eight weekly sessions, each lasting one hour. The sample comprised 188 parents who were randomised to an intervention group (n = 95) (who attended the TSP with their children immediately) or a control group (n = 93) (who were offered the TSP after four months of follow-up). Data were collected by self-administered questionnaires at baseline and at four-month follow-up.

Results

The majority of participants were mothers (88%) with a partner (88%) and white European (82%); 40% worked full time or part time and 34% had health problems (e.g. chronic fatigue, cancer or arthritis). The TSP demonstrated statistically significant positive effects on parental self-efficacy for managing children's psychosocial wellbeing and depressed mood (0.004 and 0.007). There were trends towards improvement on parental satisfaction with life (p = 0.053), global health (p = 0.065) and parental ratings of children's sleeping (p = 0.074) and mobility (p = 0.012). Effect sizes were small (0.11–0.23). Levels of anxiety, depression and perceived stress were all higher than published norms.

Conclusion

The TSP is an effective means of improving parental self-efficacy and depressed mood. Additional means of supporting parents need to be investigated.

QUALITATIVE RESEARCH

Qualitative research proposes that there is no objective reality as assumed by the quantitative positivist paradigm. It is a constructivist approach in which the individual constructs the meaning and interpretation of reality from their own experience. Nevertheless, like quantitative studies, qualitative research utilises a range of methods and methodologies that facilitate the exploration of different phenomena, meaning and experience.

In qualitative research, data are collected from observation and interview within a population and describe the range of responses, as well as variation between responses. Narrative data are collected as opposed to numerical data in quantitative research and, thereby, a *depth* of understanding about the issue under investigation is provided in contrast to the *breadth* of understanding sought in quantitative research.

Examples of qualitative methodologies include:

- *symbolic interactionism* – that seeks to understand the social meaning that shapes human behaviour (see Beard & Fox 2008)

- *phenomenology* – that seeks the *discovery* of a phenomenon (European philosophical tradition) or the *experience* of a phenomenon or its *meaning* (North American / empirical tradition) (see Ranse & Arbon 2008)

- *ethnography* – that seeks to discover cultural meaning from a *native* perspective (see Larun & Malterud 2007)

- *grounded theory* – that uses induction to develop theory (see Bahora et al 2009).

Methods for collecting data in a qualitative study include but are not limited to: focus groups; unstructured or semi-structured interviews; participant observation; ethnography; case studies; and document analysis.

Focus on qualitative research: phenomenology

Phenomenology began as a philosophical mode of inquiry in continental Europe around the turn of the 20th century. Its acknowledged founder is the German philosopher Edmund Husserl (1859–1938). Throughout the latter part of the 20th century and early 21st century phenomenology was adapted as an approach in health research inquiry, particularly by nurse researchers (Dowling 2007). The goal of phenomenological health research is to understand a human or social issue by examining the human experience of the phenomenon under investigation, whereas the goal of philosophical phenomenology is to examine the phenomenon itself (Aspers 2010, Crotty 1996, Flood 2010).

Consequently, phenomenology is both a philosophy and a research method. As a philosophy it is interested in the person's perception of a phenomenon, that is, the subjective understanding of the meaning of the phenomenon being investigated, such as the phenomenon of sadness. And, as a research approach, phenomenology is interested in understanding the human (or lived) experience of a particular phenomenon, such as what it is like to be sad. It is the latter form of phenomenology that is prevalent in the health research literature. This type of phenomenological research generally takes the form of interviewing participants, followed by analysis of the data and the development of themes from which conclusions and recommendations are drawn.

Controversy surrounds the use of phenomenology as a method in health research. Crotty (1996) refers to the study of the lived experience as 'new' phenomenology, which he argued differs from philosophical phenomenology because it attempts to draw objective conclusions from subjective data. Paley (2005), too, is critical of phenomenological health research, stating that in attempting to make sense of subjective data, nurse researchers draw objective conclusions and in doing so 'mimic science' in assuming that an objective reality exists.

Aspers (2010), however, does not see a problem with there being two approaches. While he distinguishes *philosophical* phenomenology from what he calls *empirical* phenomenology, he describes the two approaches as having different purposes. Philosophical phenomenology seeks to understand the phenomenon itself, while empirical phenomenology is interested in the social meaning of the person's experience of the phenomenon. Finlay (2010) also observes that a variety of research methods and techniques are conducted under the banner of phenomenology. She argues that rather than debating the difference in approaches, the important issue for researchers should be to be clear about which philosophical and research traditions they are using and why. Nevertheless, despite the methodological debate surrounding phenomenological health research, phenomenological studies contribute to the body of knowledge about individuals' experiences of health and illness issues and thereby can influence healthcare practices.

Research focus

Karlsson, A., Arman, M., Wikblad, K., 2008. Teenagers with type 1 diabetes – a phenomenological study of the transition towards autonomy in self-management. International Journal of Nursing Studies 45, 562–570.

ABSTRACT

Background

Becoming autonomous is an important aspect of teenagers' psychosocial development and this is especially true of teenagers with type 1 diabetes. Previous studies exploring the everyday problems of teenagers with diabetes have focused on adherence to self-care management, how self-determination affects metabolic control and the perception of social support.

Objective

The aim of the study was to elucidate lived experiences, focusing on the transition towards autonomy in diabetes self-management among teenagers with type 1 diabetes.

Design and method

Data were collected using interviews and a qualitative phenomenological approach was chosen for the analysis.

Participants

Thirty-two teenagers (18 females and 14 males) were interviewed about their individual experiences of self-management of diabetes.

Findings

The lived experiences of the transition towards autonomy in self-management were characterised by the overriding theme 'hovering between individual actions and support of others'. The findings indicate

Cont... ▶

that individual self-reliance and confirmation of others are helpful in the transition process. Growth through individual self-reliance was viewed as a developmental process of making one's own decisions; psychological maturity enabled increased responsibility and freedom; motivation was related to wellbeing and how well the diabetes could be managed. The theme 'confirmation of others' showed that parental encouragement increased the certainty of teenagers' standpoints; peers' acceptance of diabetes facilitated incorporation of daily self-management activities; and support from the diabetes team strengthened teenagers' self-esteem.

Conclusion

In striving for autonomy, teenagers needed distance from others but still to retain the support of others. A stable foundation for self-management includes having the knowledge required to practise diabetes management and handle different situations.

Critical thinking

- Is Karlsson et al's research basic or applied?
- What is the rationale for your decision?
- Based on the findings of this study what advice would you give to the parents of a teenager with type 1 diabetes? Why?

QUANTITATIVE OR QUALITATIVE?

In the planning phase of an investigation a decision is made early in the research process concerning which methods or methodology to use, namely, quantitative or qualitative, or whether to use multiple methods or methodologies – *triangulation*. Choosing a method is best addressed by considering the question to be investigated and the methodology that best informs the research question. For example, if a researcher wants to investigate the *incidence* of asthma in the community, then epidemiological (quantitative) data will provide that information. However, if the researcher wants to know *what is the experience of a person living with asthma?* then a semi-structured interview or focus group is an appropriate (qualitative) method for data collection. Table 6.2 summarises the similarities and differences between quantitative and qualitative research.

TRIANGULATION

Triangulation, or the use of mixed methods and/or methodologies in psychological and social research, is a process whereby various forms of data are collected from different sources. Its justification is that no single method can provide a comprehensive explanation for the phenomenon under investigation and that collecting data from different sources provides multiple perspectives and enables better understanding (Denzin 2009, Torrance 2012). Triangulation may be applied to one or more of the following: methodology, method, data and/or investigator. It can

Table 6.2		
TYPES OF RESEARCH		
Types of research		
	Quantitative	Qualitative
Methodology	Scientific Positivist	Philosophical Sociological Post-modern
Purpose	Explanation Prediction Objective truth	Interpretive Critical Subjective understanding
Methods	Experimental Measurement Statistical analysis	Interview Observation Narrative analysis
Sample size	Usually large	Usually small
Research evaluation	Reliability Validity Correlation	Rigour Credibility Auditability
Ethics	Beneficence not harm Informed consent Confidentiality Right to withdraw from research Merit and integrity of the research	

utilise both quantitative and qualitative paradigms and methods for data collection, for example, by obtaining data from key informant interviews (qualitative) and questionnaires (quantitative). It can also include collecting data using different methods within the same research paradigm, for example, focus group and participant observation, which are both qualitative.

The purpose of triangulation is to validate the findings by collecting data on the same phenomenon from different sources (Howe 2012). Collecting data from various sources enables researchers to corroborate their findings, or not. And if both quantitative and qualitative methods are used, a broad *and* deep understanding of the issue is obtained. For example, in determining the needs of parents who have a child with a disability, a researcher could interview key informants (qualitative research) and use this data to design a questionnaire to canvass the opinions of a wider selection of the target population (quantitative research).

In summary, the question of whether to use quantitative or qualitative methods to conduct research relates not to what is the better method but to what is the more appropriate method of providing the information sought. If the identification of the magnitude – or the extent – of an issue is sought or a hypothesis is to be tested, then quantitative methods are required. On the other hand, if the researcher is concerned with understanding human experience from an informant's perspective, then a qualitative method is called for. Furthermore, by utilising both quantitative and qualitative methods – as in triangulation – researchers can obtain a greater understanding of the research question under investigation.

Health professionals as consumers of research

While most health professionals do not *conduct* research in their day-to-day work, all will use research findings on a daily basis. Schneider et al (2013 p 289) refers to this as being a consumer of research. Being a consumer of research requires health professionals to understand and utilise research evidence in clinical practice. Specifically this means being able to:

- access contemporary research reports related to your area of intended healthcare practice
- analyse and critique research findings and conclusions
- underpin clinical practice with an evidence base, that is, articulate the evidence base for clinical practices
- know the processes required to translate research findings into new clinical practices
- know the processes required to change clinical practices that are not supported by contemporary evidence
- observe ethical issues of research participation (and advocate on behalf of participants should this be required).

Accessing research findings

The findings of research studies need to be disseminated before they can influence practice. Research reports are published in a variety of genres including: as an article in a refereed journal; as an article in a non-refereed journal; as a systematic review; as a monograph; as a conference presentation or poster; as a report on an internet specialist website; or in the popular media, including newspapers, television and the internet.

Where a research report is published can be indicative of the degree of confidence the reader can place in the claims made by the researcher. For example, the conclusions drawn by the author of an article published in a scholarly refereed journal can be accepted with more confidence than claims posted on a news-based website or reported in a daily newspaper.

REFEREED JOURNALS

Articles submitted to a refereed journal undergo peer review prior to being accepted for publication. This involves a process of subjecting the author's work to scholarly review by experts in the field of the study. For an article reporting on research findings the peer review process aims to ensure the research design is sound and ethical, and that the conclusions drawn and claims made by the authors can be substantiated by the process and results presented. One drawback, however, of disseminating research findings through the peer review process is that it can take months or even years for an article to be accepted by a scholarly journal, thereby delaying the time taken for the research findings to influence practice.

SYSTEMATIC REVIEWS

A systematic review of the literature identifies a single question and examines all of the published quality literature that relates to the question. They are commonly used to examine cause and effect and clinical effectiveness studies (Schneider et al 2013), for example, to identify risk factors for cancer or to ascertain the most effective drug treatment for osteoarthritis. In the health field systematic reviews are considered to provide the highest level of evidence.

The Cochrane Collaboration is the most widely known publisher of systematic reviews. The collaboration aims to provide independent evidence to inform healthcare decision making. Cochrane reviews combine the results of the world's best medical studies and are recognised as the 'gold standard in evidence-based health care' (Cochrane Collaboration 2011). In assessing systematic reviews Hagger (2012) suggests that the features of a 'good' review article are that it:

- is **original** – makes a unique contribution to the literature and field of study

- **advances thinking and knowledge** – challenges previous ideas and contributes to new and existing understandings of the issue

- is **theory-based** – takes into consideration what has gone before, and uses current thinking and evidence to develop new ideas

- is **evidence-based** – takes into consideration previous research findings when developing new ideas

- is **accurate, comprehensive and rigorous** – uses the highest methodological standards when conducting the review, and includes all important studies in the field or **provides justification for their exclusion**

- **provides recommendations for future research** – diligent in generating new questions to be addressed, and fosters future research enquiry and empirical work

- **stimulates debate** – values scholarly debate between researchers and theorists on key questions related to theory, research and practice.

OTHER PUBLICATIONS

Research findings can also be disseminated through conference presentations and posters that may or may not be peer assessed and may or may not be published. As with journal articles that have been accepted through a review process, conference material will have met criteria with regard to methodological and interpretive soundness and, hence, the reader can place greater confidence in the conclusion(s) drawn by the researcher.

Another source of research reports is the popular media that, in the main, are not peer reviewed. Included in this category are newspaper articles, television programs and the internet. Less confidence can be placed in the reliability, validity and credibility of claims made in such reports if they have not undergone the scrutiny of professional review.

Government departments and non-government organisations frequently publish reports as a monograph, which is a small book or treatise on a particular subject. Governments, academics and organisations also publish reports and policies in hard copy and on the internet in what has become known as the 'grey literature'. The credibility of these reports is influenced by who is the author and who published it. Non-refereed journals and newsletters are another source for research reports or updates. However, as these publications have not been subjected to the scrutiny of review by experts they do not carry the same authority as a report published in a scholarly refereed journal. Nevertheless, they can be informative and a discerning reader can critically evaluate the conclusions drawn by the authors just as they also would for a refereed article.

Access to research information by the general public has increased exponentially in recent years, principally through the internet but also through current affairs programs on television and from the print media. Many patients now research their conditions on the internet prior to visiting their general practitioner (GP). While this enables patients to be more informed about their condition and treatment options it is important to stress that any information sourced from the popular media must be critically assessed before being accepted as valid. To conclude, before accepting claims made by researchers the responsibility rests with readers to critically appraise the veracity of those claims, regardless of whether the research findings are peer assessed or not but particularly if they are not.

Analysis and critique of research reports

In analysing and critiquing research articles and reviews some questions apply to both quantitative and qualitative studies such as 'how were ethical considerations addressed?'. There are also separate questions to be asked due to the different approaches of the two paradigms regarding research design, data collection, analysis, interpretation and conclusions drawn. The questions in Boxes 6.1 and 6.2 (adapted from Schneider et al 2013) provide a template for critically appraising quantitative and qualitative research reports.

Adapted from Schneider Z & Whitehead D, 2013 Nursing & midwifery research, 4th edn. Elsevier, Sydney

Box 6.1 Critical review of quantitative studies

Article details	Record the author name(s), publication date, article title and journal details. Is the article published in a scholarly journal and has it been through a peer review process? Is the title consistent with the stated aim of the study? Is the abstract a succinct summary of the study, its findings and recommendations?

Cont... ▶

Aim of the study	Is the hypothesis and/or purpose clearly stated? What is the research question?
Method	Does the literature review demonstrate a need for the study? Has relevant literature been consulted? What is the study design? Is it appropriate for the hypothesis or question under investigation? Is the data collection process, including participant recruitment, and method (e.g. questionnaire), clearly described? What statistical tests are used? Were they descriptive, correlational or inferential? Are the statistical tests used appropriate for the question/issue under investigation?
Findings	Was the hypothesis confirmed/refuted? Are the findings statistically significant? Have the findings been interpreted in relation to the research question and aims? Were there any unexpected findings?
Significance of findings	What is the significance of the findings? Why are they important? To whom are they important? What are the implications of the findings for clinical practice? What are the implications of the findings for further research?
Limitations/rigour	Are the limitations of the study reported? Is the sample size sufficient for the statistical tests used in the study? Can the findings be generalised, or are they limited to the population studied? Is there a conflict of interest (e.g. who funded the study)? Is sufficient detail provided to allow replication of the study?
Conclusion	Can the conclusion logically be drawn from the data analysis and findings? Is the conclusion related to the findings and the stated aim of the study? Do the recommendations regarding clinical practice or future research logically follow from the analysis of the findings? Did the study provide new insights or a different perspective of the issue?

Adapted from Schneider Z & Whitehead D, 2013 Nursing & midwifery research, 4th edn. Elsevier, Sydney

Box 6.2 Critical review of qualitative studies

Article details	Record the author name(s), publication date, article title and journal details. Is the article published in a scholarly journal and has it been through a peer review process? Is the title consistent with the stated aim of the study? Is the abstract a succinct summary of the study, its findings and recommendations?
Aim of the study	What is the purpose of the study? What is the issue or phenomenon under investigation?
Method	Does the literature review demonstrate a need for the study? Has relevant literature been consulted? What is the study design? Is it appropriate for the issue under investigation? Is the data collection process, including participant recruitment, ethics and method (e.g. focus group), clearly described? Is the theoretical framework and the process used for data analysis clearly described? Is the data analysis method appropriate for the question/issue under investigation?
Findings	Is the phenomenon sufficiently identified? Have the findings been interpreted in relation to the research question and aims? Is a new theory developed or are the findings related to existing theory?
Significance of findings	What is the significance of the findings? Why are they important? To whom are they important? What are the implications of the findings for clinical practice? What are the implications of the findings for further research?
Limitations/ rigour	Are the limitations of the study reported? Can the findings be generalised, or are they limited to the population studied? Is there a conflict of interest (e.g. a power relationship between participants and the interviewer)? Is sufficient detail provided to allow replication of the study?

Cont... ▶

Conclusion	Can the conclusion logically be drawn from the data analysis?
	Is the conclusion related to the findings and the stated aim of the study?
	Do the recommendations regarding clinical practice or future research logically follow from the analysis of the findings?
	Did the study provide new insights or a different perspective of the issue?

Research focus

Cox, J., De, P., Morissette, C., et al., 2008. Low perceived benefits and self-efficacy are associated with hepatitis C virus (HCV) infection-related risk among injection drug users. Social Science and Medicine 66, 211–230.

ABSTRACT

Hepatitis C prevention counselling and education are intended to increase knowledge of the disease, clarify perceptions about vulnerability to infection and increase personal capacity for undertaking safer behaviours. This study examined the association of sharing drug equipment against psychosocial constructs of the AIDS risk reduction model, specifically, knowledge and perceptions related to hepatitis C virus (HCV) among injection drug users (IDUs). Active IDUs were recruited between April 2004 and January 2005 from syringe exchange and methadone maintenance treatment programs in Montreal, Canada. A structured interviewer-administered questionnaire elicited information on: drug preparation and injection practices; self-reported hepatitis C testing and infection status; and AIDS risk reduction model constructs.

Separate logistic regression models were developed to examine variables in relation to sharing syringes and sharing drug preparation equipment (drug containers, filters and water). Among the 321 participants, the mean age was 33 years, 70% were male, 80% were single and 91% self-identified as Caucasian. In the multivariable analyses, psychosocial factors linked to syringe sharing were lower perceived benefits of safer injecting and greater difficulty to inject safely. As with syringe sharing, sharing drug preparation equipment was associated with lower perceived benefits of safer injecting but also with low self-efficacy to convince others to inject more safely. Interventions should aim to heighten awareness of the benefits of risk reduction and provide IDUs with the skills necessary to negotiate safer injecting with their peers.

Cont... ▶

Classroom activity

In small groups:

1. Obtain the complete article from the Science Direct database for Cox et al's study and assess it using the critical review of quantitative studies guidelines in Box 6.1.
2. Alternatively, find another peer-reviewed article that reports on a quantitative study and assess it using the critical review of quantitative studies guidelines in Box 6.1.

Research focus

Ranse, J., Arbon, P., 2008. Graduate nurses' lived experience of in-hospital resuscitation: a hermeneutic phenomenological approach. Australian Critical Care 21, 38–47.

ABSTRACT

Aim

The purpose of this research was to explore, describe and interpret the lived experience of graduate [junior] registered nurses who have participated in an in-hospital resuscitation event within the non-critical care environment.

Method

Using a hermeneutic phenomenological design, a convenience sample was recruited from a population of graduate registered nurses with less than 12 months' experience. Focus groups were employed as a means of data collection. Thematic analysis of the focus group narrative was undertaken using a well-established human science approach.

Findings

Responses from participants were analysed and grouped into four main themes: needing to decide, having to act, feeling connected and being supported. The findings illustrate a decision-making process resulting in participants seeking assistance from a medical emergency team based on previous experience, education and the perceived needs of the patient. Following this decision, participants are indecisive, questioning their decision. Participants view themselves as learners of the resuscitation process, being educationally prepared to undertake basic life support but not prepared for roles in a resuscitation event expected of the registered nurse, such as scribe. With minimal direction participants identified, implemented and evaluated their own coping strategies. Participants desire an environment that promotes a team approach, fostering involvement in the ongoing management of the patient within a 'safe zone'.

Cont... ▶

Conclusion

Similarities are identifiable between the graduate nurses' experience and the experience of bystanders and other health professional cohorts such as: the chaotic resuscitation environment; having too many or not enough participants involved in a resuscitation event; being publicly tested; having a decreased physical and emotional reaction with increased resuscitation exposure; and having a lack of an opportunity to participate in debriefing sessions. Strategies should be implemented to provide non-critical care nurses with the confidence and competence to remain involved in the resuscitation process: first, to provide support for less experienced staff; and second, to participate in the ongoing management of the patient. Additionally, the need for education to be contextualised and mimic the realities of a resuscitation event was emphasised.

Classroom activity

In small groups:

1. Obtain the complete article from the Science Direct database for Ranse and Arbon's study and assess it using the critical review of qualitative studies guidelines in Box 6.2.

2. Alternatively, find another peer-reviewed article that reports on a qualitative study and assess it using the critical review of qualitative studies guidelines in Box 6.2.

Evidence-based healthcare practice

Evidence-based healthcare practice is premised on the notion that every clinical intervention needs to be supported by findings from contemporary research. In theory this means that health professionals will utilise effective practices, question practices that lack supporting evidence and cease practices that are harmful (Greenhalgh 2010). Such evidence needs to be both quantitative and qualitative because results, for example from RCTs alone, are not sufficient to change practice (Britten 2010, Zayas et al 2011).

Health professionals whose practice is underpinned by an evidence base, therefore, are able to articulate the rationale and refer to the research findings that support particular interventions and keep themselves up to date by regularly accessing the relevant quality literature in their area of practice or speciality. Importantly, practitioners will possess the skills to evaluate research findings and, where relevant, translate these into new practices, or cease existing practices that are not supported by contemporary evidence. Nevertheless, despite the rhetoric surrounding evidence-based best practice, barriers exist that prevent the transfer of identified best practice guidelines into everyday clinical care. Such barriers include resistance from health professionals as well as structural barriers within organisations (Avorn & Fischer 2010, Morrison et al 2012).

Research conducted by Forsner et al (2010) examining the barriers and facilitators to implementing clinical guidelines in psychiatry found there were three categories of barriers and facilitators to implementing clinical practice change: organisational resources; health professionals' individual characteristics; and perceptions of guidelines and implementation strategies. The researchers also found differences between the practitioners in the implementation team and the staff at the clinics, including: concern about control over clinical practice; beliefs about evidence-based practice; and suspicions about financial motives for introducing the guidelines. The researchers concluded that the adoption of new guidelines could be improved if staff at the local level were able to actively participate in the implementation process, and if the identified barriers were addressed at an organisational and individual level.

Earlier research by Grohl and Wensing (2004) examined the implementation of guidelines for diabetes care and found there were three categories of barriers to implementing clinical practice change, namely: individual, social and organisational/economic.

Individual factors included:

- *cognitive* – decision-making processes and risk–benefit analysis
- *educational* – learning styles
- *attitudinal* – perceived behavioural control, self-efficacy
- *motivational* – the individual's motivational stages and barriers.

Social factors included:

- *social learning* – role models
- *social network and influence* – values and culture
- *patient influence* – patient expectations and behaviour
- *leadership* – style, power and the leader's commitment.

Organisational and economic factors included:

- *innovativeness of the organisation* – specialisation, decentralisation and professionalism
- *quality management* – culture and leadership
- *complexity* – interaction between system parts
- *organisational learning* – capacity and arrangements for ongoing learning
- *economic* – rewards and incentives for change or maintaining the status quo.

The authors concluded that while the research identifies a range of factors that pose barriers to clinical practice change, the findings do not specify which of the factors are the most influential, nor in which circumstances they might have the most influence. Regardless, the findings are important because they highlight the complexity involved in bringing about change in clinical practice – even when there is evidence to support the change. Additionally, the findings identify areas for future research to explore these contributing factors further.

In summary, research provides the evidence on which best practice can be based. However, while health professionals are responsible for ensuring their practice is based on the available evidence, the responsibility for this does not rest with individual health professionals alone because the transfer of the research findings into clinical practice change is complex, political and influenced by social and organisational factors. Evidence-based practice, therefore, is not and cannot be merely an individual health professional's responsibility.

Research ethics in healthcare practice

Throughout the world any research conducted on humans must conform to ethical codes or guidelines. The primary ethical consideration of any research involving humans is that of beneficence, or the principle that on balance the potential good resulting from research participation must outweigh the potential harm.

Ethical codes and guidelines are intended to protect the rights of vulnerable people. The first code of medical ethics, the Nuremburg code, was developed subsequent to the Nuremburg Tribunal that investigated the human rights violations of the medical experiments carried out by doctors in Germany during the Second World War. In 1949 the World Medical Association released an international code of medical ethics, based on the Nuremburg code, which became known as the *Declaration of Helsinki*. The Helsinki declaration is a statement of ethical principles that provides guidance to physicians and other participants in medical research involving human subjects (World Medical Association 2008) and is the foundation on which worldwide codes of health research ethics are based.

AUSTRALIAN AND NEW ZEALAND CODES OF ETHICS

In Australia the body that oversees the ethical conduct of research involving human subjects is the National Health and Medical Research Council (NHMRC) and in New Zealand it is the Health Research Council (HRC). Both councils have developed guidelines for the ethical conduct of research involving human subjects, namely the NHMRC *National Statement on Ethical Conduct in Human Research* (NHMRC et al 2009) in Australia, and HRC *Guidelines on ethics in health research* (2005) in New Zealand.

In 2007 (and updated in 2009) the NHMRC, Australian Research Council (ARC) and the Australian Vice-Chancellors' Committee (AVCC) released the *National Statement on Ethical Conduct in Human Research*, which contains Australia's primary guidelines for ethically conducting research involving human participants. The purpose of the statement is to: promote ethical human research; ensure that participants are accorded respect and protection; and foster research that benefits the community. The statement is based on four values that the design and conduct of all research involving human participants must follow. The central theme of these values is respect for all human beings and beneficence is the value that underpins the other three. The values are:

- respect for human beings
- research merit and integrity
- justice
- beneficence (NHMRC/ARC 2009).

RESEARCH WITH INDIGENOUS PEOPLE

Following a history of colonisation and injustice Indigenous people are sensitive to the ethics of health research (Baum 2008 p 154). Hence further issues need to be considered for research that includes Indigenous people. Therefore, in addition to heeding the ethical principles outlined in the *Guidelines on ethics in health research*, New Zealand researchers, for example, must also take into consideration additional issues for Māori developed by the HRC (2010). The council directs that all research proposals involving Māori must observe the principles of the Treaty of Waitangi and incorporate this in the proceedings and processes of ethics committees; particularly relevant are the principles of:

- **partnership** – working together with *iwi, hapu, whanau* and Māori communities to ensure Māori individual and collective rights are respected and protected

- **participation** – involving Māori in the design, governance, management, implementation and analysis of research, especially research involving Māori

- **protection** – actively protecting Māori individual and collective rights, Māori data, Māori culture, cultural concepts, values, norms, practices and language in the research process (HRC 2010).

Australia, too, has developed guidelines for research with Indigenous people. In collaboration with the NHMRC the National Aboriginal and Islander Health Organisation developed guidelines for research in Indigenous communities. Key principles of the guidelines include:

- **community engagement** – consultation and negotiation with Aboriginal and Torres Strait Islander people and involvement of community members in the research

- **benefit** – the potential health benefit for Aboriginal and Torres Strait Islander people is evident in the research proposal

- **sustainability and transferability** – how the result of the research can lead to achievable and effective health gains for Aboriginal people, beyond the research project is demonstrated in the proposal

- **building capacity** – how Aboriginal communities, researchers and others will develop relevant capabilities and retain ownership of data and publication is demonstrated

- **priority** – the research and potential outcomes are a priority for Aboriginal communities

- **significance** – the research addresses important public health issues for Aboriginal people and takes account of the history of Indigenous colonisation, Indigenous values and respect for culture (NHMRC/ARC 2003, 2010).

HEALTH PROFESSIONALS AS PATIENT ADVOCATES

As well as conducting research, health professionals also engage in health research either as participants or because the patients they care for are participants. Consequently, it is crucial that health professionals are aware of the 'rights' of research participants, including themselves (Schneider et al 2013 p 95).

With regard to caring for patients who are research participants, a health professional's role includes: ensuring: the patient fully understands what they are consenting to (informed consent); that the rule of beneficence applies; that the patient's anonymity, privacy and dignity is respected; and that the patient is aware that they can withdraw from the research at any time. At times this may involve acting as an advocate for the patient such as providing additional information to the patient or explaining the patient's right to not participate in the research should they not want to.

Extreme examples of the need to advocate on behalf of patients include the 1980s RCT of cervical cancer, conducted at the National Women's Hospital in Auckland, New Zealand, in which conventional cancer treatment was withheld from some participants in the study without their consent (Paul 1988, Skegg 2011) and the United States army-sponsored AIDS research in Thailand in the 1990s that tracked the natural course of vertical transmission of HIV in children born to sero-positive mothers. The infants were not given the antiretroviral drug (ARV) zidovudine (AZT) despite the drug being proven to be effective in reducing vertical HIV transmission in American and French studies. Thirty-seven children in the Thai study contracted the HIV virus (Hassani 2005, Robb et al 1998). Similar controversy surrounded trials of AZT in Africa in the 1990s, in which control groups were given a placebo, despite the results of other trials that convincingly demonstrated the effectiveness of ARV drug treatment, thereby making a control group unethical (Brewster 2011). Haire (2011) further argues that the debate that ensued following the exposure of the ARV trials in developing countries was important because it highlighted the need for health equity and access to care to redress health disparities. Researchers, she argues, have a duty of care and a moral responsibility to ensure that treatments for the diseases under investigation must be made available to the populations participating in the study, regardless of where they live.

In summary, codes of ethics and ethical research guidelines serve the purpose of protecting participants in health research. It is the responsibility of health professionals to ensure these principles are adhered to and to take action on behalf of themselves or the patient in their care should the health professional become aware that this is not the case.

Classroom activity

In United States army research, reported by Robb et al (1998) and Praphan (1998), the researchers argued that AZT was not deemed standard treatment in Thailand for individuals at risk of contracting HIV (although it was at that time in Western countries) therefore it was not unethical to withhold the drug from infants born to HIV-positive mothers. Brewster (2010), reporting on African ARV trials, disagrees and argues that once an intervention is proven to be effective it is unethical to include a placebo group in drug trials.

Debate the ethics of researchers withholding a known effective treatment because it is not a standard treatment in the country where the research is conducted.

Cont... ▶

Do you agree or disagree with Haire's view that researchers have a duty of care and a moral responsibility to provide treatment for the disease under investigation to participants of the study, regardless of where they live, or the cost of the treatment (Haire 2011)?

- Explain your reasons for this view.

Research focus

Aldridge, J., Charles, V., 2008. Researching the intoxicated: informed consent implications for alcohol and drug research. Drug and Alcohol Dependence 93, 191–196.

ABSTRACT

This article considers the informed consent process in relation to carrying out research with intoxicated participants in 'field' research settings. There is little discussion in the literature of the potential problems that the intoxication of research participants may pose to research. Intoxication is a potential problem for all researchers but is heightened in field research that takes place in settings where participants are likely to be intoxicated, such as licensed venues, in drug consumption rooms or police custody suites. The risks to research participants that intoxication poses should not be resolved by electing not to do research with intoxicated participants; it is argued that these risks can be managed to some extent and are offset by the benefits of such research. Moreover, intoxication (and the impairment of cognitive functions relevant to valid informed consent) may not always be identifiable through behavioural or biochemical methods of detection. The search for accurate and field-practical methods for identifying intoxication among participants is useful but not the only strategy for researchers who want to ensure the validity of the consent process. Suggestions are provided for devising research protocols that acknowledge and accept intoxication of research participants and attempt to protect them. One solution is to sidestep identification of intoxication per se as a strategic objective in the consent process and turn instead to established methods for ensuring that information has been understood by potential research participants.

Critical thinking

What is your view of the recommendation made by Aldridge and Charles (2008) to ensure that information has been understood by potential research participants and to sidestep identification of intoxication per se as a strategic objective in the consent process when obtaining informed consent from intoxicated people?

Cont... ▶

- Identify the ethical issues in this recommendation.
- Can an intoxicated person give informed consent?
- If yes, in what circumstances?
- If no, what are the implications for research involving intoxicated people?

Conclusion

In this chapter, the two major research paradigms – quantitative and qualitative – were presented. Differences and similarities of the two approaches were highlighted and the conclusion drawn that the selection of a particular research paradigm is influenced not by the intrinsic merits of either a positivist or a critical approach but by the question under investigation and the best way to seek an answer to the question.

The importance of research in the everyday practice of psychologists and health professionals was emphasised, including the notion that research provides the evidence on which all healthcare practice is based. The complexities of translating research findings into practice were recognised and the role of health professionals as consumers of research was emphasised. Finally, the important role played by health professionals in the ethical conduct of research was highlighted.

REMEMBER

- Research is fundamental to the clinical practice of psychologists and health professionals because it provides the evidence on which healthcare practice is based.
- Skills as a research consumer are essential in healthcare practice.
- Research findings can identify healthcare practices that are effective and efficient, thereby identifying 'best practice'.
- Research findings can identify healthcare practices that are not effective or efficient and thereby provides evidence to facilitate change.
- Health professionals play a key role in the ethical conduct of research.

Further resources

Bragge, P., 2010. Asking good clinical research questions and choosing the right study design. Injury, International Journal Care of Injured 41S, S3–S6.

Brewster, D., 2011. Science and ethics of human immunodeficiency virus/acquired immunodeficiency syndrome controversies in Africa. Journal of Paediatrics and Child Health 47, 646–655.

Ministry of Health, 2006. Operational standard for ethics committees: updated edition. NZ Ministry of Health, Wellington.

National Health and Medical Research Council, Australian Research Council & Australian Vice-Chancellors' Committee, 2007. National Statement on Ethical Conduct in Human Research. NHMRC, AVCC and ARC, Canberra.

Schneider, Z., Whitehead, D., LoBondio-Wood, G., et al 2013. Nursing and midwifery research: methods and appraisals for evidence based practice, fourth ed. Elsevier, Sydney.

Weblinks

Cochrane Library

http://www3.interscience.wiley.com/cgi-bin/mrwhome/106568753/HOME

The Cochrane Library contains high-quality, independent evidence that can inform healthcare decision making. It includes reliable evidence from Cochrane and other systematic reviews, clinical trials and more. It includes the combined results of the world's best medical research studies, which are recognised as the gold standard in evidence-based healthcare.

Health Services Consumer Research

www.hscr.co.nz

The HSCR website provides accurate, reliable and insightful information on consumers and providers of healthcare services in New Zealand to help monitor and improve healthcare service delivery.

Joanna Briggs Institute

www.joannabriggs.edu.au

The Joanna Briggs Institute is an international not-for-profit research and development organisation specialising in evidence-based resources for health professionals in nursing, midwifery, medicine and allied health. The institute is a recognised global leader in evidence-based healthcare.

National Health and Medical Research Council

www.nhmrc.gov.au

The NHMRC is Australia's peak body for health and medical research, health advice and for ethics in healthcare and in health and medical research.

New Zealand Health Research Council/Te Kaunihera Rangahau Hauora o Aotearoa

www.hrc.govt.nz

This is the New Zealand Government's main funding agency for health research. Its mission is to benefit New Zealand through health research, with the goal of improving health for all.

Science Direct

www.sciencedirect.com

Science Direct is operated by the publisher Elsevier. It is one of the world's largest collections of published scientific research, including health and social sciences.

References

Aldridge, J., Charles, V., 2008. Researching the intoxicated: informed consent implications for alcohol and drug research. Drug and Alcohol Dependence 93, 191–196.

Aspers, P., 2010. Empirical phenomenology: a qualitative research approach (The Cologne Seminars). The Indo-Pacific Journal of Phenomenology 9 (2), 1–12.

Avorn, J., Fischer, M., 2010. Bench to behaviour: translating comparative effectiveness research into improved clinical practice. Health Affairs: At the intersection of health, health care and policy 29 (10), 1891–1900.

Bahora, M., Sterk, C., Elifson, K., 2009. Understanding recreational ecstasy use in the United States: a qualitative inquiry. International Journal of Drug Policy 20 (1), 62–69.

Barlow, J., Powell, L., Gilchrist, M., et al., 2008. The effectiveness of the training and support program for parents of children with disabilities: a randomized controlled trial. Journal of Psychosomatic Research 64, 55–62.

Baum, F., 2008. The new public health. Oxford University Press, Australia.

Beard, R., Fox, P., 2008. Resisting social disenfranchisement: negotiating collective identities and everyday life with memory loss. Social Science and Medicine 66, 1509–1520.

Bragge, P., 2010. Asking good clinical research questions and choosing the right study design. Injury, International Journal Care of Injured 41 (Suppl 1), 3–6.

Brewster, D., 2011. Science and ethics of human immunodeficiency virus/acquired immunodeficiency syndrome controversies in Africa. Journal of Paediatrics and Child Health 47, 646–655.

Britten, N., 2010. Qualitative research and the take-up of evidence-based practice. Journal of Research in Nursing 15 (6), 537–544.

Cochrane Collaboration, 2011. Cochrane Handbook for systematic reviews of interventions. Online. Available: www.cochrane-handbook.org 19 Sep 2012.

Cox, J., De, P., Morissette, C., et al., 2008. Low perceived benefits and self-efficacy are associated with hepatitis C virus (HCV) infection-related risk among injection drug users. Social Science and Medicine 66, 211–230.

Crotty, M., 1996. Phenomenology and nursing research. Churchill Livingstone, Melbourne.

Denzin, N., 2009. The research act: a theoretical introduction to sociological methods. Transaction Publishers, New Jersey.

Dowling, M., 2007. From Husserl to van Manen. A review of different phenomenological approaches. International Journal of Nursing Studies 44, 121–142.

Finlay, L., 2010. Debating phenomenological research methods. Phenomenology and Practice 3 (1), 6–25.

Flood, A., 2010. Understanding phenomenology. Nurse Researcher 17 (2), 7–25.

Forsner, T., Hansson, J., Brommels, M., et al., 2010. Implementing clinical guidelines in psychiatry: a qualitative study of perceived facilitators and barriers. BMC Psychiatry 10 (8), 1–20.

Greenhalgh, T., 2010. How to read a paper: the basics of evidence-based medicine. Wiley-Blackwell, Chichester.

Grohl, R., Wensing, M., 2004. What drives change? Barriers to and incentives for achieving evidence-based practice. Medical Journal of Australia Supplement 180, 57–60.

Hagger, M., 2012. What makes a 'good' review article? Some reflections and recommendations. Health Psychology Review 6 (2), 141–146.

Haire, B., 2011. Because we can: clashes of perspective over researcher obligations in the failed PrEP trials. Developing World Bioethics 11 (2), 63–74.

Hassani, B., 2005. Trials by fire: the case of unethical clinical trials in the countries of the south. University of Toronto Medical Journal 82 (3), 212–216.

Health Research Council of New Zealand (HRC), 2005. Guidelines on ethics in health research. HRC, Auckland.

Health Research Council of New Zealand (HRC), 2010. Guidelines for researchers on health research involving Māori. HRC, Auckland.

Howe, K., 2012. Mixed methods, triangulation and causal explanations. Journal of Mixed Methods Research. Sage, Thousand Oaks, pp. 1–8.

Karlsson, A., Arman, M., Wikblad, K., 2008. Teenagers with type 1 diabetes – a phenomenological study of the transition towards autonomy in self-management. International Journal of Nursing Studies 45, 562–570.

Larun, L., Malterud, K., 2007. Identity and coping experiences in chronic fatigue syndrome: a synthesis of qualitative studies. Patient Education and Counseling 69, 20–28.

Morrison, V., Bennett, P., Butow, P., et al., 2012. Introduction to health psychology in Australia, second edn. Pearson Education, Sydney.

National Health and Medical Research Council, Australian Research Council & Australian Vice-Chancellors' Committee, 2009. National Statement on Ethical Conduct in Human Research, 2007. (updated 2009). NHMRC, AVCC & ARC, Canberra.

National Health and Medical Research Council, Australian Research Council (NHMRC/ARC), 2003. Values and ethics – guidelines for the ethical conduct in Aboriginal and Torres Strait Islander research. NHMRC, Canberra.

National Health and Medical Research Council, Australian Research Council (NHMRC/ARC), 2010. Criteria for health and medical research of Indigenous Australians. NHMRC, Canberra. Online, Available: http://www.nhmrc.gov.au/your-health/indigenous-health 19 Sep 2012.

Paley, J., 2005. Phenomenology as rhetoric. Nursing Inquiry 12 (2), 106–116.

Paul, C., 1988. The New Zealand Cervical Cancer Study: could it happen again? British Medical Journal 297 (6647), 533–539.

Praphan, P., 1998. Ethical issues in studies in Thailand of the vertical transmission of HIV. The New England Journal of Medicine 338 (12), 834–835.

Ranse, J., Arbon, P., 2008. Graduate nurses' lived experience of in-hospital resuscitation: a hermeneutic phenomenological approach. Australian Critical Care 21, 38–47.

Robb, M., Khambaroong, C., Nelson, K., 1998. Studies in Thailand of the vertical transmission of HIV. New England Journal of Medicine 338 (12), 843–844.

Schneider, Z., Whitehead, D., LoBondio-Wood, G., et al 2013. Nursing and midwifery research: methods and appraisals for evidence based practice, fourth ed. Elsevier, Sydney.

Skegg, P., 2011. A fortunate experiment? New Zealand's experience with a legislated code of rights. Medicine and Law Review 19, (Spring), 235–266.

Swanwick, T., 2010. Quantitative research methods in medical education, Ch 21. In: Norman, G., Eva, K. (Eds.), Understanding medical education: Evidence, theory and practice. Wiley Online Library. Online. Available: http://onlinelibrary.wiley.com/doi/10.1002/9781444320282.ch21/summary 19 Sep 2012.

Torrance, H., 2012. Triangulation, respondent validation, and democratic participation in mixed methods research. Journal of Mixed Methods Research. Sage, Thousand Oaks, pp. 1–23.

World Medical Association, 2008. World Medical Association Declaration of Helsinki: ethical principles for medical research involving human subjects. Online. Available: http://www.wma.net/en/30publications/10policies/b3/ 19 Sep 2012.

Zayas, L., Drake, B., Jonson-Reid, J., 2011. Overrating or dismissing the value of evidence-based practice: consequences for clinical practice. Clinical Social Work 39, 400–405.

Chapter 7
Behaviour change

PATRICIA BARKWAY

Learning objectives

The material in this chapter will help you to:

- describe and understand the dominant psychological approaches that aim to explain health behaviours, namely
  » behavioural/learning theory
  » cognitive theory
  » the health belief model
  » the theory of planned behaviour
  » the transtheoretical model of behaviour change
  » motivational interviewing
  » the health action process approach
- utilise the above theories and models to explain the initiation and the continuation of health-enhancing and health 'risk' behaviours
- utilise the above theories and models to modify health behaviours
- identify the limitations of psychological theories and models as predictors and moderators of health behaviours.

Key terms
- Behavioural/learning theories
- Cognitive theories
- Health belief model
- Theory of planned behaviour
- Transtheoretical model of behaviour change
- Health action process approach
- Motivational interviewing

Introduction

How healthy is your lifestyle? Do you regularly follow the health practices identified in Chapter 4 regarding nutrition, physical activity, cigarette smoking and alcohol consumption? Have you ever made a decision regarding one of these health behaviours but not continued with the activity as you intended, for example, to exercise regularly? Or perhaps you did follow through with your intention and maintained the activity. Why might there be different outcomes to these scenarios when your intention was the same in both? What other factors might influence the outcomes in these two scenarios?

Such questions underpin psychological health research and contribute to the development of theories and models that can explain and predict an individual's health-related behaviours. Additionally, psychological theories propose models of behaviour change and identify interventions that can change unhealthy behaviours. This chapter will examine a range of psychological approaches that propose explanations as to how internal (within the person) and external (within the environment) factors influence an individual's health behaviours and lifestyle.

Health-enhancing behaviours: what are they?

Health behaviours are actions that enhance, maintain or threaten an individual's health. They are activities that an individual practices or abstains from in order to maintain health or to reduce the risk of illness or accident. Health behaviours can be either positive or negative and include such practices as: following a healthy diet and eating in moderation; not driving a car while under the influence of alcohol or drugs; keeping immunisations up to date; and regular health screening such as for dental health and breast or prostate cancer. When practised regularly (such as daily teeth brushing) a health behaviour is called a health *habit*, while clusters of health behaviours are referred to as *lifestyle*.

Health-enhancing behaviours: why focus on them?

Up until the mid-20th century global public health threats were mainly from infectious and communicable diseases. However, in developed countries, a shift occurred over the past one hundred years whereby the major health threats are now posed by diseases in which lifestyle plays a role in the aetiology and/or management of illness (Frieden 2010). For example, the modifiable risk factors for coronary heart disease, a leading cause of disease burden, are tobacco smoking, high blood pressure, high cholesterol level, insufficient physical activity, overweight/obesity, poor nutrition and diabetes (AIHW 2010), all of which are linked to health behaviours and lifestyle.

Disease burden is measured by disability adjusted life years (DALYs), which comprises years of life lost (YLLs) (mortality) and years lived with disability (YLDs) (morbidity). In Australia, New Zealand and other Western nations the health conditions with the greatest disease burden (measured by DALYs and YLDs) are cancers, cardiovascular diseases, mental illness, injuries, chronic respiratory disease and diabetes (AIHW 2010). Each of these conditions, at least in part, can be attributed to lifestyle and the course of the conditions can be moderated by health behavioural practices. Hence, there is intuitive appeal in encouraging people to lead a healthy lifestyle to thereby reduce their disease risk and to improve quality of life for people with chronic health conditions. There is also abundant research evidence about the relationship between health behaviours and health from research evidence to support lifestyle interventions (Chiu et al 2011, Cox et al 2008, Harvey et al 2008).

From the individual's perspective the reasons to change health behaviours include prevention (to avoid the risk of a health problem), management (treatment of an identified health problem) recovery (living well with an ongoing health problem) and for general wellbeing. From the health professionals' and health services' perspectives additional motives include reducing the incidence and burden of the health issue in the community and the best utilisation of resources.

Critical thinking

- What factors do you think influence an individual to engage in a healthy or unhealthy lifestyle?
- Does an individual choose his/her lifestyle? Explain your answer.
- Is willpower alone sufficient to ensure an individual will cease a harmful behaviour or commence a positive one? Explain your answer.
- Is knowledge alone sufficient to ensure that an individual will cease a harmful behaviour or commence a positive one? Explain your answer.

Health psychology: theories and models

Health psychology is interested in factors that influence the initiation, continuation, cessation and modification of behaviours that impact on health and health outcomes. To this end psychological theories propose hypotheses to explain and predict behaviour, while models (which are derived from theories) detail the processes and stages of how the behaviour under observation is enacted. In addition to observable behaviours the health beliefs held by individuals and the impact these beliefs have on their health-related behaviours are investigated. Finally, health psychology is interested in finding effective strategies to help people to overcome resistance to change their behaviour and prevent relapse.

Psychological theories and models of health behaviour attempt to explain or predict an individual's engagement in behaviours that influence the risk for illness or injury and the maintenance of health. Psychological theories of health behaviour fall into two broad categories: behavioural/learning theories and cognitive theories. Behavioural/learning approaches include operant conditioning, classical conditioning and modelling or imitation (see below and Ch 1). Cognitive approaches include the health belief model, the transtheoretical model of behaviour change and motivational interviewing. The theory of planned behaviour introduces social influences to a cognitive model as does the health action process approach. These behavioural and cognitive approaches to behaviour change will now be examined.

Learning theories

Learning (also called behavioural) theories propose that personality is determined by prior learning, that human behaviour is changeable throughout the lifespan and that changes in behaviour are generally caused by changes in the environment. They are concerned only with behaviour that is observable, and not mental or affective processes. Specifically, learning theories focus on the conditions that produce behaviour, factors that reinforce behaviour and vicarious learning through watching and imitating the behaviour of others. The three main learning approaches are:

- *classical conditioning* – learning by association
- *operant conditioning* – learning by reinforcement
- *social learning theory* – vicarious learning (modelling/observation and copying).

CLASSICAL CONDITIONING

As outlined in Chapter 1, classical conditioning was first described by the Russian physiologist Ivan Pavlov who observed the relationship between stimulus and response through demonstrating that a dog could be conditioned to salivate (respond) to a non-food stimulus (a bell) (Pavlov 1927). For example, a patient may be receiving intravenous chemotherapy for cancer, which has the side effect of nausea. Over time the patient may experience nausea when the chemotherapy nurse enters the room, and before the injection is given. The feeling of nausea when the nurse is present has been learned through classical conditioning.

OPERANT CONDITIONING

B F Skinner formulated the notion of instrumental or operant conditioning in which reinforcers (rewards) contribute to the probability of a response being either repeated or extinguished. Skinner's research demonstrated that the contingencies on which behaviour is based are external to the person, rather than internal. Consequently, changing contingencies could alter an individual's behaviour (Skinner 1953). For example, if a child throws a tantrum when told it is bedtime, and the parent relents and allows the child to stay up later, the child learns that they can get what they want by throwing a tantrum. To reverse this behaviour the parent would need to ignore the child's tantrum and firmly insist that it is bedtime.

OBSERVATIONAL LEARNING THEORY

Observational learning theory (also called modelling or social learning theory) was proposed by Bandura (1969, 2006) who asserts that observational learning has a more significant influence on how humans learn than intrapsychic (psychoanalytic) or environmental (behavioural/learning) forces alone. Bandura proposed that human behaviour results from the interaction between the environment and the person's thinking and perceptions. He also asserted that humans can learn from observing – not just by doing. Observational learning differs from operant conditioning in that it is not the learner who is rewarded for the behaviour; rather, the learner observes the other person being rewarded and learns vicariously through this. New behaviours are acquired by observing others being rewarded for performing a behaviour, and then imitating that behaviour.

Observational learning is particularly important for children's learning because it is easier to influence a behaviour while it is being acquired rather than changing an established behaviour. Hence parents, family and schooling play a significant role in the health habits that children acquire. These habits can be both positive health behaviours, such as participating in sport and cleaning their teeth, or negative practices such as tobacco smoking. For example, in a 12-month study of 1237 seventh and eighth grade students in Germany, Krahé and Möller (2010) found that watching violent media was predictive of aggressive behaviour.

LEARNING THEORY APPROACHES

Have you ever received a parking fine, a speeding ticket, lost your driver's licence, been locked out of a concert until interval because you arrived late or been refused borrowing rights at your library until you paid your fine for late returns? Do you feel motivated after your boss tells you that he is impressed with your work or smile back at someone who has just smiled at you? Most of us, without realising it and without being able to use the technical terminology of behavioural change programs, actually practise behaviour modification in our everyday lives and have it practised on us. In your various roles as citizens, partners, parents, friends and health professionals, you will, by the end of this chapter, be surprised to discover how much of your own behaviour is governed by the fundamental principles of learning theory, on which behavioural change programs are based, and how much of the behaviour of those around you is at least partly determined by your own behavioural change strategies.

BEHAVIOURAL CHANGE PROGRAMS

Behavioural change programs aim to change behaviour, not attitudes, beliefs, motivation, personality or other unobserved characteristics of individuals. Behaviour may be defined as anything that a person does or says; that is, behaviour is any action or response to an environmental event that is observable and measurable. Behaviours can be overt (readily observed and counted) or covert (not readily observed but can still be counted and changed, such as thoughts and feelings using the principles described in this chapter). Regardless of the orientation of specific programs, all behavioural change programs operate on the following four tenets:

- Behaviour can be explained by the principles of learning and conditioning.
- The same laws of learning apply to all behaviour, both normal and abnormal.
- Abnormal behaviour is the normal response to abnormal learning conditions.
- Behaviour can be 'unlearned' and changed.

These four tenets underpin the four major theoretical models that have been derived from learning theory, namely, classical conditioning, operant conditioning, observational (imitation) learning and cognitive behaviourism (Beck 1976, Ellis 1984, Meichenbaum 1974).

Historically, behaviour therapy referred to the techniques based on classical conditioning, devised by Wolpe (1958) and Eysenck (1960) to treat anxiety; behaviour modification was used to describe programs based on the principles of operant conditioning devised by Skinner (1953) to create new behaviours in children who had an intellectual disability and patients experiencing psychotic symptoms.

In current practice, the terms behaviour therapy, behavioural change programs and behaviour modification are used interchangeably to describe therapeutic programs based on the principles of behavioural/learning theory. The term 'behavioural change program' will be used in this chapter. The following outlines the principles a clinical psychologist would use when designing a behavioural program.

Functional analysis of behaviour

The principles of operant conditioning (learning by reinforcement) describe the relationship between behaviour and environmental events, both antecedents and consequences that influence behaviour. This relationship, referred to as a contingency, consists of three components:

- antecedents (i.e. stimulus events that precede or trigger the target behaviour)
- behaviours (i.e. responses, usually the identified problem behaviour)
- consequences (outcomes of the behaviour, i.e. what actually happened immediately after the problem behaviour occurred).

Specifying these contingencies forms the basis of a functional analysis of behaviour. The aim of a functional analysis is to identify factors that influence the occurrence and maintenance of a particular (problem or desired) response. This process should not be confused with other explanatory models that may seek to explain behaviour in terms of a medical diagnosis or a personality trait. Behavioural change programs are more concerned with the nature of our interactions with the environment than with our nature per se.

Conducting a functional analysis of behaviour is the first step in designing a behavioural change program. It consists of the three components outlined below.

1. Selecting the target behaviour

The target behaviour must be specified in such a way that it can be readily observed and measured. The behaviour of interest may be a behavioural excess (e.g. tantrums, exceeding the speed limit, driving while intoxicated) or a behavioural deficit (e.g. an eight-year-old who cannot tie his shoelaces, an adult who does not complete recommended physiotherapy exercises, a well elderly person who does not perform self-care activities). From the examples given, it will be clear that behavioural deficits are of two types: behaviours that exist in the behavioural repertoire of the individual but which the individual does not perform, and behaviours that are not in the behavioural repertoire of the individual and must be developed. It is important to distinguish among these different groups of target behaviours as each requires the application of different behavioural change strategies.

Behaviour must never be viewed in isolation. The behavioural change agent considers the setting in which the behaviour occurs, the nature of the task and the characteristics of the client. Behaviour may be appropriately performed in one setting and not another. For example, it would be appropriate for a three-year-old child who has just learned to take his clothes off to do so in the bathroom in his home, but not in a busy shopping centre. A behavioural change program in this instance would aim to teach the child the appropriate setting for performing this newly acquired behaviour. Behaviour may also be considered problematic due to its rate, duration or intensity rather than the behaviour itself. For example, taking a shower is a common behaviour that may become problematic if the person spends one hour doing so or showers multiple times through the day. In this case, the behavioural change program would aim to reduce the amount of time spent in the shower or the frequency of showers.

2. Identifying current contingencies

This process involves two steps. The first is identifying the stimulus event(s) (i.e. antecedents) that precede(s) an occurrence of the problem behaviour. This includes an assessment of the physical (where the behaviour occurs) and social (who is present) environment in which the behaviour occurs. Certain behaviours will frequently occur at a high rate in one setting and be absent or occur at a low rate in others. For example, parents may complain about their child throwing tantrums and being argumentative at home to the child's teacher, who reports that the child is compliant and polite in the classroom. Alternatively, the teacher may notice that the child stays on task in some subjects and not in others or during the morning session but not during the afternoon. In the hospital setting, two nurses may discover that a particular patient rings the buzzer for nursing assistance twice as often for one nurse compared with another, or that a child with cerebral palsy is more likely to persist with his physiotherapy exercises when his mother is not in the treatment room. These observations provide important information about the stimulus events that may be controlling the target behaviour.

The second step requires identifying the consequences that follow the problem behaviour; that is, what happened after the behaviour was performed? To follow through with our examples above, did the parents respond to the child's tantrum by giving the child what she wanted or did they ignore her tantruming behaviour? Did they engage in a verbal debate with the child when she talked back or did they calmly state their rule that talk backs would not be answered? In an aged care setting two nurses notice that an elderly resident rings the buzzer twice as often for one nurse compared with another—were there any differences in each of the two nurses' responses to the buzzer ringing? A child does not cooperate with physiotherapy exercises when his mother is in the room—what was the mother doing in the treatment room during her child's physiotherapy sessions? Answers to these questions are essential for effective behavioural management to occur.

3. Measuring and recording behaviour

There are five basic methods of measuring behaviour in healthcare settings:

- narrative recording
- counting or frequency data
- timing or duration recording (temporal data)
- checking or interval recording (categorical data)
- rating (magnitude data).

Once you have specified the target behaviour and identified the setting in which this behaviour occurs, it is necessary to obtain a baseline of the frequency or length of its occurrence. The way you measure frequency or length depends on the nature of the target behaviour and what you wish to find out about the behaviour.

Narrative recording

Narrative recording involves the observation and recording of behaviour in progress. It is often used in the early stages of the functional analysis of behaviour as a way of identifying possible antecedents and consequences of a given problem behaviour. Figure 7.1 provides an example of a narrative recording chart, for example, for a child with type 1 diabetes mellitus who refuses to take and record their blood sugar levels while at school.

```
Time, date, year: _____

Child's name: _____

Child's sex: _____ Child's age: _____ School grade: _____

Relevant details e.g. ethnicity, social background: _____

Observer(s): _____

Setting: _____

Description of behaviour: _____

Behavioural consequences: _____

Possible determinates of behaviour: _____
```

Figure 7.1 Narrative recording sheet for assessing a child's problematic behaviour

Counting

Counting is the method of choice if the target behaviour is discrete (i.e. an observer can identify the beginning and end of each instance of behaviour). Behaviours such as head banging, exercising and incontinence are examples of discrete, countable behaviours. Simple tally sheets or frequency counters can be used to record countable behaviours. One can also count the number of tasks completed or the percentage of items correct. These are examples of counts of the product or outcome of behaviour. They do not require continuous observation of the behaviour per se. Figure 7.2 provides an example of a recording chart for counting responses. In this case, the number of times the person awoke in the night is recorded.

Name:............................. Monitored from:.../.../... to.../.../...Behaviour: Awakenings per night		
	Week 1	Week 2
Monday		
Tuesday		
Wednesday		
Thursday		
Friday		
Saturday		
Sunday		

Figure 7.2 Counting chart for (self) monitoring sleep disturbance over a two-week period

Timing (duration)

When a behaviour becomes a problem because of the length of time it takes to complete the task, or when you are interested in increasing the duration of a particular behaviour, you may choose to collect temporal data. Examples of behaviours for which temporal data are appropriate are length of time it takes for a doctor to perform a given task such as a surgical procedure, the length of time it takes for a hospitalised patient to shower in the morning or the amount of time a person spends in the gym practising physiotherapy exercises. Figure 7.3 provides an example of a chart for timing the duration of a target behaviour, in this case performing rehabilitation exercises in the gym over a four-week period.

Exercise record				
Name:				
Date monitoring began:				
Period commencing	Week 1	Week 2	Week 3	Week 4
Monday				
Tuesday				
Wednesday				
Thursday				
Friday				
Saturday				
Sunday				

Figure 7.3 Chart for recording the amount of time spent in the gym over a four-week period

Checking

Checking or interval recording is used when you want to know whether an individual performs a specified task or not. In such cases your code requires a simple yes–no response. By checking on groups of related behaviours, you can quickly build up a picture of the individual's current level of functioning. For example, you may wish to increase the self-care behaviours of a patient with advanced dementia. When he arrives at breakfast each morning, you can check whether he has combed his hair, shaved, dressed in day clothes (as opposed to pyjamas) and is wearing shoes. After you obtain a baseline following several days of checking, you will be ready to design a behavioural change program to address any outstanding deficits in self-care. Figure 7.4 is an example of a checklist, for example, for assessing how well a person with dementia manages their personal hygiene and grooming.

Assessment of self-care behaviour

Name:				
Date:				
Hair neat/ combed				
Clean shaved				
Face clean				
Dressed appropriately				
Clothes clean				
Wearing shoes				
Hands and nails clean				

✓   Satisfactory
X   Not present or unsatisfactory
N/A Not applicable

Figure 7.4 Checklist for assessing self-care behaviour

Rating

Rating is a method of assessing the quality of a response and, as such, requires a subjective judgment on the part of the observer. You may wish to assess the intelligibility of the speech of a person who is dysarthric. One quick measure of intelligibility is to ask the nursing staff and family members to rate the person on a five-point scale ranging from 1 = very difficult to understand to 5 = very easy to understand.

In summary, a functional analysis of behaviour can identify the antecedents (what triggers the behaviour) and the consequences (outcomes of the behaviour). Consider one of your own health behaviours from a behavioural/learning perspective and monitor this for one week using the 'Health behaviour monitoring exercise' in Figure 7.5, then complete the *Classroom activity*.

Health behaviour monitoring exercise

Select one of your health behaviours e.g. eating, drinking alcohol, cigarette smoking, physical activity. Monitor this behaviour for a week and record the following:

Behaviour:

Date	Time	Place	Antecedents ★	Consequences ☐	Reflection/comments

★ **Antecedents:** Where were you? Who else was present? What were your preceding thoughts or feelings? What events preceded/coincided with the behaviour?

☐ **Consequences:** What was the outcome? What were your subsequent thoughts or feelings?

Figure 7.5 Health behaviour monitoring exercise

Classroom activity

Make a copy of the health behaviour monitoring exercise and record one or more of your health behaviours for a week.

In small groups discuss the following questions:

1. Do you notice a pattern regarding this behaviour? Describe.
2. What influences the maintenance (or not) of this behaviour?
3. What role do antecedents and consequences play in the initiation and continuation of this behaviour?
4. Does anything surprise you? Expand.
5. What understandings has this activity provided for you regarding working with people who need to cease, initiate or maintain a health-enhancing behaviour?

Cognitive theories of health behaviour

Cognitive psychological theories propose that people actively interpret their environment and cognitively construct their world. Therefore, behaviour (including health-related behaviour) is a result of two factors, namely:

- internal (within the person) events, which are the individual's thoughts and perceptions about themselves, the world and their behaviour in the world

■ external (within the environment) events, which are the stimuli and reinforcements that regulate behaviour.

While cognitive psychology emerged as a field of study and therapy in the 1970s the notion that one's thinking influences one's behaviour is not new. Epictetus, the Greek Stoic philosopher, is attributed to making the statement that 'we are disturbed not by the things but by the view we take of them' and Buddha observed that 'we are what we think' (Wood 2012 p 172). Consider the following scenario that exemplifies how different outcomes can result from different thoughts about the same situation or event.

Critical thinking

While applying sunscreen Ben noticed a black mole on his left thigh. What feelings would Ben have and what action might he take if his thoughts about this were:

■ This is just another freckle.

■ Oh no! I have a fatal cancer like my cousin Jarrod who died last year.

■ I don't remember seeing this before.

HEALTH BELIEF MODEL

The health belief model (HBM) (Fig 7.6) was the first cognitive explanatory model in health psychology and continues to be used today. It was developed in the 1950s by Hockbaum and Rosenstock to explain the unexpected low levels of participation in health screening and illness prevention programs (Rosenstock 1966, 1974, 1991).

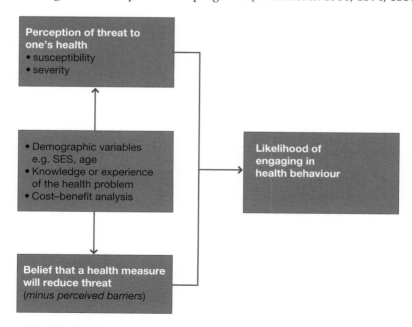

Figure 7.6 Health belief model

Since the 1970s the HBM has been widely utilised in health education and health promotion programs. This cognitive model predicts the seeking of treatment or the changing of health behaviours on the basis of two factors:

- the individual's perception of threat to his/her health, including susceptibility and severity

- the degree to which the individual believes that a particular health action or behaviour will influence the health outcome and be effective in reducing the threat. It includes an assessment of the perceived benefits of the behaviours and the perceived barriers to carrying out the new behaviour.

When the model was devised it was assumed that increased knowledge through health education programs would lead to greater participation in public health programs. However, the expected outcome of changed health behaviours following exposure to health education did not always eventuate. For example, in a study of sexual risk taking among American college students ($n = 71$), Downing-Matibag and Geisinger (2009) found that situational characteristics such as 'spontaneity' interfered with students being able to engage in 'safe sex' despite the student being aware of the possibility of acquiring a sexually transmitted infection.

Initially health education strategies utilising the HBM do increase the individual's motivation to engage in health-enhancing behaviours, but this does not necessarily translate into action. The knowledge that a particular behaviour is beneficial or harmful to one's health is insufficient, on its own, to change many people's health practices or behaviour. This is because the HBM identifies *what* to change but not necessarily *how* to make the required changes, nor does the HBM teach the skills required to make and sustain the change.

Consider the current concern being expressed about rising obesity rates in Western nations. The majority of obese people know that being overweight poses health risks and understand that to lose weight they need to eat a healthy diet and be physically active – that is, to balance kilojoule intake and expenditure. Yet obesity levels continue to rise. Therefore, while the HBM is useful in predicting some health behaviours, such as regular breast screening by a woman with a family history of breast cancer, the model is not universally applicable for all people or all health issues.

Critical thinking

Consider the health behaviour of annual dental examinations recommended by dentists as a preventive strategy to identify any dental problems early. Use the HBM to explain who, in the following two scenarios, is more likely to have annual dental examinations and why.

- Adam is a recent school leaver who has commenced employment as an apprentice electrician. Throughout his school years he attended annual dental checkups through the school dental scheme. Two years ago he experienced severe toothache that was diagnosed as an abscess and

Cont... ▶

cracked tooth. Treatment involved root canal therapy and capping of the tooth. Adam's parents' private health insurance will cover his dental expenses until he is 25 years old.

■ Carrie is a recent school leaver who is currently a full-time university student. Throughout her school years she attended annual dental checkups through the school dental scheme. Apart from the annual checkups Carrie never underwent any other dental treatment. Neither Carrie nor her parents have private health insurance.

THEORY OF PLANNED BEHAVIOUR

The theory of planned behaviour (TPB) was first proposed by Ajzen and Maddern (1986) to seek understandings of behaviours that behavioural and cognitive theories had failed to explain, particularly the non-uptake of healthy behaviours. The TPB is based on the premise that using cognitive and behavioural models alone is insufficient to understand health behaviours or to produce change. It proposes that social processes must also be taken into account. It, therefore, introduces 'social cognitions' to the previously developed cognitive models like the HBM.

The TPB (see Fig 7.7) proposes that three beliefs are predictive of the individual's health behaviour or behavioural outcomes. These are:

■ the individual's attitude to the behaviour

■ the subjective norm

■ the individual's perceived behavioural control.

Overall, the TPB is a better predictor of health behaviour change than previous cognitive models because it takes account of the individual's belief in their capability

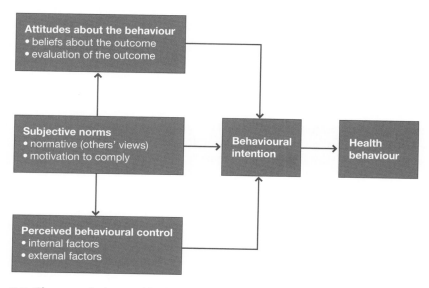

Figure 7.7 Theory of planned behaviour

to achieve the desired outcome (self-efficacy) and the social context in which the behaviour occurs. For example, in a high school where binge drinking is an accepted 'norm' it can be predicted that many adolescents will engage in this behaviour, despite being aware that this practice is harmful. This is because an individual may not have the confidence to be different and is motivated to comply with the subjective norm. Furthermore, research suggests that it is not just intention that leads to performing a certain behaviour but that environmental factors also play a role. Norman's (2011) study of binge drinking among undergraduate students found that while binge drinking was influenced by the student's intention to drink, contextual cues such as how much others were drinking also influenced whether they engaged in binge drinking or not. The researcher concluded that in addressing binge drinking as a health issue it is important to focus on both the motivational intentions of the individual as well as environmental factors.

Classroom activity

In small groups:

Use the TPB to identify and discuss the attitudes, subjective norms and perceived behavioural controls that an individual might hold when they engage in the following health behaviours:

- wearing a bicycle helmet
- a teenager with asthma not using her preventer 'puffer' at school
- driving a car while intoxicated.

TRANSTHEORETICAL MODEL OF BEHAVIOURAL CHANGE

The transtheoretical model of behaviour change (TTM) utilises both behavioural and cognitive strategies. The model was developed by Prochaska and DiClemente (1984) from their research in addiction studies. It was further refined by Prochaska et al (1992) and Prochaska (2006).

TTM proposes that lasting behaviour change can be achieved using this cognitively based therapy to assist people to move towards the maintenance stage of a positive health behaviour such as gambling cessation. While the authors present the stages in a sequential manner they stress that movement through the stages is not linear. An individual will move backwards and forwards through and between the stages before maintenance is established (see Fig 7.8). It is not uncommon for an individual who has reached the maintenance stage to relapse and revert to an earlier stage before achieving stable maintenance. When relapse occurs the person is encouraged to view this as part of the cycle of change, not failure – a challenge not a catastrophe.

The five stages of change of the TTM are:

1. *Precontemplation* – The stage in which the person does not recognise that the behaviour poses health risks and therefore does not perceive a need to change. This may be due to lack of knowledge or information, or the person

may be using denial. For example, a person with osteoarthritis may be unaware of the role of exercise in maintaining joint mobility and consequently reduce their physical activity as a strategy to manage pain. A tobacco smoker who rationalises that, 'My grandfather smoked until he was 80 years old and never suffered any ill effects' may be utilising denial regarding the risks associated with smoking.

2. *Contemplation* – The stage in which the person is aware that the behaviour potentially causes health problems but is ambivalent about making a commitment to change. A shift to this stage from precontemplation may be triggered by an event such as when a smoker or a close family member is diagnosed with a smoking-related health problem.

3. *Preparation* – In this stage the individual acknowledges the risk inherent in the behaviour and makes a commitment to change such as purchasing nicotine patches, tells others of their intention or seeks professional assistance.

4. *Action* – This is the stage at which intervention is most effective. This is when the individual takes action to change a health behaviour such as the smoker who purchases nicotine replacement patches and enrols for a Quit smoking course.

5. *Maintenance or termination* – Maintenance is the stage in which the person sustains the desired health behaviour (e.g. smoking cessation), while termination applies to the health behaviours that do not need to be ongoing such as vaccination or health screening.

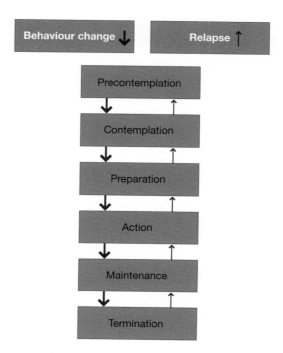

Figure 7.8 Transtheoretical model

Transtheoretical model in clinical practice

A strength of the TTM is that it suggests strategies to work with unmotivated clients who previously were not considered amenable to intervention or treatment (Prochaska 2006, Di Clemente et al 2011). This enables the therapist to facilitate movement towards a stage of readiness. After identifying the stage at which the client is at, the therapist can then initiate interventions to facilitate the client moving to the next stage. For example, if the individual is at the precontemplation stage and is unaware of the risk the behaviour poses for their health the therapist can present the relevant health education information to the client to facilitate movement to the next stage. However, if the patient is using denial in this stage, intervention is extremely difficult, whereas intervening at the action stage is more effective because the person is motivated to make changes. This is the stage at which intervention is most likely to be effective in bringing about the desired change in behaviour.

Providing intervention based on an individual's stage of cessation is the principle behind the Australian Quit Now and New Zealand Quitline Me Mutu smoking cessation campaigns. Graphic images of the consequences of smoking on cigarette packets and in television commercials aim to shift smokers from the precontemplation to the contemplation and ultimately action stages. The Quit programs also provide information about access to strategies and support services to assist smokers to move from the contemplation stage through to the action and maintenance stages.

It is important to note that once the person reaches the maintenance stage relapse is still possible, as it is at any of the preceding stages. Should relapse occur the individual's thoughts regarding the relapse will influence what happens next. For example, a person who views relapse as a *setback* or *challenge* can plan to return to the stage previously achieved, whereas a person who views relapse as a *failure* or *catastrophe* will not be motivated to persevere with the behaviour change.

In summary TTM identifies the stages an individual goes through when making health behaviour changes. It identifies internal and external influences, thereby identifying opportunities for intervention. It is particularly effective for changing addictive (e.g. alcohol and gambling problems) and other behaviours that pose health risks (e.g. unsafe sex).

MOTIVATIONAL INTERVIEWING

Miller and Rollnick initially developed motivational interviewing as a therapeutic intervention for use with people who had addictive behaviours such as drug, alcohol or gambling problems, but it is now used for a wide range of health issues (Rollnick & Miller 1995, Rollnick et al 2007). It evolved from the person-centred counselling approach of humanistic psychologist Carl Rogers (Hettema et al 2005) and shares similarities with the TTM in that both interventions aim to encourage the individual to recognise the need for change and then to take action to bring about change. Both models also stress the importance of the individual taking responsibility for initiating and implementing the behaviour change.

In a motivational interview the person is encouraged to explore all the beliefs and values they hold for and against a behaviour that requires change – to thereby create a state of cognitive dissonance (conflict) for the person. The person is asked to make a list of the positive and negative consequences of the behaviour. For example, eliciting statements like 'gambling gives me a buzz when I win' and 'my relationship with my partner is suffering because of my gambling' are conflicting outcomes of continuing to gamble. The person is then encouraged to make a decision regarding whether or not they wish to stop gambling. If they decide to make the behavioural change (i.e. cease gambling) the therapist then assists the person to develop and implement a plan to facilitate the behaviour change. The key points of the motivational interviewing counselling approach are (Rollnick & Miller 1995, Rollnick et al 2007):

- Motivation to change is elicited from the client, and not imposed externally.
- It is the client's task, not the counsellor's, to articulate his or her ambivalence.
- Direct persuasion is not an effective method for resolving ambivalence.
- The counselling style is generally a quiet and eliciting one.
- The counsellor is directive in helping the client to examine and resolve ambivalence.
- Readiness to change is not a client trait but a fluctuating product of interpersonal interaction.
- The therapeutic relationship is more like a partnership or companionship than expert/recipient roles.

Four principles underpin a motivational interviewing counselling approach: empathy expression, whereby the counsellor conveys understanding of the person's situation and perspective; non-confrontation, to allow the person to identify the discrepancies for themselves; accept resistance as a part of the process of change; and encourage self-efficacy and optimism regarding the person's ability to change (Rollnick et al 2007).

A significant component of the motivational interviewing approach is for the therapist to resist telling the person what they should or should not do and to not lead the person to a decision by coercion as this can lead to resistance (Palmer 2012). Rather, the role of the therapist is to assist the person to come to their own decision and to assist them in developing and implementing an action plan. See the *Research focus* for an example of using motivational interviewing to facilitate medication adherence by adolescents with asthma.

Critical thinking

Using the motivational interviewing approach make a list of the positive and negative consequences of tobacco smoking.

Research focus

Riekert, K., Borrelli, B., Bilderback, A., et al., 2011. The development of a motivational interviewing intervention to promote medication adherence among inner-city African-American adolescents. Patient Education and Counseling 82, 117–122.

ABSTRACT

Objective

To develop and assess the feasibility of a motivational-interviewing-based asthma self-management program for inner-city, African-American, adolescents with asthma.

Methods

Thirty-seven African-American adolescents (aged 10–15 years) recently seen in an inner-city emergency department for asthma and prescribed an asthma controller medication participated in the newly developed program consisting of five home visits. Adolescents and their caregivers completed phone-based surveys before and after the intervention.

Results

Ninety-five per cent of the adolescents completed all five sessions; 89% of caregivers and 76% of adolescents believed other families would benefit from the intervention. Caregivers were more likely to report 100% adherence post-intervention compared with pre-intervention and reported a trend for adolescents taking greater responsibility for their asthma. There were no pre–post differences in adolescent-reported medication adherence, but adolescents did report increased motivation and readiness to adhere to treatment. Caregivers and adolescents each reported statistically significant increases in their asthma quality of life.

Conclusions

The findings from this pilot study suggest that motivational interviewing is a feasible and promising approach for increasing medication adherence among inner-city adolescents with asthma and is worthy of further evaluation in a randomised trial.

Practice implications

Incorporating motivational interviewing into disease management programs may enhance their effectiveness.

Critical thinking

Reikert et al's 2011 research demonstrated that a psychological strategy (motivational interviewing) can positively influence a physical behaviour.

- List other physical health problems for which motivational interviewing could be used to bring about health behavioural change.
- Identify the desired behavioural change for each of these health problems.

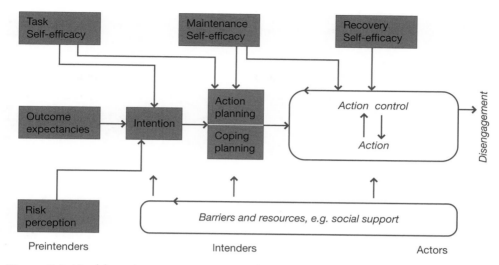

Figure 7.9 Health action process approach model

Schwarzer R 2011 Health action process approach. Online: http://userpage.fu-berlin.de/health/hapa.htm

HEALTH ACTION PROCESS APPROACH

The health action process approach (HAPA) is a social cognition model that highlights the role of self-efficacy and addresses the 'intention–behaviour gap' (Schwarzer 1992, 2011) or why people do or do not complete a behaviour that they intend to complete. The model (see Fig 7.9) adds a social dimension to previous cognitive models.

Schwarzer developed the model from research that identified that self-efficacy played a role in the individual's intention to change and subsequently whether change occurred or not. The model makes a distinction between the three stages, being: intention, decision making and motivation; planning and action; and maintenance and recovery. It proposes there are three precursors to change:

- self-efficacy or the individual's belief in their ability to action the change
- outcome expectations or the belief as to whether the intended action will improve health or not
- risk perception or whether or not changing will affect health.

Of the three precursors Schwarzer suggests that self-efficacy is the best predictor of behavioural outcomes (Schwarzer 2011). Like the TPB, the HAPA proposes that the individual's belief in their ability to carry out the desired behaviour is predictive of the individual's success in doing so. For example, the model would predict that the person who believes he can comply with a recommended dietary change will be more successful in making the change than a person who believes that making the change is too difficult.

COGNITIVE BEHAVIOURAL THERAPIES

Cognitive behavioural therapies refers to a range of interventions that utilise both cognitive and behavioural strategies to bring about changes in an individual's

CASE STUDY: TAMARA

Tamara is a 33-year-old physical education teacher who has smoked since she was 15 years old. Both her parents smoke and, while her mother has not experienced any ill effects from smoking, her father has just been diagnosed with early-stage emphysema. Initially, Tamara commenced smoking because most of her friends smoked and she did not want to be the 'odd one out'. Later, when she started clubbing, she realised that smoking helped her to maintain her weight because she wasn't tempted to snack if she smoked while drinking, even though she now has to go outside the venue to do so.

While studying for her education degree Tamara became aware of the potential for harm to her health should she continue to smoke. On two occasions she gave up, once for 12 months. She found social occasions to be the most difficult because people around her smoked and she longed for a cigarette in her hand when she drank alcohol. At first she allowed herself to only smoke on weekends when she was out with her friends but very soon she had resumed smoking daily. Since her father's recent diagnosis Tamara has decided to give up smoking 'for good'.

Classroom activity

In small groups:

1. Identify internal factors that influence Tamara's smoking.
2. Identify external factors that influence Tamara's smoking.
3. Explain Tamara's behaviour using
   - HBM
   - TPB
   - TTM
   - HAPA.
4. Suggest what needs to happen for Tamara to be successful in giving up smoking.
5. Suggest the conditions required for Tamara to give up smoking.

behaviours and to treat some mental illnesses (including but not limited to depression, anxiety, phobias and schizophrenia) and chronic illness (e.g. chronic fatigue syndrome), and to manage behavioural problems such as addictive behaviours. The underlying premise behind cognitive behavioural therapies is that thoughts, feelings and behaviours are interrelated and changes in one or more will bring about change in one or all of these. Key elements of cognitive behavioural approaches are a focus on:

- the present rather than the past, and identifying the problem and its extent (history is acknowledged for its contribution to the present problem but is not the focus of treatment)

- setting goals that are achievable and measurable
- collaboration between the person and the therapist to set goals and test strategies
- bringing about changes in thoughts, feelings, behaviour and physiological responses (Meadows et al 2007).

Critical thinking

Change is easier to initiate than sustain.

- Consider this statement in relation to a health-enhancing behaviour of your own that you have tried to modify, in other words, taking up a new behaviour or discontinuing an existing one.
- Which model best explains your success or otherwise regarding this health behaviour?

Classroom activity

Carol is a problem gambler who states sincerely that she wishes to cease gambling because of the impact on her life, her relationships and her health. Nevertheless, she regularly attends the local hotel where she plays the 'pokies'. Away from the hotel Carol states she will no longer gamble. Her goal is to be a non-gambler; she is aware of the risks associated with gambling for her and she believes she can stop.

In small groups:

1. Discuss why willpower has not been sufficient to enable Carol to curb or cease gambling.
2. Identify which theories explain her behaviour.
3. Suggest strategies that could assist Carol to succeed in curbing her gambling.
4. Which theories/models underpin these suggested strategies?

Limitations of psychological models

While behavioural and cognitive approaches to initiating and maintaining health behaviours can be effective, they do not provide a universal explanation for all people in all situations. Commentators suggest this is because relying on an individual's behavioural response and cognitive process is a narrow approach to understanding human behaviour (Crossley 2000, Murray 2010, Norman 2011). Cognitive and behavioural models of health behaviour do not take into consideration other psychological and social factors that influence the initiation, continuation or cessation of health behaviours.

The models also assume rational decision making and fail to take into account unconscious processes as identified in psychoanalytic theory, such as the defence mechanism of denial. Nor do they acknowledge the contribution of affective states such as fear or the physiological component of some practices such as nicotine addiction in tobacco smoking or genetics. Significantly, the models do not take into account where the person is located in the lifespan or the social contexts of individuals' lives. Social factors (which are examined in more detail in Ch 4) that are not specifically considered in psychological behavioural change theories include:

- *Socioeconomic status (SES).* Does the person have access to the resources required to make the change required?

- *Social connectedness.* Does the person have sufficient social supports to carry out the activity?

- *Gender.* Do men and women respond in the same way to similar health challenges?

- *Ethnicity.* What role does ethnicity play in health behaviours?

- *Culture.* How applicable are psychological theories developed in Western cultures to people from non-Western cultures?

Finally, cognitive and behavioural models are better predictors of behavioural *intention* than they are of behavioural *outcomes* (Morrison et al 2012). They are, therefore, more effective in predicting who is at risk of health problems but not particularly useful in predicting who will be successful in engaging in health-enhancing behaviours, or who will be successful in changing unhealthy behaviours.

Conclusion

This chapter presented a range of psychological theories and models that propose explanations as to how internal and external factors influence an individual's health behaviours and lifestyle. These theories and models provide useful insights into the motivators and reinforcers regarding why an individual does or does not engage in health-enhancing behaviours or why an individual engages in behaviours that pose health risks. These understandings also identify possibilities to change health behaviours; however, this knowledge needs to be utilised within a framework that also takes account of the social contexts of the person's life.

REMEMBER

- Health behaviours are influenced by a range of physical, psychological and social factors.
- Psychological theories and models can predict an individual's health behaviours.
- Psychological theories and models identify strategies whereby individuals can change health behaviours.
- While psychological theories and models provide useful insights for understanding, predicting and changing health behaviours they, nevertheless, have limitations and are not necessarily universally applicable.

Further resources

Chiu, C., Lynch, R., Chan, F., et al., 2011. The health action process approach as a motivational model for physical activity self-management for people with multiple sclerosis. Rehabilitation Psychology 65 (3), 171–181.

Cooper, D. (Ed.), 2011. Interventions in mental health-substance use. Radcliffe, London.

Dempsey, A., 2011. Predicting oral contraception continuation using the transtheoretical model of behaviour change. Perspectives on Sexual and Reproductive Health 43 (1), 23–29.

Norman, P., 2011. The theory of planned behavior and binge drinking among undergraduate students: assessing the impact of habit strength. Addictive Behaviors 36, 502–507.

Rollnick, S., Miller, W., Butler, C., 2007. Motivational interviewing: helping patients change behavior. Guilford, New York.

Weblinks

Australian national tobacco campaign

www.quitnow.info.au

The Australian national tobacco campaign is part of the Australian Government's continuing efforts to reduce the level of tobacco use among Australians and is aimed directly at smokers, both youth and adults.

Flinders University Human Behaviour and Health Research Unit

www.flinders.edu.au/medicine/sites/fhbhru

The Human Behaviour and Health Research Unit is a centre for research, evaluation and development of chronic condition management. The website contains links to the centre's programs, research and publications that focus on coordinated care, care planning, behavioural change and self-management.

Information on self-efficacy

www.des.emory.edu/mfp/self-efficacy

This website provides resources and publications about self-efficacy including the writings and video interviews of Albert Bandura.

The health action process approach

http://userpage.fu-berlin.de/~health/hapa.htm

This website provides an overview of research and publications relating to Schwarzer's (2011) health action process model.

The Quit Group

www.quit.org.nz

QUIT Me Mutu is the Quit Group New Zealand website that provides support and information for people who wish to cease smoking.

References

Ajzen, I., Maddern, M., 1986. Predictions of goal directed behaviour: attitudes, intentions and perceived behavioural control. Journal of Experimental Social Psychology 22, 453–474.

Australian Institute of Health and Welfare, 2010. Australia's health 2010. AIHW, Canberra.

Bandura, A. (Ed.), 2006. Psychological modeling: conflicting theories, second ed. Aldine Transaction, New Jersey.

Bandura, A., 1969. Principles of behaviour modification. Holt, Rhinehart & Winston, New York.

Beck, A.T., 1976. Cognitive therapy and emotional disorders. International Universities Press, New York.

Chiu, C., Lynch, R., Chan, F., et al., 2011. The health action process approach as a motivational model for physical activity self-management for people with multiple sclerosis. Rehabilitation Psychology 65 (3), 171–181.

Cox, J., De, P., Morissette, C., et al., 2008. Low perceived benefits and self-efficacy are associated with hepatitis C virus (HCV) infection-related risk among injection drug users. Social Science and Medicine 66, 211–230.

Crossley, M., 2000. Rethinking health psychology. Open University Press, Buckingham.

DiClemente, C., Schumann, K., Greene, A., et al., 2011. A transtheoretical model perspective on change: process-focussed intervention in mental health-substance use. In: Cooper, D. (Ed.), Interventions in mental health-substance use. Radcliffe, London.

Downing-Matibag, T., Geisenger, B., 2009. Hooking up and sexual risk taking among college students: a health belief model perspective. Qualitative Health Research 19 (9), 1196–1209.

Ellis, A., 1984. Rational-emotive therapy and cognitive behaviour therapy. Springer, New York.

Eysenck, H.J., 1960. Behaviour therapy and the neuroses. Pergamon, London.

Frieden, T., 2010. A framework for public health: the health impact pyramid. American Journal of Public Health 100 (4), 590–595.

Harvey, P., Petkov, J., Misan, G., et al., 2008. Self-management support and training for patients with chronic and complex conditions improves health related behaviour and health outcomes. Australian Health Review 32 (2), 330–338.

Hettema, J., Steele, J., Miller, W., 2005. Motivational interviewing. Annual Review of Clinical Psychology 1, 91–111.

Krahé, B., Möller, I., 2010. Longitudinal effects of media violence on aggression and empathy among German adolescents. Journal of Applied Developmental Psychology 31, 401–409.

Meadows, G., Singh, B., Grigg, M., 2007. Mental health in Australia: collaborative community practice. Oxford University Press, Melbourne.

Meichenbaum, D.H., 1974. Cognitive behaviour modification: an integrative approach. Plenum, New York.

Morrison, V., Bennett, P., Butow, P., et al., 2012. Introduction to health psychology in Australia, second ed. Pearson Education, Sydney.

Murray, M., 2010. Health psychology in context. The European Health Psychologist 12, 39–41.

Norman, P., 2011. The theory of planned behavior and binge drinking among undergraduate students: assessing the impact of habit strength. Addictive Behaviors 36, 502–507.

Palmer, C., 2012. Therapeutic interventions. In: Elder, R., Evans, K., Nizette, D. (Eds.), Practical perspectives in psychiatric and mental health nursing, third ed. Elsevier, Sydney.

Pavlov, I.P., 1927. Conditioned reflexes: an investigation of the physiological activity of the cerebral cortex. Trans. G.V. Anrep. Oxford University Press, London.

Prochaska, J., 2006. Moving beyond the transtheoretical model. Addiction 101 (6), 768–778.

Prochaska, J., DiClemente, C.C., Norcross, J.C., 1992. In search of how people change: applications to addictive behaviors. American Psychologist 47, 1102–1114.

Prochaska, J., DiClemente, C., 1984. The transtheoretical approach: crossing traditional boundaries of therapy. Dow Jones/Irwin, Chicago.

Reikert, K., Borrelli, B., Bilderback, A., et al., 2011. The development of a motivational interviewing intervention to promote medication adherence among inner-city African American adolescents. Patient Education and Counseling 82, 117–122.

Rollnick, S., Miller, W., 1995. What is motivational interviewing? Behavioural and Cognitive Psychotherapy 23, 325–334.

Rollnick, S., Miller, W., Butler, C., 2007. Motivational interviewing: helping patients change behaviour. Guilford, New York.

Rosenstock, I., 1966. Why people use health services. Milbank Memorial Fund Quarterly 44, 94–124.

Rosenstock, I., 1974. Historical origins of the health belief model. Health Education Monographs 2, 1–8.

Rosenstock, I., 1991. Health belief model: explaining health behavior through expectancies. In: Glanz, K., Lewis, F.M., Rimer, B.K., (Eds.), Health behavior and health education: theory research and practice. Jossey-Boss, San Francisco, pp. 39–58.

Schwarzer, R., 1992. Self-efficacy: thought control of action. Hemisphere, Washington.

Schwarzer, R., 2011. Health action process approach. Online. Available: http://userpage. fu-berlin.de/~health/hapa.htm 17 Sep 2012.

Skinner, B.F., 1953. Science and human behaviour. Macmillan, New York.

Wolpe, J., 1958. Psychotherapy by reciprocal inhibition. Stanford University Press, Stanford.

Wood, J., 2012. Interpersonal communication: everyday encounters, seventh ed. Cengage Learning, Wadsworth.

Chapter 8
Communication in healthcare practice

DEB O'KANE

Learning objectives

The material in this chapter will help you to:

- describe basic interpersonal communication principles
- understand the importance of person-centred communication
- identify the key skills of active listening to facilitate effective communication
- identify important ethical communication issues
- understand the process of cultural safety and intercultural communication
- understand the role of communication within a multidisciplinary team
- identify communication issues between health professionals such as horizontal bullying
- understand the role of health professionals in health education and client advocacy.

Key terms

- Person-centred communication
- The health professional–client relationship
- Active listening
- Professional boundaries
- Self-disclosure
- Intercultural communication
- Client education and advocacy
- Multidisciplinary teams

Introduction

Communication is vital in all parts of healthcare interactions, but none more so than in the health professional–client relationship where it is a key requirement for safe and effective practice. Being able to communicate effectively will assist you in working together with the client, family and carers, supporting them in shared responsibility and decision making about their health and lifestyle. Effective communication is not just about being able to talk clearly; it is also about listening and understanding what has been communicated. Listening is critical when working with other people, and a health professional who can listen well will find people more willing to talk openly and honestly about their health issues.

Health psychologists are interested in knowing how health professionals communicate in practice and what can be done to improve this in order to enhance the relationship between all parties involved. This chapter will examine the fundamental aspects of communication in healthcare practice, focusing on the challenges and variables health professionals need to consider when working with other people in care delivery. In the next chapter the partnerships that can be developed from effective communication are examined.

Person-centred communication

Person-centred communication (PCC) is one of the most important dimensions of health professional–client communication. In the past, clients have often been seen as a 'diagnosis' ('the broken leg in bed 1') with a focus on assessment and symptom management. Lack of attention to other factors such as the social, psychological and behavioural aspects of the person's life has left the client without a context for their health issue and often feeling 'unheard'. Research in a number of clinical settings has demonstrated that people who are provided client-centred care experience better health outcomes (Di Blasi et al 2001) and greater client satisfaction (Venetis et al 2009). Research in the United States and the United Kingdom also demonstrates a strong correlation between client satisfaction and the interpersonal skills of the health professional (Boudreaux et al 2004, Toma et al 2009), making it even more vital for health professionals to develop effective communication skills and behaviours in their daily practice. So with this in mind, what is PCC?

PCC is a collection of skills used by health professionals that are respectful and responsive to the individual's needs, values and preferences (Bertakis et al 2009, Levinson 2011). It is not always easy to define the exact level or type of communication required for each client because the variation in people's needs and experiences are unique and different for each individual. What is important is to remember that PCC is not limited to verbal communication but embraces all forms of communication that can affect client care such as written and non-verbal elements. Success is dependent on both parties (the client and the health professional) being able to speak, question and listen. It is a two-way process in which the language and meaning in the message is correctly understood by both, enabling an accurate exchange of information, thus enabling the client to participate in their own care (The Joint Commission 2010).

SKILLS OF COMMUNICATION

In providing appropriate healthcare it is important for all health professionals to consider their own communication style by examining the skills they already possess and those they need to develop in order to communicate effectively with clients, families and other health/service providers. It also helps to have a personal awareness of the likely barriers of communication in practice because inadequate communication can cause distress for clients and their families. Confusion, uncertainty and being unsure of what's being said can leave clients feeling unclear of their illness, diagnosis, treatment or management plan.

The majority of communication textbooks focus on the process of communication or identify groups of different behaviours and qualities that are collectively known as communication skills. The essence of good communication lies within the skills required to deliver and receive the message effectively and include such skills as active listening, reflection, empathy, body language and vocal style. Some authors refer to these as attending behaviours (Ivey et al 2010) while others call them micro skills (Egan 2010). The key element of good communication is to extract the unique experiences and preferences of the client and respond appropriately and effectively.

FACILITATING THE INTERACTION

Ways of encouraging the person to speak about their experience may vary. Ivey et al (2010) write about the importance of 'open invitations to talk' or open-ended questions in encouraging communication in comparison with closed questions. Open-ended questions provide emotional space and often encourage longer responses: 'Tell me what it's been like to have rheumatoid arthritis'; 'Could you tell me ...?'; 'I'm wondering ...'; 'Some people have experienced ... do you?'. Closed questions are often effective when requiring factual content and shorter responses: 'How many years have you had rheumatoid arthritis?'; 'What is your date of birth?'; 'Do you have a regular doctor?' Both have a place in healthcare but sometimes closed questions get in the way of two-way interaction and open-ended questions don't always yield clear information (Balzer Riley 2011). Of course, the response will also depend on the individual. It is not a satisfactory experience for the client to be asked repeated closed questions, with no other comments. There is also the danger that continued open-ended questions yield little concrete information and annoy the client. A variety of different types of questions and comments will often not only yield more in-depth responses, it will also help build rapport and encourages the client to be more cooperative (Balzer Riley 2011). Practise will help in developing these skills. Reflecting on your everyday communication, it may be surprising to find how often each of these kinds of questions are already used. The following are micro skills that facilitate effective communication:

- minimal encouragers
- empathy
- reflection
- summarising.

MINIMAL ENCOURAGERS

Minimal encouragers can indicate to the individual that the helper understands what they are saying. These can be non-verbal, such as the occasional eye contact, leaning forward or nodding the head, or verbal, such as: 'Oh?'; 'So?'; 'Then?'; 'And?'; 'Uh-huh', or a restatement of the same words spoken by the other person: 'So you feel that the treatment was a waste of time ...'. Sometimes silence is very effective, showing the client that you are listening and allowing the person to gather their thoughts and say more about a particular topic (Blonna et al 2011). It is useful to observe how other people show their interest in what someone is saying to them and how different behaviours encourage or discourage a conversation continuing. The important skill is to be aware of how the interaction is flowing and how the client is responding to what the health professional is saying. If the client seems anxious or annoyed, or showing other feelings, it is better to explore their feelings: 'You seem a bit anxious. Are you happy to continue with the interview?' This demonstrates concern and also helps build rapport. There are a variety of ways of showing clients that you understand what is being said and that also help you organise your own thoughts.

EMPATHY

An important aspect of communication is the use of empathy whereby the health professional lets the person know he or she is sensing the person's emotions. Rogers (1961) would consider it a quality inherent in the individual – the ability to feel with the other person in their situation. 'Reflection of feeling can be taught as a cognitive skill ... sensitive empathy, with all its intensity and personal involvement, cannot be so taught' (Rogers 1987). It is true that there is a difference between a learned skill and an inherent quality and it is important to differentiate between them. A naturally empathic person will probably find that they gently reflect or 'mirror' the person's feelings back to them: 'You seem really stressed at the moment'.

REFLECTION

As a beginning health professional, it is often helpful to practise reflection of feelings, that is, reflecting back the person's feelings and listening and responding to the emotions being expressed, not just the content of what they have said (Blonna et al 2011). The actual words used will vary, but it may simply mean repeating back what the other person has said such as, 'So you were at that hospital for a week?'.
Or, it might be more supportive to the client to say, 'I get the feeling it was quite a frightening time for you'. Of course, while this can be supportive to clients, some may find it threatening because they might not wish to divulge their feelings. Another useful technique is paraphrasing. At intervals during the interaction it can help to sum up what has been said so far: 'So you have had joint and muscle pain and you have had problems with your balance for 20 years.'

SUMMARISING

At the end of the interview summarising can also be helpful. This is similar to paraphrasing but sums up the whole conversation. 'So, if I've got it right, what you have been telling me is ...'. Sometimes this can help clients review what they have told

Table 8.1	
EFFECTIVE COMMUNICATION IN A HEALTHCARE SETTING	
Engage	Establish eye contact to show interest.
	Ask both open and closed questions to encourage clients to be exact about their health concerns/behaviour.
Listen	Use 'active listening' such as clarifying, paraphrasing and responding to verbal and non-verbal cues to help ascertain what the client is concerned about.
Clarify/ reflect	Summarise information to show clients they have been heard.
	Constantly check if the client has understood the information and provide opportunities to question what's being said to avoid misunderstandings.
Enquire	Enquire about all areas of the person's life not just the problem area. This ensures you get an accurate description of not only the physical problem but the social and psychological impact it may be having on the client and family.
Convey empathy	Be empathic by reflecting and verbalising your sense of the client's feelings and meanings of the problem behaviour. This will show you are trying to see things from their point of view and are offering support.

Adapted from Maguire P, Pitceathly C 2002 Key communication skills and how to acquire them. British Medical Journal Vol 325 No 7366, p 697–700

you and help health professionals check they have understood what the client said (Balzer Riley 2011). In a busy clinical environment summarising may take additional time, but it can frequently help improve your understanding of a situation and a client may appreciate it and feel their health issues have been understood accurately. It has been the writer's experience that international healthcare students, with English as a second language, often find summarising helpful because it provides a clarification tool to use when they aren't clear what the client has said.

In conclusion, some common identified skills for effective communication in a healthcare setting between client and provider are noted by Maguire and Pitceathly (2002) in Table 8.1.

The importance of language

Words alone do not convey meaning or understanding. It is important to remember that a layperson may have less knowledge about basic anatomy and physiology than you might assume. Medical terminology that has become part of a health professional's everyday language is useless jargon if not understood by the listener. Therefore health professionals cannot assume that everyone with whom they engage will understand their meaning.

LANGUAGE AND CULTURE

Language is a key part of a person's culture and helps them identify who they are as an individual and in society. Often a person's culture will influence the way they see and engage with the world, so it is useful for health professionals to reflect on their own culture and try to understand it in the context of their practice and communication skills. As culture is such a complex concept it should not be reduced to a particular behaviour or attribute in one particular population group but considered in light of all available information, including thoughts, beliefs, attitudes, behaviour, background, heritage and spirituality. As early as the 1900s, linguists and anthropologists Edward Sapir and Benjamin Whorf proposed that words and language are strongly influenced by culture (Otto 2006).

Colloquial language or slang words and euphemisms may be used by people who are too embarrassed to speak about personal matters. Unless familiar with the terminology it may appear to the health professional that the client is speaking a whole new language. For instance, an elderly lady may ask to 'spend a penny' to describe her need to urinate or a child may say they have a 'tummy bug' to describe a recent virus they are recovering from. In some cultures there may be several words within the language that can be used to describe one concept, whereas in other languages the existence of even one word may not be present. Ultimately, what means one thing to one person may mean something entirely different to somebody else so it is up to the health professional to avoid language that can be misleading or ambiguous by clarifying all medical terminology. If they are uncertain about what is being said, health professionals should ask the client to explain. This ensures all parties have achieved a clear understanding.

INTERCULTURAL COMMUNICATION AND CULTURAL SAFETY

There are three key elements to achieving cultural safety in healthcare practice: cultural awareness, cultural sensitivity and cultural safety (see Table 8.2). These concepts, though related, should be understood in their own right to ensure culturally safe communication with others (Eckermann et al 2009).

Table 8.2		
KEY ELEMENTS TO ACHIEVING CULTURAL SAFETY IN HEALTHCARE PRACTICE		
Cultural awareness	**Cultural sensitivity**	**Cultural safety**
A beginning step towards understanding there is difference. Many people undergo courses designed to sensitise them to formal ritual and practice rather than the emotional, social, economic and political context in which people exist.	Alerts health professionals to the legitimacy of difference and begins a process of self-reflection on the powerful influences from their own life experiences that may impact on their interaction with others.	Achieved when the client perceives their healthcare was delivered in a manner that respected and preserved their cultural integrity.

Ramsden IM: Cultural safety and nursing education in Aotearoa and Te Waipounamu. Unpublished PhD thesis, 2002, Victoria University of Wellington, available at www.cultural safety.massey.ac.nz, 19 February 2008.

Strongly linked with cultural safety is the process of *intercultural communication*. Kiesling and Bratt Paulson (2004) define this as the ability to utilise a range of tools and skills to enhance the communication process with people who speak languages other than the dominant local language. Though English is the official language of Australia and New Zealand, it is not a first language for a significant number of Indigenous Australians, Māori or other citizens. Australia and New Zealand have a growing multicultural population with a huge diversity of first, second and subsequent generations who each may have distinctive cultural and linguistic needs, especially if they are from non-English-speaking backgrounds. Intercultural communication is an important aspect of maintaining cultural safety and if not addressed can contribute to a breakdown in communication and ultimately have a significant impact upon the effectiveness of healthcare. For instance, Australian research has identified ineffective communication as one of the main factors leading to poor health outcomes in Indigenous Australians (Cass et al 2002, Coulehan et al 2005, Lawrence et al 2009). To provide culturally safe clinical services, health professionals need to be aware of differences in intercultural communication and be able to identify factors that impede or enable communication in health service delivery, particularly for those living in rural and remote areas.

Some areas to consider when engaging with people from culturally diverse backgrounds are as follows (ACT Health 2012):

- Speak clearly and simply without being simplistic or patronising.
- Place yourself in the client's situation and think how you would like to be treated.
- Clarify meaning: both yours and others.
- Be aware of your own non-verbal behaviour and the way you interpret that of others.
- Monitor your own style and the way you respond to difference.
- Relate to others as individuals, recognising similarities rather than only differences.
- Ensure you understand your clients' living arrangements, relationships and accessibility to health services.
- Ask questions if you do not understand (if in doubt, ask).

Remember, it is a health professional's responsibility to recognise the unique differences in people. Cultural safety may be different for each person. Maintain cultural awareness and sensitivity to the client's needs and be willing to engage in dialogue to enhance culturally safe communication. Most health services now offer the use of interpreters and either Aboriginal liaison officers or Māori health liaison officers, so recognise when this would be beneficial to the communication process.

Critical thinking

- Have you had experience learning a second language? What were the challenges and benefits from doing this?

Cont... ▶

- Think of a time when you tried to convey a particular verbal message but the recipient did not understand you. What reasons may have caused this misunderstanding?
- How did you resolve the issue? Did this help or hinder the situation?
- How is language different in personal and professional relationships? How may this impact on the relationships?

The health professional–client relationship

In identifying the skills needed for effective communication, it is easy to see them as mere lists made up of concrete, discrete behavioural actions without considering the importance of relationship development and the connection needed between clients and health professionals. The importance of caring and humanity is emphasised by Chochinov (2007) when he cites a seminal paper by Francis Peabody:

One of the essential qualities of the clinician is interest in humanity, for the secret of the care of the patient is in caring for the patient.
(1927 cited in Chochinov 2007 p 187)

Similarly, Jean Watson, a pioneer in developing 'caring theory', identified several essential elements originally known as 'carative factors' but recently redefined as 'caritas processes' (Watson 2008). These elements support factors such as commitment, trust and continuity that are central to caring practice, communication and the healthcare relationship. Through the helping relationship, health professionals and clients may share a sense of two individuals working together – to have a sense of shared humanity that is essential to the spiritual, psychological and humanistic dimensions of the relationship (Stein-Parbury 2009). Although clinical skills and knowledge are very important in being a safe and competent health professional, it must never be forgotten that the tasks and procedures are being implemented on real people with real feelings of pain, fear and a wide range of other emotions and sensations. To be able to enter into their experiences is not simply a right for health professionals but a privilege that clients have given through their consent and trust.

INTERPERSONAL RELATIONSHIPS, ETHICS AND COMMUNICATION

Interpersonal relationships can be both personal and professional, with interpersonal interactions being central to both (Balzer Riley 2011). Personal relationships may include friendships, intimate or romantic relationships, whereas a health professional–client relationship, though therapeutic, is a professional relationship established to meet the needs of the client. What, then, is the best way to relate to clients? How do they want health professionals to relate to them? You can begin by being sensitive to how a client behaves in interactions and modify responses in line with this. Sitting in different health professionals' waiting rooms you may observe the approaches of various receptionists to clients. Some vary their style depending on the client. They may address them using their first name or title; they know their clients and how to communicate with them. Others don't vary in their approach, always using the first name or a colloquial term such as 'darl' and it is interesting to see how some clients are quite relaxed about this, while others visibly bristle. Being an effective communicator means trying to 'read' clients and how they respond to what you say and do (Balzer Riley 2011). Of course, the task will often dictate the interaction; you might be assessing the individual's health status, taking a blood specimen or consulting them about their dietary needs, while at the same time engaging in a conversation about the weather or their interests outside the healthcare situation. Conversation may act as a means of lessening the client's (and sometimes the health professional's) anxiety or generally defusing the tension of a situation. Again, the focus should always be on the client and what their needs are.

Ethical behaviour is essential for delivering high-quality healthcare. As a health professional there are explicit ethical obligations related to communication that are fundamental to developing and maintaining a professional relationship (Duncan 2009). These can include informed consent, confidentiality and conflict to name a few. Each brings with it fresh challenges the health professional may face on a daily basis. Let's look at three common ethical issues of communication in more detail. These are power imbalance, professional boundaries and self-disclosure.

POWER IMBALANCE

When health professionals are consulted it is more often than not because they are seen as an expert in a particular area and the client is seeking help from someone who they deem has the skill and knowledge to help them. Though not necessarily perceived by the health professional, having the skills, knowledge, influence and authority that the client requires inadvertently leads to an inherent power disequilibrium between the two parties. The practitioner is in a position of power, while the client may feel vulnerable.

It is important for the client to feel comfortable in confiding their concerns or health issues with the health professional without feeling they are relinquishing their own responsibility and control over any decisions concerning them. A health professional who provides information encourages the client to be an active partner in the therapeutic alliance. Using micro skills during communication will go some way to alleviating this power imbalance, whereas a misuse of this power is considered abuse.

PROFESSIONAL BOUNDARIES

In today's healthcare environment, roles are much less differentiated than in previous years and health workers might now be more open and reveal more of their own personalities than before (Nelson & Gordon 2006). For example, in many public hospitals, doctors do not wear white coats; health professionals might wear more casual-looking clothes rather than formal white or green uniforms so a client might be confused about which role the person assisting them has. At a time when roles are more blurred and many express the need to be treated as equals, developing a relationship with the appropriate professional boundaries can be an uncertain road to navigate.

Ultimately, the relationships we form with clients differ from those we form with friends and family. At times it may be appropriate to be informal and engage in social conversation with some clients, but it is important to first be sensitive to the individual you are caring for and be prepared to work at establishing a helping relationship. For example, it might be preferable to address someone by their title and surname until it is established that the person is comfortable to be called by their first name.

While some boundaries are very clear and inviolable (e.g. physical, verbal or sexual abuse) others can be blurred (e.g. when the client asks about your marital status or invites you on a date), and require the health professional to be aware of when the professional relationship may be crossing the boundary or moving into a 'grey' area. This requires self-reflection, and the willingness to discuss the relationship dilemma with a manager or supervisor who will be able to consider the context of the relationship and offer advice. Remember it is the health professional's responsibility at all times to establish and maintain a professional relationship by setting clear boundaries regardless of how the client has behaved.

One particular 'grey' area to consider is the possibility of a dual relationship, which can become even more apparent in small communities, such as in rural and remote areas. Due to the population size, it may be that the health professional has both a personal and a professional relationship with the client; that is, they are a close friend as well as the practitioner caring for them. It is therefore of paramount importance that all aspects of the relationship such as role and boundary shifts are clarified by articulating what your role and responsibilities will include while working with the person as a health professional. Communicating in such a transparent manner helps protect client confidentiality and ensure the client's needs are a priority.

SELF-DISCLOSURE

There are invisible boundaries that all individuals erect around themselves, depending on the situation. This impacts on who we choose to disclose personal information to. Self-disclosure (revealing personal information about our lives to others) is generally accepted as a valuable tool in personal relationships and can be just as valuable in a professional relationship if used appropriately and in moderation. While health professional to client self-disclosure is unacceptable in most contexts, it may be acceptable and appropriate in special circumstances. For example, a mother who has recently experienced a 28-week gestation pregnancy loss and is struggling to grieve for the child may find it useful to hear about what proved helpful in the grieving process from a health professional who has gone through a similar experience. This kind of select and limited disclosure may be judged helpful in meeting the therapeutic needs of the client.

It is never acceptable for a health professional to disclose information that is self-serving or intimate. To avoid blurring boundaries, the required skill is to know what is considered suitable personal information to discuss and to ask the question 'Is it appropriate to do so?', while remaining within the scope of the professional relationship. Therefore it is the responsibility of health professionals to direct their attention to their clients' needs as being first and foremost, rather than their own. In reflecting on this you can ask yourself the question: 'Whose needs are being served by my self-disclosure?'

Critical thinking

Consider the behaviours, language and beliefs that define a professional relationship.

- How does this differ from a personal one?
- How is this decided?

Classroom activity

In small groups address the questions posed by the given scenarios.

Discuss the key issues identified and the implications each may have on health professionals and their communication practice with clients.

SCENARIO 1:

You are a doctor providing primary healthcare for a small Aboriginal community. While you are at the post office collecting your mail on your day off, the wife of a client who is under your care asks for your opinion on her husband's latest blood results. What ethical issues arise in this situation? How would you respond and why?

SCENARIO 2:

You are the nurse on a surgical ward preparing a 50-year-old woman for a hysterectomy. She is very anxious and tearful, saying she is afraid that she will no longer feel 'whole' or like a woman. You are of a similar age and have gone through the same surgical procedure. Do you think it would be helpful to share your experience with her? Explain why.

Other influences on communication in healthcare settings

Individual health professional and client interactions may not always be successful. Some health professionals, as well as clients, are not easy to work with and may behave in unreasonable ways, be uncooperative, or be physically or verbally aggressive at times. Particularly, but not just in large healthcare organisations, status can be an issue. Some health professionals within the service may be considered, or consider themselves, to have higher status than others. Furthermore, administrators you may not know or ever communicate with, make decisions affecting the work situation. This may give the feeling of a narrow span of control, which may in turn lead to a high level of informal communication or gossip between staff such as, 'Did you hear about ...?'

The diverse educational backgrounds of professionals and staff in a healthcare service may contribute to communication problems. Various disciplines may have jargon or specialised language that other health professionals (or clients) may not understand. Different staff will have varying qualifications, which can make for rivalry between the different disciplines. An individual may be an excellent health professional but have little or no administrative skills but, because of their seniority, may have leadership responsibilities. Decisions they make may not always be the right or popular ones.

A growing concern emerging in healthcare, and particularly in the nursing literature, is the issue of horizontal violence or bullying, sometimes called lateral violence. Though horizontal violence takes many forms, one of its common characteristics includes 'overt and covert non physical hostility' (Roy 2007). Such communication from one or more people towards an individual can be disrespectful, offensive or undermining, leading to feelings of helplessness, humiliation and being harassed or bullied. One group highlighted as frequently, but not exclusively, exposed to horizontal violence are new nursing graduates (Roy 2007), though the problem can manifest between any team members irrespective of gender, age, experience or discipline.

In the light of this issue and the others above, it is important to consider ways of dealing with challenging situations or trying to avoid them happening, and to promote better communication between all staff levels. Various ways of sharing decision making and promoting consultation are to be encouraged within organisations and teams. This should include ensuring there is provision for down–up as well as up–down communication between all areas of the hierarchy through regular meetings and social contact. Another way of enhancing staff-to-staff communication and providing for professional growth and development is to encourage and provide clinical supervision, support and mentoring. And finally, ideally, any organisation should also have a good mix of staff from a variety of cultural and ethnic backgrounds.

Client education

Although much of a health professional's time centres on treatment, an important role in working with clients is that of providing information and health promotion to individuals and groups. Apart from professionals who work full time in health promotion, many health professionals may think their role in client education is limited to handing out a booklet or showing a DVD to a client before they are discharged. However, with increasingly short lengths of stay in hospital and people being more knowledgeable about health matters, it is an area of increasing importance in clinical practice and research. In spite of this, there is frequently little time allowed for this significant aspect of care (Leino-Kilpi et al 2005).

Various professional bodies emphasise the importance of educating clients about their health status. For example, the Australian Physiotherapy Council (APC) includes in its standards the importance of providing education to clients (APC 2008). For Australian nurses, client education is a core competency (Australian Nursing and Midwifery Council (ANMC) 2006). Education is important in helping clients gain knowledge and, therefore, empowerment in managing their problem (Chang & Kelly 2007). It will depend on whether a health professional is working in the community or in a hospital setting as to the approach taken. A healthcare worker in the community may work with individuals, groups, families or carers implementing planned and programmed education sessions, whereas in the hospital setting you are more likely to work with the individual client and their particular needs.

So what are the communication skills needed for successful client education? According to Chang and Kelly (2007), any education must be based on sound approaches with proper understanding of clients' requirements and ability and motivation to learn, including aspects of culture and literacy. You can first find out what the client already knows by asking questions such as, 'What do you think is going on?' and then move towards questions that address the gaps. It is useful to predict questions the client may ask or information they might wish to know. Questions such as, 'What will happen to me?', 'Will it be painful?' and 'When will I know the results?' are common to many areas in healthcare practice. Effective education takes time and patience on the part of health professionals. The skills of active listening once again become extremely important. The client may be anxious or fearful and unable to process any information being said, therefore the health professional will need to identify the cues to respond appropriately, whether it is a matter of reassuring the person's uncertainties or expanding their knowledge regarding the health issue. In such circumstances it can be helpful to also provide written information for the client. In other words, once the cognitive, behavioural and emotional needs of the client have been addressed and understanding is clear to all involved parties, then you can feel confident the client has learnt something. In this context not only has education occurred but also PCC.

Advocacy

The healthcare literature defines advocacy as protecting and promoting the rights of people who may be vulnerable and incapable of protecting their own interests, and though this is true it can also be argued that it has several dimensions from legal and ethical obligations to philosophical debates about the foundations of healthcare practice. For instance, it may be as straightforward as a professional representing a client by speaking to a senior health professional on behalf of a client who is too anxious to ask questions or unable to speak for themselves (Benner et al 2010). However, it may also mean different things, from counsellor to 'whistleblower' (a person who publicly exposes unsafe or illegal practices).

For the purpose of this chapter, we are interested in the more specific qualities and skills of being an advocate that enable health professionals to assure people in their care that they are the recipient of quality care, whether for the purpose of changing policy and legislation, accessing relevant health and social care information or supporting a person's decision making (Health Consumers Queensland 2010).

Various codes of conduct and professional standards underline the importance of advocacy when working with clients (Baldwin 2003). In her analysis of nursing literature Baldwin (2003) found that advocacy had three qualities: a therapeutic health professional–client relationship; the promotion and protection of the client's involvement in making decisions and informed consent; and being a mediator between clients and relatives or friends and healthcare providers, with communication being central to each. Therefore, for a health professional to act as a client advocate they must possess the skills and attributes needed for effective communication. Otherwise, how else can they ensure the client is in the position to make informed decisions about their care? The most common features of communication in the role of client advocate include the ability to involve people in all aspects of their own healthcare by listening, respecting, responding, sharing and supporting people's contributions, including their right to decline treatments (ANMC 2006, Nursing Midwifery Council (NMC) 2008).

In recognising the need for advocacy, you should also recognise that conflict may occur on some occasions. For example, possible disagreement within the team regarding a client's management plan, or the decisions made by the client and their family that conflict with those of the healthcare team may lead to differences of opinions emerging. It is essential at times like these for each party to define the area of disagreement in a safe manner and address any concerns. It may be that a resolution cannot be found but discussing the issue openly can go some way to at least helping understand each other's perspective. Remember, in such situations it is the health professional's responsibility to always keep the client's and family's best interests in mind rather than their own, while considering the consequences of how far you as a health professional might wish to take the issue.

Multidisciplinary teams

As a health professional, you may find yourself in a variety of healthcare settings, ranging from large institutions where communication passes down a hierarchy from an administration that has little to do with the everyday life of health professionals, to small teams where there may be a team leader who encourages shared or individual decision making. Up until now the chapter has focused mainly on the one-to-one relationship between a health professional and client. Yet healthcare frequently involves teamwork, requiring professionals to work effectively with each other using good communication and interpersonal skills. Having clear team communication processes enhances not only the team functioning but also an individual member's commitment to the team and its goals. However, this is not always an easy process. Teams do not suddenly start to work well together. They need to develop, grow and mature. The team dynamics will constantly change as new staff arrive and established members leave. As in any group of humans spending time together, the dynamics are often complicated, with potential for problems to arise, particularly in relation to communication between members. The more members there are in a team, the more opportunity for misunderstandings and errors being made in communication. In healthcare this can quite literally be a matter of life and death therefore the need for effective communication is critical.

Many of the problems in communication within a healthcare setting occur due to a breakdown in the listening process. Hearing and listening are distinctly different. Though a team member may hear what is being said, to truly listen requires that person to actively attend, interpret, evaluate and respond to both the verbal and non-verbal message being relayed. As previously discussed in this chapter, the use of active listening skills is important to let the sender know you are listening and understand everything being said. Repetition, clarification, paraphrasing and reflection are essential skills whether you are working with one individual or a team.

TeamSTEPPS is one of many team training programs offering structured communication tools to improve interpersonal communication between health professionals. It recommends various mnemonics to aid the communication process between team members. One such mnemonic is SBAR, which can deliver clear communication about a client's condition in a concise manner to other health professionals. SBAR stands for (TeamSTEPPS 2006):

- Situation – what is happening to the client?
- Background – what is the clinical background?
- Assessment – what do I think the problem is?
- Recommendation – what would I recommend?

Additional factors may also influence the ability to work and communicate as part of a health team. With the challenge of increased workloads, staff shortages, and the urgency of completing tasks or making decisions within a certain timeframe impacting on health professionals on a frequent if not daily basis, your ability to communicate effectively may become compromised. You may also be distracted by the tasks that need to be completed, begin to suffer stress-related behaviour, begin to question personal issues in terms of your own life and its meaning, or develop a sense of depersonalisation for both clients and staff. For example, the question: 'Are the pathology results back for bed 16?' treats the client as an object, not a person. All these factors contribute to poor communication and to treatment regimes that become focused on achieving completion of treatment in the time allowed, rather than on the client's needs.

Critical thinking

Are you part of any decision making in clinical practice? With whom? How do you find it? What's helpful, what hinders this process?

Think about a time when an important decision had to be made in your work environment regarding a client.

- Were all health professionals in the team involved in the decision? When planning beforehand and defining roles etc., who ultimately had the last word?
- Was there open communication between all members of the team in making decisions?

Conclusion

Communication is a fundamental aspect of the health professional–client relationship. As a health professional, whether introducing yourself, assessing clients or working with them to achieve treatment or educational goals, combining effective communication skills with clinical skills and knowledge can help facilitate positive working relationships between you and your client. Furthermore, an efficient multidisciplinary healthcare team requires effective communication between its members. In summary, good communication skills are an essential part of being a competent health professional.

> **REMEMBER**
>
> - Communication is a fundamental component of the relationship between health professionals and clients.
> - Maintaining ethical obligations related to communication is necessary when developing and maintaining a professional relationship.
> - Situation variables influence the quality and type of communication.
> - Language and culture play an important role in the communication process.
> - Multidisciplinary teamwork is an important aspect of healthcare delivery.
> - Client education facilitates self-management of health problems.
> - Client advocacy promotes the rights of vulnerable people.

Further resources

Bach, S., Grant, A., 2009. Communication and interpersonal skills for nurses. Transforming Nursing Practice. Learning Matters, Exeter.

Casey, A., Wallis, A., 2011. Effective communication: principles of nursing practice. Nursing Standard 25 (32), 35–37.

Eubanks, R.L., McFarland, M.R., 2010. Chapter 4: Cross-cultural communication. Journal of Transcultural Nursing 21 (4), 137–150.

Malloy, P., Virani, R., Kelly, K., et al., 2010. Beyond bad news: communication skills of nurses in palliative care. Journal of Hospice and Palliative Nursing 12, 166–174.

McCray, J., 2009. Preparing for multi-professional practice. In: McCray, J. (Ed.), Nursing and multi-professional practice. Sage, London.

McLean, M., Cleland, J., Worrell, M., et al., 2011. 'What am I going to say here?' The experiences of doctors and nurses communicating with patients in a cancer unit. Frontiers in Psychology 2 (339), 1–7.

Milan, F.B., Parish, S.J., Reichgott, M.J., 2006. Model for educational feedback based on clinical communication skills strategies: beyond the 'feedback sandwich'. Teaching and Learning in Medicine 18 (1), 42–47.

National Health and Medical Research Council, 2005. Cultural competency in health: a guide for policy, partnerships and participation. NHMRC, Canberra.

Rosenberg, S., Gallo-Silver, L., 2011. Therapeutic communication skills and student nurses in the clinical setting. Teaching and Learning in Nursing 6 (1), 2–8.

Shuang, L., Volvic, Z., Gallois, C., 2011. Introducing intercultural communication: global cultures and contexts. Sage, London.

TeamSTEPPS Clinical Handover Pilot Study, 2009. Safety and Quality Unit, Department of Health South Australia. Online. Available: http://www.safetyandquality.gov.au/wp-content/uploads/2012/01/TeamSTEPPS.pdf.

Villagran, M., Goldsmith, J., Wittenberg-Lyles, E., et al., 2010. Communicating COMFORT: a communication-based model for breaking bad news in health care interactions. Communication Education 59, 220–234.

Webb, L., 2011. Nursing: communication skills in practice. Oxford University Press, Oxford.

Weblinks

Communication for health in emergency contexts

www.chec.meu.medicine.unimelb.edu.au/resources/index.html

This site provides scenarios and information specifically related to an emergency department.

Communication skills for health professionals

www.oscehome.com/Communication-Skills

This site provides information to improve communication skills particularly related to client interviews.

Cultural connections for learning

www.intstudentsup.org/diversity/resources

This site provides international students and clinical staff valuable resources to promote resilience and effective working in the healthcare workforce.

Diversity RX

www.diversityrx.org

This website lists important issues in cross-cultural communication to promote cultural competence.

Introduction to communication skills

http://www.oup.com/uk/orc/bin/9780199582723/webb_ch01.pdf

This site, by Lucy Webb, provides a useful resource to understand the underpinning theories of communication.

Practical clinical skills

www.clinicalskillscentre.ac.uk

http://au.youtube.com/watch?v=22ckNruSnmg

These two sites have interesting written information, as well as numerous videos of healthcare students practising various clinical skills, including communication scenarios. The first is the general website, the second leads more specifically into communication skills.

Royal College of Surgeons (UK)

http://www.intercollegiatemrcs.org.uk/pdf/comms_guidance.pdf

This website contains the instructions for candidates for the Royal College of Surgeons' communication exam. It provides a good opportunity to view a variety of possible scenarios and issues that are important for beginning health professionals to consider.

Therapeutic communication skills

http://au.youtube.com/watch?v=xpFkrD02t1A&feature=related.

This video discusses the elements of basic communication and demonstrates various therapeutic communication skills.

References

ACT Health, 2012. Health information for professionals: cultural safety. Online. Available: http://www.health.act.gov.au/professionals/student-clinical-placements/cultural-safety 13 Jan 2012.

Australian Nursing and Midwifery Council (ANMC), 2006. National competency standards for the registered nurse. Online. Available: www.anmc.org.au 18 Jun 2012.

Australian Physiotherapy Council (APC), 2008. Australian standards for physiotherapy. Online. Available: http://www.physiocouncil.com.au/australian_standards_for_physiotherapy 18 Jun 2012.

Baldwin, M., 2003. Patient advocacy: a concept analysis. Nursing Standard 17 (21), 33–39.

Balzer Riley, J., 2011. Communication in nursing, seventh ed. Mosby, St Louis.

Benner, P., Sutphen, M., Leonard, V., et al., 2010. Educating nurses: a call for radical transformation. Jossey-Bass, San Francisco.

Bertakis, K.D., Franks, P., Epstein, R.M., 2009. Patient-centered communication in primary care: physician and patient gender and gender concordance. Journal of Women's Health 18 (4), 539–545.

Blonna, R., Loschiavo, J., Watter, D., 2011. Health counseling: a microskills approach for counselors, educators, and school nurses, second ed. Jones and Bartlett, Burlington.

Boudreaux, E.D., Friedman, J., Chansky, M.E., et al., 2004. Emergency department patient satisfaction: examining the role of acuity. Academic Emergency Medicine 11, 162–168.

Cass, A., Lowell, A., Christie, M., et al., 2002. Sharing true stories: improving communication between Aboriginal patients and healthcare workers. The Medical Journal of Australia 176 (10), 466–470.

Chang, M., Kelly, A.E., 2007. Patient education: addressing cultural diversity and health literacy issues. Urology Nursing 27 (5), 411–417.

Chochinov, H., 2007. Dignity and the essence of medicine: the A, B, C, and D of dignity conserving care. British Medical Journal 335, 184–187.

Coulehan, K., Brown, I., Christie, M., et al., 2005. Sharing the true stories. Evaluating strategies to improve communication between health staff and Aboriginal patients, Stage 2 report. Cooperative Research Centre for Aboriginal Health, Darwin.

Di Blasi, Z., Harkness, E., Ernst, E., et al., 2001. Influence of context effects on health outcomes: a systematic review. The Lancet 357 (9258), 757–762.

Duncan, P., 2009. Values, ethics and healthcare. Sage, Thousand Oaks.

Egan, G., 2010. The skilled helper: a problem-management and opportunity-development approach to helping, ninth ed. Thompson Brooks/Cole, Belmont.

Health Consumers Queensland, 2010. Health advocacy framework. Queensland Health, Brisbane.

Ivey, A.E., Ivey, M.B., Zalaquett, C.P., 2010. Intentional interviewing and counseling: facilitating client development in a multicultural society, seventh ed. Brooks/Cole, Cengage Learning, Belmont.

Kiesling, S., Bratt Paulson, C. (Eds.), 2004. Intercultural discourse and communication. Cambridge University Press, Cambridge.

Lawrence, M., Dodd, Z., Mohor, S., et al., 2009. Improving the patient journey: achieving positive outcomes for remote Aboriginal cardiac patients. Cooperative Research Centre for Aboriginal Health, Darwin.

Leino-Kilpi, H., Johanasson, K., Heikkinen, K., et al., 2005. Patient education and health-related quality of life: surgical hospital patients as a case in point. Journal of Nursing Care Quality 20 (4), 307–331.

Levinson, W., 2011. Patient-centred communication: a sophisticated procedure. British Medical Journal – Quality and Safety 20 (10), 823–825.

Maguire, P., Pitceathly, C., 2002. Key communication skills and how to acquire them. British Medical Journal 325 (7366), 697–700.

Nelson, S., Gordon, G., 2006. The complexities of care. ILR Press, Ithaca.

Nursing Midwifery Council (NMC), 2008. The code: standards of conduct, performance and ethics for nurses and midwives. Online. Available: http://www.nmc-uk.org/Publications-/Standards1 18 Jun 2012.

Otto, B., 2006. Language development in early childhood. Pearson Education, Upper Saddle River.

Ramsden, I.M., 2002. Cultural safety and nursing education in Aotearoa and Te Waipounamu. Unpublished PhD thesis, Victoria University of Wellington. Online. Available: www.culturalsafety.massey.ac.nz, 19 Feb 2008.

Rogers, C., 1961. On becoming a person. Houghton Mifflin, Boston.

Rogers, C., 1987. Comments on the issue of equality in psychotherapy. Journal of Humanistic Psychology 27 (1), 38–39.

Roy, J., 2007. Horizontal violence. ADVANCE for Nurses. Online. Available: http://nursing.advanceweb.com/editorial/content/editorial.aspx?cc=102740 Jun 2012.

Stein-Parbury, J.M., 2009. Patient and person: developing interpersonal skills in nursing, fourth ed. Elsevier, Sydney.

TeamSTEPPS, 2006. Pocket guide. Team strategies and tools to enhance performance and patient safety. Agency for Healthcare Research and Quality, Rockville.

The Joint Commission, 2010. Advancing effective communication, cultural competence, and patient- and family-centered care: a roadmap for hospitals. The Joint Commission, Oakbrook Terrace.

Toma, G., Triner, W., McNutt, L.A., 2009. Patient satisfaction as a function of emergency department previsit expectations. Annals Emergency Medicine 54 (3), 360–367.

Venetis, M.K., Robinson, J.D., Turkiewitz, K.L., et al., 2009. An evidence base for patient-centered cancer care: a meta analysis of studies of observed communication between cancer specialists and their patients. Patient Education Counselling 77, 379–383.

Watson, J., 2008. The philosophy and science of caring, revised ed. University Press of Colorado, Boulder.

Chapter 9
Partnerships in health

DEB O'KANE

Learning objectives

The material in this chapter will help you to:

- understand the dynamics of health professional–client partnerships
- understand the issues in client engagement with treatment
- appreciate the importance of involving clients in their own care
- gain insight into differences in treatment expectations between health professionals from different cultural backgrounds
- understand how effective partnerships impact on working with people who have chronic illness, disability or complex health issues
- appreciate the interplay between clients' and health professionals' attitudes and backgrounds in the clinical setting and the influence of these and environmental factors on successful treatment outcomes.

Key terms

- Partnership
- Compliance, concordance and adherence
- Client-centred practice
- Empathy
- Recovery
- Biomedical
- Chronic illness
- Health locus of control
- Collaborative practice

Introduction

The title of this chapter takes for granted the fact that the health professional–client relationship requires involvement of at least two people. Those two people may encounter each other in a variety of settings: in a busy acute surgical ward; in an outpatient or emergency department; in the client's own home or practice rooms; in a community health centre; or in an ambulance to give only some examples. Whatever the setting, something is happening: an encounter between two human beings, both with varying agendas, needs, attitudes and feelings.

As already discussed in Chapter 8, communication is essential to establish and maintain personal and professional relationships, from our own family and friends to the colleagues we work with or clients and families in our care. In clinical practice, it remains the responsibility of health professionals to initiate and maintain a working relationship with their clients and team members. This may prove to be easy or challenging. Not all clients are good communicators and some may exhibit challenging behaviours. However, whatever the client's personal qualities are, it is important to think about how you approach interactions with clients and what your own motivations and goals are. These are factors health professionals have control of and are responsible for.

Person-centred communication goes some way to thinking about how an alliance can be established with the people we work with and care for, but as well as being a relationship between two people, the relationship also needs to be seen as a partnership. The term partnership in healthcare is often used to reinforce the concept of a relationship where health professionals and clients both share some degree of responsibility for the treatment decisions, implementation and outcomes. However, partnerships similarly can occur across multiple sectors and include a variety of people, disciplines and organisations, all with a clear purpose or goal in mind. A partnership such as this brings together a diverse range of skills and resources, offering more opportunities to impact on health issues such as chronic illness, health prevention, health promotion and education. The following considers some of the implications in such partnerships.

Fostering partnerships

It is first beneficial to examine the language used for the people being cared for within a healthcare setting as this demonstrates how language and the power of language can influence partnerships. Historically when someone is a recipient of a health service, whether in the public or private sector, inpatient or community, they are generally known as a 'patient'. However, recently a wider variety of terms have been used in various fields of healthcare such as 'client', 'service user' or 'consumer', with the aim of trying to identify and express the relationship between the parties involved. Rusch et al (2005) argue that it is an innate human quality to place labels on people, not only in healthcare but to a population at large if there are easily recognisable traits, behaviours or characteristics to distinguish particular groups of people such as skin colour or clothes that identify someone's affinity with a particular music style. The term or label we use to describe a person can invoke different perceptions, attitudes and behaviours towards that person.

While labels can serve a purpose when they provide us with generic information about a person or population, such as people with chronic fatigue syndrome, labels are problematic when they are used to stereotype people such as 'frequent flyers' or 'drug addict'. The label is very powerful in that the use of one word can not only identify the recipient of care but also the relationship and possible power dynamics (McLaughlin 2009). Language influences the very nature of how health professionals establish and maintain a professional relationship due to the assumptions we make from the terms we use (McDonald 2006). For example, the different terms used over a number of years to refer to people who receive mental healthcare has long been in the literature, with little agreement on the particular term used nationally or internationally. Australians tend to use the term 'consumer' while Britons use the term 'service user'. Each term, though different, has the same underlying value; that is, for the person to feel empowered rather than stigmatised and to ultimately have an impact on care delivery.

PERCEPTION IS REALITY

On a similar note, how a health professional describes a person's contribution to their own health needs can affect how people perceive that person. Much of the literature concerned with health professional–client communication issues focuses on getting the client to cooperate with the health professional's treatment goals or compliance (Zolnierek & Dimatteo 2009). The word compliance seems to be used without consideration of how it might shape health professionals' attitudes to relationships with clients. If an individual is not willing or able to do what is requested of them at a particular time, they may be described, both verbally and in their client records, as noncompliant. The problem with this is that such a descriptor can frequently be taken up by other healthcare team workers, often without any thought or questioning of its origins.

The danger is the strong possibility that a client may then be perceived as such for the rest of their treatment history. It can then become a self-fulfilling prophecy, where other health professionals expect a person to have a particular attitude to treatment and relate to them in such a way that leads the client to demonstrate that attitude. Possibly, some health professionals may describe a client as noncompliant because they present a challenge of some sort, usually to do with not wishing to accept a particular form of treatment that has been prescribed for them. Sometimes it might be as straightforward as the client having very little English and not understanding what the health professional is expecting of them; it may be a well-educated person who simply questions what is being done to them; or it might also be a client who refuses to accept any kind of treatment.

TERMINOLOGY

The term *compliance* itself has been criticised because of its paternalistic or even coercive implication that all medical advice or treatments should be followed without question. Often health professionals can be quick to assume a client is being uncooperative or disobedient if they choose not to follow the recommended treatment regimen (Horne et al 2005, Horne 2006). This noncompliance, however, may at times be unintentional such as a person with significant memory problems who frequently forgets to take their medication or it may be as simple as a person being unable to afford the prescribed treatments. On the other hand, the client may intentionally be noncompliant due to their health beliefs or concerns about side effects, for example, a client who decides to stop taking their steroid medication due to weight gain.

An alternative term *adherence* has since been introduced into the healthcare literature, aiming to signify a stronger implication of choice by a client, that is, having the opportunity to decide whether to adhere to the recommended treatment or advice. However, it is debatable as to whether this is an improvement; for instance, adherence also has the implication of following rules or direction. Both compliance and adherence focus on the client's behaviour in following treatment regimens, whereas in the United Kingdom, the term *concordance* has recently been used with the purpose of defining the relationship, rather than the behaviour between a health professional and a client. It is based on collaboration and respect for each other's contributions (Horne 2006). Despite the various labels, it could be argued that it is better for none of them to be used, but instead to simply describe the client's behaviour as part of a partnership between a health professional and a recipient of care, with the emphasis on the engagement process.

Person-centred practice

Person-centred practice (PCP) is not a new concept and though significantly different to the health-professional-led biomedical model, it has been in the literature for many years exerting significant influence on policy, practice and delivery of care. Definitions vary between identifying the elements needed for individualised client care, while others look at it from an organisational perspective in order to provide best possible care. Either way at the heart of PCP is the person receiving care. It provides a model of care based on mutually beneficial partnerships among healthcare providers, clients and families, and is the foundation from which patient-centred communication stems (Ch 8). In PCP attention is paid to all elements of the person (the 'whole'), taking into account the wider context of the person's lifestyle such as those social, environmental and psychological factors that may contribute to the assessment and management of the health issue. Collaboration, therapeutic alliance, sharing power and responsibility for decision making, and the freedom of choice and autonomy, become central to the delivery of care (Department of Human Services 2006, 2008) and require commitment and considerable effort on the part of health professionals and organisations. In Australia and New Zealand many healthcare organisations have started to encourage clients, particularly those with a chronic illness, to adopt personalised care plans or self-management plans. These offer an opportunity for health professionals to collaborate with clients and develop a formal written record that respects the client's opinions in relation to their care so that control and ownership is held by the client rather than the professional.

A successful partnership between a health professional and client can go a long way to achieve PCP yet several barriers are often cited as reasons for being unable to establish the partnership or deliver PCP. The literature shows time constraints, lack of resources, differing agendas, organisational constraints and a belief they 'know best' as reasons for health professionals being unable to deliver PCP (Rabinowitz et al 2004, van Weel-Baumgarten 2010). Although some of these may seem inevitable, particularly in light of the increasing pressure to undertake the growing number of tasks, paperwork and staff shortages, you need to question if this is truly saving time and money in the longer term when evidence suggests there is a negative impact on the health outcomes including engagement in treatment regimens, pain management and client and carer satisfaction (Venetis et al 2009). While acknowledging these barriers, as a health professional there are several features of establishing a partnership that can be undertaken in practice to support PCP. McCormack (2001) identifies these as:

- getting close to the person
- providing care that is consistent with the person's values
- taking a biographical approach to assessment
- focusing on ability rather than dependency.

CASE STUDY: PATRICK

Patrick is a 19-year-old male who has recently been diagnosed with schizophrenia after a short period of hospitalisation for an acute psychotic episode. One nurse has informed him that it is highly likely he will need to take neuroleptic medications for the rest of his life. This has greatly upset him because he has found he has an increased appetite and therefore put on weight as a side effect of the medication. He describes feeling helpless and unable to see a future while living with his illness. His weight is a major issue for him because he believes it will reduce his chances of finding employment in the hospitality industry and affect his chances of finding a girlfriend.

Classroom activity

In small groups discuss:

1. As a health professional listening to Patrick, how would you respond?
2. What could you do to demonstrate PCP?
3. How could the core principles of recovery-oriented care (see below) be applied to this situation?

Recovery

As healthcare moves away from an exclusive biomedical-focused model, and embraces psychosocial aspects of care, healthcare services similarly have begun the process of examining how they deliver fundamental services. Parallel with the PCP philosophy of care is the concept of a recovery-oriented health system, which can have major implications on care delivery.

The concept of 'recovery' in health usually has an emphasis on regaining or restoring something that has been lost. For example, we often describe people as recovered after a bout of illness, implying they have regained their full strength and returned to the state of being healthy once more. But this is a limited understanding. What happens to the person who as a consequence of trauma loses a limb or the person who is diagnosed with type 1 diabetes? Some of these issues have already been discussed in previous chapters when exploring the concept of 'health', and whether people who have not returned to a previous health status are now not 'healthy'? For each individual, recovery will be a different personal experience. If we accept there are other dimensions of health then the notion of recovery likewise should support internal and external factors that may contribute to a person's journey of recovery.

Since the 1980s when people with a lived experience of mental illness began to challenge the biomedical driven model of care, the concept of recovery-oriented health has grown remarkably to the point that it now guides and underpins all mental health reform in policy and practice (Commonwealth of Australia 2009, New Zealand Ministry of Health 2005, Shepherd et al 2008). In the mental health context recovery refers to a person being able to live a full and meaningful life, despite having an ongoing mental illness. It embraces notions of hope and setting goals for the future – not just symptom management. For health professionals, working in a recovery framework involves not just working with a consumer to manage the symptoms of their mental illness, but also working with the person to enable them to live a fulfilling life (Muir-Cochrane et al 2010). However, it should not be thought of as a philosophy of care for mental health practice only. The guiding principles of recovery-oriented healthcare are universal and can be applied to a range of healthcare settings, particularly in chronic illness where the person plays a significant role in managing their illness.

RECOVERY PRINCIPLES

The principles of recovery in healthcare are not difficult to understand, though the reality of its implementation may prove more difficult in a biomedically driven healthcare system. The philosophy of recovery encompasses a range of factors that require individual, organisational and systematic change. Therefore, rather than a model in its own right, recovery should be seen as a flexible process or framework to guide health professionals in their practice. While recovery from illness and/or disability continues to be perceived as synonymous with cure or symptom relief, then those elements that also contribute to a person's health, including personal, social, vocational, family and education, become largely ignored. These elements, alongside others such as service provision, access/funding, human rights and social inclusion, can all have an impact or be affected as a consequence of illness or poor health. It is therefore important that they are not pushed aside when we consider a person's journey to recovery. Collectively, these factors constitute an individual's 'lived experience' of recovery and are the foundation to guide health professionals in delivering care to support someone to understand and come to terms with their illness. People who have experienced chronic mental illness often describe their recovery in terms of having the ability to live a satisfying and meaningful life despite their serious illness or the lasting effects the illness may have on them.

RECOVERY-ORIENTED PRINCIPLES

The past decade has seen a growing international body of literature from researchers, service providers, clinicians and service users that has developed, refined and operationalised the concept of recovery-oriented healthcare in an attempt to find commonalities that can be used to facilitate and promote recovery-oriented care in different healthcare systems. In terms of what can be done as a health professional, if the aim of recovery is for people with chronic illness or disability to develop new meaning and purpose in their lives, not just the alleviation of symptoms, then it is up to health professionals to assist in this process by developing and maintaining a collaborative partnership not just with the identified client. Family, carers, teams or agencies may need to be involved in different aspects of care and resource provision. From listening to people's stories of how they accepted and overcame the challenges of their illness or disability, several key facilitators have been identified as underpinning the philosophy of recovery and supporting clients in their journey. These include taking control of one's life through hope, empowerment, support, education, medication management, spirituality, choice, advocacy and autonomy to name a few (Davidson 2008, Deegan 1996, Mental Health Coordinating Council 2008, Roberts & Wolfson 2004, Shepherd et al 2008). Health professionals can work towards supporting a person with their health issue by helping them identify their strengths and the protective factors that promote recovery rather than focus on the changes, limitations and losses that may have occurred as a result of the illness or disability.

Shepherd (2007) provides '10 top tips' for recovery-oriented practice in mental health that could easily be applied in other healthcare settings. See Box 9.1 for how Shepherd's tips can be applied to general health issues.

Adapted from Shepherd G. 2007 Specification for a comprehensive 'Rehabilitation and Recovery' service in Herefordshire. Hereford PCT Mental Health Services. Available at www. herefordshire.nhs.uk (last accessed 10th January, 2012).

Box 9.1 '10 top tips' for recovery-oriented practice

After each interaction, the health professional should ask, did I...?

1. Actively listen to help the person to make sense of their health problems?
2. Help the person identify and prioritise their personal goals for recovery – not professional goals?
3. Demonstrate a belief in the person's existing strengths and resources in relation to the pursuit of these goals?
4. Identify stories of individuals' experiences of illness, which inspire and validate hope? (be aware, though, of confidentiality when telling another client's story and, if you recount a story of your own, be mindful of whose interests are served in telling the story i.e. the client's not your own).

Cont... ▶

5. Pay particular attention to the importance of goals that take the person out of the 'sick role' and enable them to actively contribute to the lives of others?

6. Identify non-health resources – friends, contacts, organisations – relevant to the achievement of their goals?

7. Encourage self-management of health problems (by providing information, reinforcing existing coping strategies, etc)?

8. Discuss what the person wants in terms of therapeutic interventions such as biomedical and psychological treatments, alternative therapies and joint crisis planning, respecting their wishes wherever possible?

9. Behave at all times so as to convey an attitude of respect for the person and a desire for an equal partnership in working together, indicating a willingness to 'go the extra mile'?

10. While accepting that the future is uncertain and setbacks will happen, continue to express support for the possibility of achieving these self-defined goals – maintaining hope and positive expectations?

Table 9.1 illustrates the many similarities between the philosophy of recovery and that of PCP. Ultimately the partnership established between the person receiving a healthcare service and the health professional delivering it is based on the premise that the recipient of care knows themselves better than anyone else and hence is an 'expert by experience' (Roberts & Wolfson 2004). The health professional while acknowledging and valuing the person's contributions, can offer advice and guidance via their own knowledge and experience gained through professional training to help support the person in managing their own healthcare needs (Roberts & Wolfson 2004).

If you think about the role of a health professional working with someone who has type 1 diabetes, the partnership would incorporate advice on exercise, dietary intake, medication management/administration, support groups and education regarding risk factors related to the illness. However, you need to remember that not everybody will require the same amount of support and guidance; for instance, a 19-year-old newly diagnosed person with diabetes may want very different things from the partnership compared with a 55-year-old who has managed their diabetes over a number of years. The partnership, therefore, initially needs to establish the goals for each party through an open and trustworthy relationship based on transparency and respect for each other's contributions.

Chronic illness, disability and complex health issues

Chronic illness has become a leading cause for concern worldwide, accounting for 60% of deaths, particularly in low–middle income countries (World Health Organization (WHO) 2011). Marmot and Wilkinson (2006) note several underlying risk factors such as poverty and inequality, poor nutrition, inadequate environmental health conditions, physical inactivity, alcohol misuse and tobacco smoking that are

Table 9.1

COMPARABLE PRINCIPLES IN RECOVERY-ORIENTED PRACTICE AND PERSON-CENTRED CARE

Recovery-oriented practice	Person-centred care
Recovery is fundamentally about a set of values related to human living applied to the pursuit of health and wellness.	A value base that asserts the absolute value of all human lives regardless of age or cognitive ability.
The helping relationship between clinicians and clients moves away from being expert–patient to clinicians being 'coaches' or 'partners' on an individual's journey of discovery.	The need to move beyond a focus on technical competence and to engage in authentic humanistic caring practices that embrace all forms of knowing and acting, to promote choice and partnership in care decision making.
Recovery is closely associated with social inclusion and being able to take on meaningful and satisfying roles in society.	Provides an enriched environment that can foster opportunities for personal growth.
People do not recover in isolation. Family and other supporters are often crucial to recovery and should be included as partners wherever possible.	Recognises that all human life is grounded in relationships.
Recovery approaches give positive value to cultural, religious, sexual and other forms of diversity as resources and supports for wellbeing and identity.	An individualised approach – valuing uniqueness. Accepting differences in culture, gender, temperament, lifestyle, outlook, beliefs, values, commitments, taste and interests.

From Hill L, Roberts G, Wildgoose J, Perkins R & Hahn S 2010 Recovery and person-centred care in dementia: common purpose, common practice? Advances in psychiatric treatment Vol. 16, p.288–298

Classroom activity

In small groups:

1. Using the 10 top tips identified by Shepherd (2007), identify other areas of healthcare practice in which tips could be utilised when working with a client diagnosed with:
   - juvenile arthritis
   - chronic obstructive pulmonary disease (COPD)
   - Alzheimer's disease
   - type 2 diabetes mellitus
   - motor neurone disease.
2. How would the client benefit?
3. How do you foresee yourself using these tips in daily practise?

common throughout the world. Such lifestyle-related risk factors can greatly contribute to the poor outcome of chronic illness and to the overall burden of chronic disease in today's society.

The costs of delivering healthcare for health problems that are often preventable is making the issue a forerunner in debate, policy and practice. With a predicted ageing population, a decrease in mortality and advanced practice regimens extending life expectancy (Australian Institute of Health and Welfare (AIHW) 2011) there seems little expectation that things will change, particularly in light of costs expected to continue rising and concern about how healthcare services will manage these escalating figures.

Chronic illness remains complex and difficult to define though commonly refers to any illness or disability that a person may endure permanently or over a prolonged period of time. There is a significant number of conditions that can be termed chronic, with coronary heart disease, stroke, lung cancer, colorectal cancer, depression, type 2 diabetes, arthritis, osteoporosis, asthma, COPD, chronic kidney disease and oral disease identified as major concerns for the Australian healthcare system (National Health Priority Action Council 2006). Other conditions include epilepsy, fibromyalgia, other cancers, chronic fatigue syndrome, hypertension and multiple sclerosis. Some chronic conditions deteriorate over time (e.g. Alzheimer's disease), while others such as cancer may have periods of remission. It may be that some people make a complete recovery where as for others death is an inevitable outcome. The AIHW (2011) characterises a chronic illness by the following:

- complex causality
- multiple risk factors
- long latency periods
- a prolonged course of illness
- functional impairment or disability (AIHW 2011).

In any of these given situations it can be true to say having a chronic illness will certainly have a lasting effect on the person's quality of life, affecting the emotional, physical, psychological and behavioural aspects of their daily living.

In health psychology, understanding how the biological, behavioural and social factors can influence chronic illness allows us to explore the human dimension of how a person lives with the chronic health issue and how this may influence their health behaviour and the behaviour of those around them. Larson (2011) describes this as how the illness is 'perceived, lived with and responded to by others'. She goes on to say that as health professionals, you shouldn't necessarily think about disability only in terms of severity or physical deterioration but to also think about disability and how it can be affected due to an individual's perception of the illness. The implications of how much a person's lifestyle is altered are very much related to their own understanding and health beliefs about the onset of the illness, its treatment and the outcomes (Larson 2011). As already identified there are numerous biological, psychological, social and environmental risks associated with chronic illness, but with the appropriate behavioural strategies implemented prior to the onset of problems being evident, these illnesses can be prevented. Areas to be targeted in health promotion, prevention and education include exercise, nutrition, cessation of smoking and alcohol moderation to name a few (see also Ch 13). Alongside these preventative support mechanisms the access to resources also needs to be improved if we hope to see any tangible long-term impact of enhancing a person's health and reducing the pressure on the health system.

Factors influencing partnerships

People with an existing chronic illness or disability can offer valuable insights into how the illness has affected them and how they best manage their health issue; therefore, as part of a partnership it is important to listen to the person as an expert in their own healthcare. That being said there are a variety of reasons why at least 50% of clients do not carry through with treatment prescribed for them. These include: side effects and costs; treatment difficulties; fatalism or resistance to control; forgetting to take medication; and little external support (Coulter 2011). For example, when the symptoms begin to subside they may see no need to complete their medication, or they cease because there may be no sign of improvement; they may decide that if a little works then a lot will be even better; or if suffering from a chronic illness, a client may tire of taking medication or other treatment. Sometimes when the client refuses, health professionals may see him or her as a problem client (i.e. someone who does not passively accept treatment), as uncooperative or constantly complaining, perceiving the client negatively without attempting to understand why it is happening by listening to the person's expertise in their own lived experience of the chronic illness. Horne (2006) suggests there is no such thing as a non-adherent client and that we have all been non-adherent at some point in our lives. Health professionals should therefore refrain from attempting to identify such people on factors such as behaviour, sociodemographics and dispositional characteristics but rather focus time and energy on understanding the person and their health issue.

Challenges for health professionals

A shared knowledge base and expertise developed by various client interest groups is a natural outcome of the accessibility of information on the internet and the empowerment of people with a disability or chronic illness. Following an internet community of individuals suffering from fibromyalgia, Barker (2008), a Canadian researcher, observed how members empowered each other and shared knowledge and research findings to not only validate the disorder but also to challenge the expertise of clinicians and seek out sympathetic health professionals to educate other practitioners who had less knowledge of the disorder than group members.

Furthermore, health professionals who aim to support and empower their clients may find that not all clients will necessarily follow the advice and direction they are given. Sometimes, too, health professionals will be working with people who are more knowledgeable about the health condition than they are. Such clients may contest the health professional's directions and decisions, and use a valid evidence base to support their viewpoint, which can be challenging, even threatening to the health professional. This, of course, must be balanced with the fact that not all information on the internet is reliable and people may have completely inaccurate, false information about their illness from reading various websites. Either way, patience is often required on the part of health professionals to listen and ensure clients understand all available information. It may be that further questioning is needed to address the concerns or decide on the best treatment options. It may also be necessary to offer the client an opportunity to see another health professional.

HEALTH PROFESSIONALS FROM A DIFFERENT CULTURE

Aspects of cultural safety and how to communicate with clients from various cultures have been explored in Chapter 8. We will now look at working with a health professional from another culture and how this may affect partnerships of care. As the healthcare workforce continues to become multicultural in nature, expectations about the client and the different roles and responsibilities of each team member may be quite different to the usual Western individualist tradition for some healthcare graduates from non-Western collectivist cultures.

What constitutes a partnership and the attitudes a health professional has about this health professional–client partnership can be very different from the client's perspective, particularly if there was an emphasis on a biomedical approach with little focus on the psychosocial aspects of treatment in a health professional's education. For instance, some cultures differ on the client's entitlement to consent to treatment or believe that the family should be responsible for any decisions about an individual's healthcare rather than advocating for client autonomy to be the main priority (Fogarty 2012). In other cultures, it is not acceptable for a health professional to challenge or confront a doctor's decision-making process but instead unquestioningly agree with all given medical directives (Meeuwesen et al 2009). Australian research has found it is frequently a culture shock for non-Western healthcare workers to encounter such differences and so do nothing to embrace the partnership model and true shared care in practice (Meeuwesen et al 2009). To overcome potential issues and maintain partnerships with other work colleagues, clients and carers, workplaces can offer acculturation programs to support the international workforce. Such programs can address concerns, reduce misunderstandings and identify and/or resolve potential cross-cultural issues. What may be required is not simply assistance with the English language and its colloquialisms, but how to relate to clients from another culture (Woodward-Kron et al 2007).

Making decisions about one's own health

Becker and Rosenstock's (1984) work that resulted in the health belief model (HBM) (see Ch 7) was concerned with how people make decisions about their health. They concluded that a person's motivation to engage in healthy behaviours depended on how severe they saw their problem to be, how susceptible they perceived themselves to be and whether they believed that making a change would make a difference to their health. Over time the HBM was developed and extended by social psychologists seeking to promote better preventive health (Janz & Becker 1984, Rosenstock 1974). It is still a commonly used model of health behaviour change and has been used in measuring individuals' likelihood of changing their health behaviours (Caltabiano & Sarafino 2007). Its basis is that preventive health behaviour in an individual is influenced by five factors: (1) any barriers they perceive to carrying out a particular response; (2) perceived benefits of performing the recommended response; (3) their perceived susceptibility to a health threat; (4) perceived severity of a health threat; and (5) cues to the person taking action in response (Becker & Rosenstock 1984). So it follows that it is what the client thinks is important in influencing their decision regarding the health behaviour (see also Ch 7).

The HBM raises the important question of how much health professionals should honestly and carefully explain to clients about their health status. It also implies the importance of having to consider the individual's capacity and ability to cope with these facts, understand them and to then act on them. This can often be an issue. It is important, therefore, for health professionals to attempt to engage clients in a working partnership, or alliance, while also recognising that this may at times be a challenge, due to the client having a variety of reasons for not wishing, or being able, to cooperate. Such factors include: not experiencing a significant degree of distress from the illness; not accepting the fact of being ill; having poor communication skills; the regimen of treatment being too complex; feeling embarrassed about the treatment; possible side effects; and the possible gains from being seen as ill (Coulter 2011). All of this reinforces the need for good communication skills, easy-to-comprehend treatment plans with clear instructions emphasising the positive gains of following treatment and, following from this, the client experiencing treatment successes. However, there will be times when communication may not be successful. For example, even given the best health professional communicator, the client may not possess adequate communication skills her/himself.

THE HEALTH PROFESSIONAL'S ROLE

In spite of the above challenges, it still remains for health professionals to aim at working successfully with their clients. Viewing treatment as a partnership rather than a battle of wills or a procedure to be done is one way to achieve collaboration. It should be seen as entering into interactions with clients with the goal of seeking to form a working alliance. While bearing in mind an individual's diagnosis and treatment plan, it is important to keep in mind the following: What are the client's needs here and now? How may they be assisted in making informed decisions about their treatment? How could their needs be incorporated into a treatment plan?

Many health professionals, however, still do not follow this approach. Unfortunately, the healthcare service industry is still largely based on medical diagnosis and treatment of disorders, rather than the client (Lyons & Chamberlain 2006). In spite of this *medically driven* model still being common, research now seems quite conclusive that, where health professionals use a *patient-based* approach to care rather than a diagnosis basis, clients are more likely to cooperate in their care (Coulter 2011). Caltabiano and Sarafino (2007) believe there is a danger in making health professionals totally responsible for the interaction, in that it may make the client seem to occupy the passive role and not able to be responsible. However, it is true that how a health professional responds to a client can influence the interaction, even though all clients should be treated equally, whether liked or not (Lyons & Chamberlain 2006).

'UNCOOPERATIVE' CLIENTS

All of the above is not to deny the existence of individual clients who do not cooperate with any form of treatment regimen, no matter how much a health professional attempts to explore their reasons and to empathise with them. Not all clients desire to be active in their treatment and some may simply require the health professional to make them better, with no ability or motivation to change behaviours that are harmful to their health. Others have no desire to improve their health status (Taylor 2006). Some may have previously been treated by health professionals who did not explain about their condition or who did not emphasise a working alliance with them, or were disinterested or even rude to them. Some clients may be actively antagonistic to accepting treatment that the evidence has shown is best for them (Lyons & Chamberlain 2006). It can sometimes require a great deal of explanation and education to enlist the client's cooperation (Downie et al 2003, Falvo 2011). Even then a health professional may not succeed with gaining the cooperation of a client.

Beliefs and perceptions

At this point it may be worth thinking about how a person's belief system may influence their behaviour in developing partnerships with health professionals. As already discussed in Chapter 7, how a person perceives illness and health will affect their ability to cope and manage their own health behaviour, therefore one model worth exploring further is the health locus of control (HLOC). This model allows us to examine a person's perception of how much degree of control they possess over their personal health, which in turn affects their behaviour, beliefs and attitudes towards their health. Though Julian Rotter originally developed the social learning theory of locus of control in the 1950s, it was the 1970s that saw the concept being developed significantly in healthcare practice, with various tools emerging that had been specifically designed to measure a person's HLOC in areas such as drug dependency, mental health and chronic pain (Wallston et al 1976).

HLOC is concerned with how much a person believes their health is controlled by internal factors or external factors. For instance, if a person believes their personal health is the result of their own behaviour and sees themselves as having control of their lives, internal factors are said to be at play. On the other hand an external explanation results when the person believes their personal health is controlled by other causes such as health professionals, social forces or even plain luck. Recent research, such as Baker et al (2008), Knappe and Pinquart (2009) or Cavaiola and Strohmetz (2010), demonstrates that assessing a person's perception of control over their health helps to better understand their engagement in healthcare practice. The higher a person's internal HLOC, the more likely they are to see themselves as able to manage their own health and bring about change independently, whereas those with a lower internal HLOC see themselves as powerless to bring about any change, believing their health is being influenced by things beyond their control (Wallston et al 1976).

Whatever model is used, the importance of a person being assisted to make an informed decision and take as much responsibility as possible for their own health reinforces the concept of the client as an active participant in the healthcare team. This is now an accepted aspect of most health service policies.

A rather different way of seeing the issue of client engagement argues that not engaging in treatment may sometimes seem like the sensible thing to the client, that is, it is a rational decision. When looking at the HBM (Becker & Rosenstock 1984), the client may not, for instance, believe that what the doctor has suggested is in their best interest and have what they see as a reasonable explanation for their belief. This is called *rational* or *intentional non-adherence* (Lehane & McCarthy 2007). The main reasons for rational non-adherence are side effects that are worrying, unpleasant or reduce the quality of life, practical barriers such as cost or changes to lifestyle and confusion about when and how much of the treatment to take. Others may choose not to accept treatment on philosophical, religious or cultural grounds.

Critical thinking

- Reflect on a time when you have been prescribed medication or some other treatment. Did you remember all the health professional's instructions? Did you do everything the health professional told you to do? If you didn't, what were your reasons?
- Following from this, imagine if you were concerned about a client of yours. How would you attempt to ensure they followed the treatment that was ordered for them? If you looked at it from their point of view, could there be possible reasons for their attitude and behaviour?
- Thinking about the concept of HLOC, what internal and external factors may impact on a client who has decided to not accept treatment? How might you as a health professional attempt to engage with them?

The context of the health professional–client partnership

It follows from the preceding discussion that another factor to be considered is the treatment context (Lyons & Chamberlain 2006). Usually most health professionals are employees of a health service or organisation. It is possible that an employer may disagree with your values or that their actions contrast with their stated policy. Words spoken and printed claiming that holistic, person-centred care will be provided may not, unfortunately, always fit with actual practice. A service may state that these concerns underpin their provision of care but there might not be adequate funding or facilities for such quality of care to be provided. There is a danger that services and health professionals can be consumed with more efficient, quicker, more economical approaches to treating clients and lose sight of the person. Diagnostic-related categories and treatment/care plans, where interventions are planned according to type and length of treatment usually required for a particular disorder, are useful to assist the efficient management of care in health agencies. But the risk is of quality of care being dependent on a budget that emphasises numbers of clients treated rather than the quality of care delivered.

So, given the above, how should a healthcare student or recent graduate approach their professional practise? It can be somewhat disillusioning for people who have a passion for helping others to encounter colleagues who are cynical or seem to lack any ability to care for their clients. In spite of these problems, there are many individual health professionals and agencies that are genuinely committed to the importance of PCP and building partnerships. It is therefore important for individual health professionals to consider what they believe about the helping relationship and how they wish to practise their profession. As you begin to practise your profession, you will begin to discover the challenges and rewards of helping people in a variety of situations.

CASE STUDY: SYLVIA

Sylvia is an 80-year-old widow who is soon to be discharged from hospital after a recent hip replacement operation. She lives alone and has no family members living in the local area. She was previously living independently but will require some short-term support for the first few weeks after discharge. Sylvia is frightened that a decision will be made to place her in a residential nursing home.

Critical thinking

You are the health professional who is responsible for Sylvia's discharge planning.

- What support do you think Sylvia will need?
- Who do you need to establish a partnership with? Provide your rationale for this.
- How will you establish and maintain the partnerships?
- What do you foresee your role to be as a health professional?
- What obstacles do you think may prevent the partnerships being effective? How would you overcome these?

Partnerships and collaborative practice

The chapter has largely focused on the partnership between two key parties, the client and the health professional, yet for effective and quality care to be delivered health professionals are often not working alone. Person-centred care packages for people with chronic or complex issues will need to rely on other disciplines, services and organisations to play a vital role in the care delivery if they are to achieve optimal healthcare that allows the person to function to the best of their ability. With this in mind, partnerships need to be initiated and sustained with people other than the client at the centre of care. Essential to an effective partnership with others is the skill of working in a cooperative and integrated way through professional collaboration in a multidisciplinary healthcare team.

Health professionals who work with others in an open and honest manner with the goal of providing care directly related to the client's needs may not always achieve the intended outcome. Evidence has shown several barriers that hinder interdisciplinary partnerships, with the most common being miscommunication and misunderstanding of each other's role and responsibility. Others include lack of trust, rivalry, stereotyping of professionals, conflicting opinions and role insecurity (Freshman et al 2010). Partnerships that promote collaborative care require time and effort by all key parties. It may be that, as a health professional, terms commonly used in one service are unfamiliar or are misunderstood due to the same word being used in a different way in another service. In this situation as in all situations when working with other professionals, clarification needs to be sought so that mutual understanding can occur just as each key player in the partnership needs to clarify their role and what they perceive their responsibility in the care package to be. Clear direction of who will do what task, expectations of each other, time management, and the overarching aim of the care package, if communicated clearly to all parties will go some way to avoid the previously mentioned barriers. Recent evidence from WHO suggests that one way of achieving effective partnerships and collaborative practice is by delivering interprofessional education. By different professionals learning together, they are able to learn 'from and about each other' (WHO 2010 p 7); this, in turn, will enhance their partnerships in practice, leading to improved health outcomes for the person at the centre of care.

Conclusion

The chapter has considered the various issues involved in relationships between health professionals, clients and others. Successful health outcomes depend on the key people involved in care, including health professionals, families, carers and communities working together to create an effective partnership. We discussed the meanings and implications in the terms health professionals use on a daily basis and the importance of the client being involved in their own care based on the philosophy of person-centred practice and recovery-oriented care, particularly in chronic and complex health issues. Cultural differences may cause challenges, misunderstandings or negative reactions between health professionals and clients. Similarly, creating partnerships with other disciplines can bring a different set of challenges. An understandings of the factors involved in healthcare partnerships helps identify possibilities health professionals can utilise to create and maintain effective partnerships throughout their career.

REMEMBER

- Successful health outcomes require a partnership between health professionals and clients.

Cont... ▶

- Terms such as compliance/adherence versus partnership, and patient/client versus consumer/service user impact differently on the health partnership relationship.
- A partnership approach enables a person to be involved in their own healthcare. This can be achieved by embracing philosophies such as person-centred and recovery-oriented practice.
- Clients may not always 'comply' with or accept the advice of a health professional.
- Cultural differences may influence the success or otherwise of health professional–client interactions.
- Factors in the healthcare agency may raise challenges in establishing effective partnerships.

Further resources

Bathgate, P., Romios, T., 2011. Consumer participation in health: understanding consumers as social participants. Institute for Social Participation Seminar Series. Online. Available: http://www.healthissuescentre.org.au/documents/items/2011/04/367933-upload-00001.pdf.

Clark, N.M., Cabana, M.D., Nan, B., et al., 2008. The clinician–patient partnership paradigm: outcomes associated with physician communication behavior. Clinical Pediatrics 47 (1), 49–57.

Coulter, A., Parsons, S., Askham, J., 2008. Where are the patients in decision-making about their own care? Policy Brief. World Health Organization, Geneva.

Hinton, K., 2011. A person-centred care mental health workshop. Online. Available: http://www.healthissuescentre.org.au/documents/detail.chtml?filename_num=384450.

Joosten, E.A., DeFuentes-Merillas, L., de Weert, G.H., et al., 2008. Systematic review of the effects of shared decision-making on patient satisfaction, treatment adherence and health status. Psychotherapy and Psychosomatics 77 (4), 219–226.

van Dulmen, S., Sluijs, E., van Dijk, L., et al., 2008. International Expert Forum on Patient Adherence. Furthering patient adherence: a position paper of the international expert forum on patient adherence based on an internet forum discussion. BMC Health Services Research 8 (47).

Weblinks

AlignMap

http://alignmap.com/the-state-of-the-art/the-verdict/

Compliance (adherence) is considered on this site, pooling a variety of research findings that question the effectiveness of strategies suggested to increase adherence by patients. It also asks if many health professionals even consider it as an issue in their clinical work.

Health issues centre – patient-centred care

http://www.healthissuescentre.org.au/subjects/list-library-subject.chtml?subject=35

This site is a resource library with publications and presentations linked to patient-centred care.

Respecting people's choices

http://www.respectingpatientchoices.org.au/index.php?option=com_content&view=articl
e&id=30&Itemid=31

Information for clients and health professionals on advanced care planning

The Royal Australian College of General Practitioners

http://www.racgp.org.au/runningapractice/relationships

This helpful article asks health professionals to consider that relationships, rather than
clients, may be a 'difficult' factor in clinical relationships.

Patient-centred care – indigenous health

http://www.racgp.org.au/afp/200812/200812nguyen1.pdf

This is an excellent resource to consider cultural safety in Indigenous health.

Transforming patient experience – the essential guide

http://www.institute.nhs.uk/patient_experience/guide/home_page.html

This site offers useful resources for health professionals who have responsibility to
improve the experience of those using a health service.

References

Australian Institute of Health and Welfare (AIHW), 2011. Chronic diseases. Online.
Available: www.aihw.gov.au/chronic-diseases 10 Jan 2012.

Baker, T.A., Buchanan, N.T., Corson, N., 2008. Factors influencing chronic pain intensity in
older black women: examining depression, locus of control and physical health.
Journal of Women's Health 17, 869–878.

Barker, K., 2008. Electronic support groups, patient-consumers and medicalization: the
case of contested illness. Journal of Health and Social Behavior 49 (1), 20–36.

Becker, M.H., Rosenstock, I.M., 1984. Compliance with medical advice. In: Steptoe, A.,
Mathews, A. (Eds.), Healthcare and human behaviour. Academic Press, London.

Caltabiano, M.I., Sarafino, E.P., 2007. Health psychology: biopsychosocial interactions, an
Australian perspective, second ed. John Wiley, Milton.

Cavaiola, A.A., Strohmetz, D.B., 2010. Perception of risk for subsequent drinking and
driving related offenses and locus of control among first-time DUI offenders.
Alcoholism Treatment Quarterly 28, 52–62.

Commonwealth of Australia, 2009. Fourth national mental health plan – an agenda for
collaborative government action in mental health 2009–2014. Australian Government,
Canberra.

Coulter, A., 2011. Engaging patients in healthcare. Open University Press, Maidenhead.

Davidson, L., 2008. Recovery – concepts and application. The Devon Recovery Group.
Online. Available: www.scmh.org.uk 8 Feb 2012.

Deegan, P., 1996. Recovery as a journey of the heart. Psychiatric Rehabilitation Journal
11, 11–19.

Department of Human Services, 2006. What is person-centred health care? A literature
review. State Government of Victoria, Melbourne.

Department of Human Services, 2008. Person-centred practice guide to implementing
person-centred practice in your health service. State Government of Victoria,
Melbourne.

Downie, G., Mackenzie, J., Williams, A. (Eds.), 2003. Pharmacology and medicines management for nurses, third ed. Elsevier, Edinburgh.

Falvo, D.R., 2011. Effective patient education: a guide to increased adherence, fourth ed. Jones and Bartlett, Burlington.

Fogarty, J., 2012. Time to watch our language. The Medical Independent 19 Apr 2012. Online. Available: http://www.medicalindependent.ie/page.aspx?title=time_to_watch_our_language 1 Sep 2012.

Freshman, B., Rubino, L., Reid Chassiakos, Y., 2010. Collaboration across the disciplines in health care. Jones and Bartlett, Burlington.

Hill, L., Roberts, G., Wildgoose, J., et al., 2010. Recovery and person-centred care in dementia: common purpose, common practice? Advances in Psychiatric Treatment 16, 288–298.

Horne, R., 2006. Compliance, adherence, and concordance. Implications for asthma treatment. Chest 130 (1 suppl), 65S–72S.

Horne, R., Weinman, J., Barber, N., et al., 2005. Concordance, adherence and compliance in medicine taking. Report for the National Co-ordinating Centre for NHS Service Delivery and Organisation R & D (NCCSDO). December 2005. University of Leeds, School of Healthcare. Online. Available: www.medslearning.leeds.ac.uk/pages/documents/useful_docs/76-final-report%5B1%5D.pdf May 2012.

Janz, N., Becker, M.L., 1984. The health belief model: a decade later. Health Education Quarterly 11, 1–47.

Knappe, S., Pinquart, M., 2009. Tracing criteria of successful aging? Health locus of control and well-being in older patients with internal diseases. Psychology Health and Medicine 14, 201–212.

Larson, P., 2011. Chapter 1 'Chronicity'. In: Lubkin, I., Larson, P. (Eds.), Chronic illness. Impact and Intervention, eighth ed. Jones and Bartlett, Burlington.

Lehane, E., McCarthy, G., 2007. Intentional and unintentional medication non-adherence: a comprehensive framework for clinical research and practice? A discussion paper. International Journal of Nursing Studies 44 (8), 1468–1477.

Lyons, A.C., Chamberlain, K., 2006. Health psychology: a critical introduction, third ed. Cambridge University Press, Cambridge.

Marmot, M., Wilkinson, R.G. (Eds.), 2006. Social determinants of health, second ed. Oxford University Press, Oxford.

McCormack, B., 2001. Autonomy and the relationship between nurses and older people. Ageing and Society 21, 17–46.

McDonald, C., 2006. Challenging social work: the context of practice. Palgrave Macmillan, Basingstoke.

McLaughlin, H., 2009. What's in a name: 'client', 'patient', 'customer', 'consumer', 'expert by experience', 'service user' – what's next? British Journal of Social Work 39, 1101–1117.

Meeuwesen, L., van den Brink-Muinen, A., Hofstede, G., 2009. Can dimensions of national culture predict cross-national differences in medical communication? Patient Education and Counseling 75 (1), 58–66.

Mental Health Coordinating Council, 2008. Mental health recovery – philosophy into practice: a workforce development guide. MHCC, Rozelle.

Muir-Cochrane, E., Barkway, P., Nizette, D., 2010. Mosby's pocketbook of mental illness. Elsevier, Sydney.

National Health Priority Action Council, 2006. National chronic disease strategy. Australian Government Department of Health and Ageing, Canberra.

New Zealand Ministry of Health, 2005. Te Tāhuhu: Improving mental health 2005–2015: The second New Zealand mental health and addiction plan. Online. Available: http://www.health.govt.nz/publication/te-tahuhu-improving-mental-health-2005-2015-second-new-zealand-mental-health-and-addiction-plan 1 Sep 2012.

Rabinowitz, I., Luzatti, R., Tamir, A., et al., 2004. Length of patients monologue, rate and completion, and relation to other components of clinical encounter: observational intervention study in primary care. British Medical Journal 328 (7438), 501–502.

Roberts, G., Wolfson, P., 2004. The rediscovery of recovery: open to all. Advances in Psychiatric Treatment 10, 37–49.

Rosenstock, I., 1974. Historical origins of the health model. Health Education Monographs 2, 328–335.

Rusch, N., Angermeyer, M., Corrigan, P., 2005. Mental illness stigma: concepts, consequences, and initiative to reduce stigma. European Psychiatry 20 (8), 529–539.

Shepherd, G., 2007. Specification for a comprehensive 'rehabilitation and recovery' service in Herefordshire. Hereford PCT Mental Health Services. Online. Available: www.herefordshire.nhs.uk 10 Jan 2012.

Shepherd, G., Boardman, J., Slade, M., 2008. Making recovery a reality. Sainsbury Centre for Mental Health, London.

Taylor, S.E., 2006. Health psychology, sixth ed. McGraw-Hill, New York.

van Weel-Baumgarten, E., 2010. Person centered clinical practice. International Journal of Integrated Care 10, 83–85.

Venetis, M.K., Robinson, J.D., Turkiewitz, K.L., et al., 2009. An evidence base for patient centered cancer care: a meta analysis of studies of observed communication between cancer specialist and their patients. Patient Education Counselling 77, 379–383.

Wallston, B.S., Wallston, K.A., Kaplan, G.D., et al., 1976. Development and validation of the health locus of control (HLC) scale. Journal of Consulting and Clinical Psychology 44 (4), 580–585.

Woodward-Kron, R., Hamilton, J., Rischin, I., 2007. Managing cultural differences, diversity and the dodgy: overseas-born students' perspectives of clinical communication in Australia. Focus on Health Professional Education 9 (3), 30–43.

World Health Organization (WHO), 2010. Framework for action on interprofessional education and collaborative practice. Online. Available: http://whqlibdoc.who.int/hq/2010/WHO_HRH_HPN_10.3_eng.pdf 10 Jan 2012.

World Health Organization (WHO), 2011. Chronic diseases and health promotion. Online. Available: www.who.int/chp/en 12 Feb 2012.

Zolnierek, K.B., Dimatteo, M.R., 2009. Physician communication and patient adherence to treatment: a meta-analysis. Medical Care 47 (8), 826–834.

Chapter 10
Stress and coping

PATRICIA BARKWAY

Learning objectives

The material in this chapter will help you to:

- distinguish between stress as a stimulus, a process and a response
- describe the stress reaction
- understand the effects of stress on health and illness
- understand how cognitive appraisals and personality styles influence an individual's coping response
- identify external moderators of stress.

Key terms

- Stress response
- Stress as a stimulus
- Stress as a transaction
- Psychoneuroimmunology
- Cognitive appraisal
- Acute and chronic stress
- Coping strategies and resources

Introduction

Stress is a term that is used in everyday conversation and frequently featured in the popular media and press. It has also been the focus of psychological research for decades. The concentration of stress research has principally been in three areas, namely to examine stress as: (1) a response – the individual's reaction; (2) a stimulus – the event or stressor that prompted the reaction; or (3) a process – the transaction between the individual and the environment.

While stress is generally considered to be a state to be avoided, the experience and outcomes of stress are, nevertheless, not always negative. At times a stressful occurrence may even be welcome. Desired events like a promotion at work and getting married produce similar physical and psychological reactions, as do unwelcome events like redundancy and divorce. Furthermore, events that are ambiguous, uncontrollable, unpredictable or unrelenting are stressful, as are multiple demands that tax the individual's ability to cope (Taylor 2012).

Consider the statement 'I am feeling *stressed*'. How often have you heard or said this? What does this statement mean? What causes stress and how is it experienced? Does everyone experience stress in the same way? Is stress always harmful and how can it be managed when it is excessive? The answers to such questions will be explored in this chapter. The concept of stress will be considered and factors that make an event stressful will be identified. The health consequences of stress will also be examined and finally moderators of stress will be examined.

What is stress?

Stress is a physical, cognitive, emotional and behavioural reaction of an individual (or organism) to a stressful event – *stressor* – that threatens, challenges or exceeds the individual's internal and external coping resources. The threat may be actual (e.g. being robbed at knife point) or perceived (e.g. a student who believes he will fail a forthcoming exam). The threat or stressor can be physically or emotionally challenging, or both. It may also be perceived as either a positive or negative event by the individual. See Table 10.1 for examples of physical and emotional stressors.

Stress prompts the individual into action. The precipitating stressor may be a major life event like a disaster such as a tsunami, or a minor life event such as daily hassles like being late for an appointment because you were caught up in traffic. Additionally the precipitating event can be viewed as negative, harmful and threatening, or challenging and exciting by the individual. Moreover, the same event may be perceived differently by different people, as evidenced by the scenario in the *Classroom activity* on page 224.

Stress as a response, stimulus or process

Stress is a topic of interest not only to health professionals but also to the general public, as evidenced by the number of publications on the topic in the popular

Table 10.1	
EXAMPLES OF STRESSORS	
Physical stressors	**Emotional stressors**
Undergoing surgery	Diagnosis of a chronic disease
Insomnia	Marriage
Loss of eyesight	Overseas travel
Heat stress	Redundancy
Physical trauma	Relationship breakup
Pain	Moving house
Illness	Winning the lottery

Classroom activity

Imagine you are given a gift voucher for a parachute jump from an aeroplane as a birthday present.

1. Would you be excited by the prospect of this adventurous opportunity or terrified at the very thought of doing this?
2. Pair up with a student whose perception is opposite to yours (negative or positive) and discuss the reason for your view.
3. Listen to the other person's explanation to gain an understanding of their view.
4. List reasons why one event might produce different reactions in different people.

psychology literature such as in self-help books, the internet and health and lifestyle magazines. Furthermore, stress is the most investigated phenomenon in health psychology research with regard to examining the relationship between psychology and disease (Contrada & Baum 2010). Despite this, not all researchers use the concept in the same way. Research that investigates the relationship between stress and health falls into three main categories that view stress as one of the following:

- *response* – the individual's physical and psychological reaction to the stressor
- *stimulus* – a stressor in the environment that precipitates a stress reaction
- *process* – a transaction between the individual and the environment.

STRESS AS A RESPONSE

Stress as a response refers to the individual's physiological and psychological reactions to a perceived threat or stressor, such as a student who discovers that the hard disc on their computer is corrupted and they do not have another copy of an assignment that is due that day. Physical symptoms include dry mouth, palpitations, appetite changes and insomnia, while psychological responses can include anxiety and forgetfulness and, in extreme circumstances, burnout or post-traumatic stress disorder (PTSD). Physiologists in the first half of the 20th century such as Cannon and Selye were the first researchers to describe the stress response and pioneered research in this field.

Fight or flight

Walter Cannon (1932) was a physiologist and early stress researcher who first described the *fight or flight* response – a primitive, inborn protective mechanism to defend the organism against harm. The response is a physical reaction by an organism (including humans) to a perception of threat. Cannon observed that when an organism was threatened the sympathetic nervous system and the endocrine system were aroused, preparing the organism to respond to the anticipated danger by either reacting aggressively (fight) or by fleeing (flight).

The physiological mechanism of this involves arousal of the sympathetic nervous system that stimulates the adrenal glands to secrete catecholamines (adrenaline and noradrenaline), which then elevate blood pressure, increase the heart rate, divert blood supply from internal organs to muscles and limbs and dilate pupils to enable the organism to take action in the face of a threat (see Fig 10.1). Activation of the endocrine system prompts the adrenal glands to secrete cortisol, which provides a quick burst of energy, heightens alertness and memory, and increases the organism's pain threshold. Together they enable the organism to confront or withdraw from the threat.

The fight or flight response is adaptive when arousal enables the individual to take action: to either address or escape the threat. However, prolonged arousal, which is unrelenting or for which adaptation does not occur, is potentially harmful and can

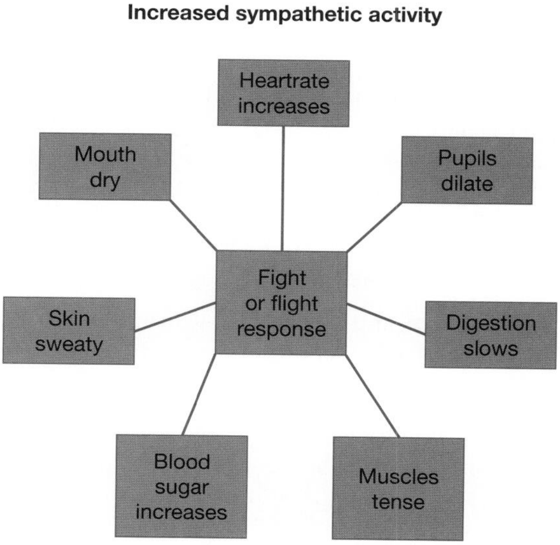

Figure 10.1 Fight or flight response

lead to long-term health consequences. For example, when caught speeding by a radar and pulled over by a police officer, neither fight nor flight is an adaptive response.

In the landmark Whitehall I and II studies, British civil servants in lower level jobs experienced greater stress due to having less control of their workload than higher level employees (Marmot et al 1997). Also, the final report of the World Health Organization's (WHO) Commission of Social Determinants of Health states that 'stress at work is associated with a 50% excess risk of coronary heart disease and there is consistent evidence that high job demand, low control and effort–reward imbalance are risk factors for mental and physical health problems' (WHO 2008 p 8).

General adaptation syndrome

Hans Selye (1956) was another pioneer stress researcher who identified the relationship between stress and illness in a model he called the general adaptation syndrome (GAS). The GAS provides a biomedical explanation of the stress response and how it influences health outcomes. The theory identifies a pattern of reaction to a threat or challenge and proposes that stress is the individual's non-specific response to the specific environmental stressor. Selye defined this as a demand on the body

Research focus

Marmot, M., Kogevinas, M., Elston, M., 1987. Social economic status and disease. Annual Review of Public Health 8, 111–135.

Bosma, H., Marmot, M., Hemingway, H., et al., 1997. Low job control and risk of coronary heart disease in Whitehall II (prospective cohort) study. British Medical Journal 314, 558–565.

WHITEHALL I AND II

The first Whitehall study (1967–1976) examined the health of 18,000 male British civil servants aged between 20 and 64 years over a period of 10 years. The findings of Whitehall I identified that there was an inverse gradient between the position participants held in the hierarchy of the civil service and mortality. In other words, people in senior positions lived longer than those in the lower employment grades. Low-grade workers experienced higher rates of coronary heart disease and three times the mortality rates of workers in the highest grades, and this finding was statistically significant. Additionally, the researchers also identified social determinants that were associated with these adverse health outcomes.

Whitehall II followed up on the findings of Whitehall I with a prospective cohort study of more than 10,000 men and women, aged 35–55 years, employed in the British civil service between 1985 and 1998 with the purpose of identifying the relationship between occupational and psychosocial factors in the workplace and risk for coronary heart disease for both men and women. The researchers concluded that 'low control in the work environment is associated with an increased risk of future coronary heart disease among men and women employed in government offices' (Bosma et al 1997 p 558).

Classroom activity

In small groups:

1. Consider the health profession that your present education is preparing you for, such as physiotherapy, paramedic practice, nursing or social work.
2. Identify potential work-related stressors for this professional group and classify them as 'able to be controlled by the health professional' or 'over which health professionals have low control'.
3. Discuss how events classified as being low control can be made less stressful.

If possible, before the tutorial:

1. Interview a health professional working in the field and ask them to identify controllable and uncontrollable stressors in their work life.
2. Compare and discuss the stressors identified by the health professional with those on lists compiled by other students in the group.

Critical thinking

Imagine you are driving from your home in the hills to your university to sit a health psychology exam when a cat suddenly darts in front of your car. You brake quickly, swerve and, fortunately, avoid hitting the cat. You are not injured but your car came to a halt against a fence post and sustained significant damage to the front end. Water is now leaking from the damaged radiator. When you try to call for assistance you discover your mobile phone is out of range. The road is quiet and traffic infrequent. You know that the nearest house is about five kilometres further on. Consider:

- What might your physical response be?
- How you might feel at this point?
- What are your thoughts?
- What might you do?

that induces the stress response – the individual is required to adapt (Selye 1956). GAS is non-specific in that the response is the same regardless of stimuli; that is, whether the stressor is physical or emotional or whether it is viewed as positive or negative.

The GAS includes three phases:

1. *alarm reaction* – in which the organism is alerted to a perceived threat
2. *resistance stage* – in which the body attempts to regain equilibrium and adapt to the stressor
3. *exhaustion stage* – occurs when the body's attempts to resist the stressor are unsuccessful.

When a threat is perceived the body's reaction is one of *alarm* and the individual is mobilised to take action. In this phase nervous system arousal and alterations to hormone levels prepare the individual for action. Initially this includes the activation of the autonomic nervous system, leading to adrenaline and noradrenaline being secreted by the adrenal medulla. Subsequently, the pituitary gland produces adrenocorticotrophic hormone, which stimulates the release of corticosteroids by the adrenal cortex.

With continued exposure to the threat *resistance* occurs. In this phase hormones remain raised and the immune system aroused as the individual takes further action to cope with the stressor. The *exhaustion* phase follows if the individual is unsuccessful in adapting to or overcoming the threat. Exhaustion weakens the body's defences, making the individual vulnerable to disease due to depleted physiological resources.

Despite the influence of Selye's stress response model on stress research it does not escape criticism. First, that it describes a physiological process and overlooks the role of cognitive appraisal as identified by Lazarus and Folkman (1984); second, not all individuals respond in the same physiological way to stress; and third, Selye's model refers to responses to *actual* stress, whereas an individual can experience the stress response to an *anticipated* stressor (Taylor 2012). For example, in agoraphobia the person fears the anxiety they might experience if they leave their 'safe place', usually their home.

In summary, the stress response is an automatic reaction that enables a person to take action in order to adapt to, or make changes in response to, a perceived or actual threat or stressor. The stress response is most effective for stressors that are of short-term duration and where adaptation is possible. However, should adaptation not be achievable or the stress prolonged, the individual is at risk of developing health problems as a consequence.

STRESS AS A STIMULUS

Another approach to stress research is to view it as a stimulus that produces a reaction. According to Yerkes and Dodson (1908) stress is the stimulus that prompts action and the amount of stress experienced predicts how well the individual performs. The stimulus can be a major life event such as those identified by Holmes and Rahe in 1967 (see Table 10.2). Alternatively the stimulus may be an accumulation of minor life events or hassles as described by Kanner and colleagues in a study that compared the stress from daily hassles and uplifts with the stress produced by major life events (Kanner et al 1981).

The Yerkes–Dodson law

Yerkes and Dodson (1908) hypothesised that a relationship exists between arousal and performance and that stress is a stimulus that prompts an individual to take action. According to the Yerkes–Dodson law, when stressed (aroused) an individual's performance increases to a maximum point after which performance reduces. The relationship is represented graphically as an inverted 'U' (see Fig 10.2).

The model proposes there is an optimal level of arousal (stress) at which an individual is challenged and thereby performs at their best. With too little arousal the individual is not sufficiently motivated to take action in response to the stimulus and

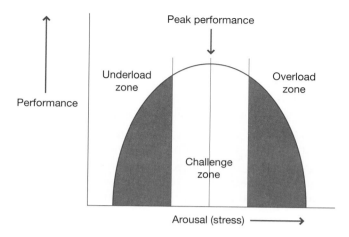

Figure 10.2 Yerkes–Dodson law

hence performance is minimal. Increasing arousal energises the individual to take the action required to achieve a goal such as study to pass an exam. However, excessive arousal can result in the individual being overloaded and, consequently, performance deteriorates, such as in the case of a student who is highly anxious about a forthcoming exam and loses concentration or becomes ill.

MAJOR LIFE EVENTS

The theory that major life events are a stimulus for stress emerged from the research of Holmes and Rahe who hypothesised that major or frequent changes in one's life predisposes the individual to illness due to the cumulative effect of the life stressors. This hypothesis was proposed by the researchers after they observed that tuberculosis infection commonly followed a major crisis or multiple life crises. They subsequently developed a tool to measure the impact of life changes on health and to predict individual vulnerability to illness: the social readjustment rating scale (SRRS) (Holmes & Rahe 1967).

This tool consists of 43 items: 17 are rated as desirable such as going on vacation; 18 are rated as undesirable such as the death of a close friend; and eight are classified as neutral such as 'major change in responsibilities at work' (Holmes & Rahe 1967 p 214). Such a change may be the consequence of a promotion that is desirable but it could be the result of a restructure and reduction of staff at the workplace, which would be undesirable because there would be fewer people to undertake the workload.

Items in the SRRS are given a weighting that reflects the magnitude of the stressful stimulus (see Table 10.2). For example, the death of a spouse was found to be the most stressful life event and was given a score of 100. A score of 150–299 for the preceding year places the individual at moderate risk for illness, whereas a score of 300 in the preceding six months or more than 500 in the preceding year places the individual at high risk of developing a stress-related illness.

Since its development in the 1960s the Holmes–Rahe SRRS is one of the most widely cited tools in stress research. Thirty years later Scully et al (2000) replicated the research to examine the usefulness of the tool as an indicator of health risk and to consider the validity of criticisms raised in the literature in relation to the tool. Scully et al's research found that the relative weightings and rank order of the selected life events remained valid and concluded that SRRS continues to be 'a robust instrument for identifying the potential for the occurrences of stress-related outcomes (Scully et al 2000 p 875). Table 10.2 compares weight and rank order for selected life events in Holmes and Rahe's seminal study and the replication by Scully et al.

Not everyone experiences or responds to major life events in the same way, though. In a study of coping following multiple negative life events Armstrong et al (2011) found that participants were more resilient following a stressful event if they had a high score on scales for emotional self-awareness, emotional expression, emotional self-control and emotional self-management.

Table 10.2

SCULLY ET AL'S UPDATED SOCIAL READJUSTMENT RATING SCALE

Holmes and Rahe 1967		Selected life events	Scully et al 2000	
Rank order	Weight		Rank order	Weight
1	100	Death of a spouse	1	100
2	73	Divorce	2	58
3	65	Marital separation	4	51
4	63	Jail term	5	50
5	63	Death of a close family member	8	45
6	53	Personal injury or illness	3	57
7	50	Marriage	6	50
8	47	Fired at work	13	34
9	45	Marital reconciliation	15	28
10	45	Retirement	29	18
11	44	Change in health of family member	7	46
12	40	Pregnancy	16	27
13	39	Sex difficulties	10	36
14	39	Gain of new family member	23	21
15	39	Business readjustment	40	12
16	38	Change in financial state	9	43

Cont... ▶

Holmes and Rahe 1967			Scully et al 2000	
Table 10.2 (continued)				
SCULLY ET AL'S UPDATED SOCIAL READJUSTMENT RATING SCALE				
Rank order	Weight	Selected life events	Rank order	Weight
17	37	Death of a close friend	12	35
18	36	Change to different line of work	14	30
19	35	Change in number of arguments with spouse	17	26
20	31	Mortgage more than $51,000	18	30

Source: Scully J, Tosi H, Banning K 2000 Life events checklist: revisiting the social readjustment rating scale after 30 years. Educational and Psychological Measurement Vol 60 No 6, p 864–876, American College Personnel Assocation, Science Research Associates, copyright Sage Publications, Inc.

Critical thinking

Despite Scully et al's conclusion that life change events are 'useful predictors of stress related symptom scores' (2000 p 875) three life events did lower their rank order by more than nine places. These were:

- retirement
- gain of new family member
- business readjustment.

Consider why these three life events may be perceived as less stressful in the 21st century than they were in the 1960s.

MINOR LIFE EVENTS

Kanner and his colleagues were interested to see if minor as well as major life events had health consequences for an individual. The researchers defined minor stressful events that were irritating or frustrating as *hassles*. Minor life events would cause inconvenience for the individual rather than require a major adjustment as is required with major life events (Kanner et al 1981). Examples of such stressful events include: discovering that your mobile phone battery is flat when you want to make a phone call; arriving late to watch a soccer grand final and being told that you cannot enter the stadium until half-time; or finding that an ATM machine is out of order when you need to withdraw cash. Findings from Kanner et al's research demonstrated that hassles can impact on health. This occurred when multiple hassles occurred at once or when minor life events occurred concurrently with a major life event and when minor stressful events were prolonged or repeated such as a person who was late for work three times in one week due to traffic congestion.

In summary, it is evident that both major and minor events may stimulate a stress reaction in humans that, in turn, can affect health. Nevertheless, the presence of a stressful stimulus is not predictive of how someone will respond to the stressor. Different people will respond differently to the same stressor and the same event can lead to positive or negative outcomes in different people. For example, a person who has a dog phobia will react differently from a dog lover when a dog is present. This observation prompted psychologists studying stress to examine the relationship between the individual, their perceptions and their environment, that is, stress as a process.

STRESS AS A PROCESS

The notion of stress as a process was first introduced by Richard Lazarus and later refined in collaboration with his colleague Susan Folkman (Lazarus 1966, Lazarus & Folkman 1984). Lazarus's theory proposed that stress was a transaction between the individual and their environment. The transaction involves the individual making a cognitive assessment (appraisal) of the demands of the stressor and the coping resources available to him or her. Lazarus distinguished between stressors that are negative (*distress*) and positive (*eustress*).

In appraising an event or situation an individual will ask one of three questions. Is the event:

- relevant or irrelevant (to the individual)?

- benign or positive (eustress)?

- threatening or harmful (distress)?

Lazarus's theory proposes that distress is experienced when a person perceives that a stressor is potentially negative and also believes that his or her available resources are insufficient to meet the demands of this particular stressor. *Cognitive appraisal* is the term used to describe the process of perceiving the stressor and of judging one's ability to manage or respond to the stressor.

Cognitive appraisal occurs at two levels: primary and secondary. Primary appraisal refers to an individual's judgment as to whether this event or situation is negative (poses a threat), positive (provides opportunity/challenge) or benign (neutral/irrelevant). Secondary appraisal refers to a person's assessment of their personal (internal) and environmental (external) resources to respond to the stressful event or situation (Lazarus & Folkman 1984). These two processes are carried out simultaneously as the person assesses the threat and their ability to manage (see Table 10.3).

Table 10.3	
COGNITIVE APPRAISAL	
Primary	Is the event challenging, irrelevant or threatening? Is the significance of the event positive, neutral or negative?
Secondary	What are my coping resources? ■ Internal (within the individual) ■ External (within the environment) How adequate are my coping resources?

CASE STUDY: JENNI

Jenni is a third-year social work student who was awarded the grade of high distinction (95%) for her health psychology essay. The lecturer recommended that Jenni submit an abstract of the paper for presentation at a forthcoming international psychology conference.

Critical thinking

Identify Jenni's thoughts. Should she appraise this event as:

- positive
- neutral
- negative.

Identify possible secondary appraisal for each of the above scenarios.

Stress myths

Finally, that stress is an unavoidable consequence of modern life that produces negative outcomes is a commonly held view that is not correct. Stress is only problematic if it is perceived as such and/or has negative consequences. According to the Yerkes–Dodson law moderate stress motivates a person to make adaptive responses (see Fig 10.2). Nevertheless, myths abound about the causes, consequences and how one should respond to stress. The American Psychological Association (APA) (2012) identifies and challenges the six most common stress myths, as outlined in Box 10.1.

Critical thinking

- Consider the six myths in Box 10.1. Do you agree that all are myths?
- Explain the reason for your answer.
- Why might someone believe that any of these myths are true?

EFFECTS OF STRESS ON HEALTH

Stress can impact on a person's health physically or psychologically (or both) and can have short- or long-term consequences. Physical outcomes include impaired immunity, vulnerability to infection and increased risk for cancer and cardiovascular and autoimmune diseases. Psychological consequences of excessive and prolonged stress include cognitive, emotional and behavioural problems, and in extreme circumstances can lead to disorders such as anxiety, depression or risky health behaviours like drug and alcohol abuse. Let us examine these effects in more detail.

Box 10.1 Six myths about stress

Dispelling the six myths about stress enables us to understand our problems and then take action against them. Let's look at these myths individually.

MYTH 1: STRESS IS THE SAME FOR EVERYBODY.

Completely wrong. Stress is different for each of us. What is stressful for one person may or may not be stressful for another; each of us responds to stress in an entirely different way.

MYTH 2: STRESS IS ALWAYS BAD FOR YOU.

According to this view, zero stress makes us happy and healthy. Wrong. Stress is to the human condition what tension is to the violin string: too little and the music is dull and raspy; too much and the music is shrill or the string snaps. Stress can be the kiss of death or the spice of life. The issue, really, is how to manage it. Managed stress makes us productive and happy; mismanaged stress hurts and even kills us.

MYTH 3: STRESS IS EVERYWHERE, SO YOU CAN'T DO ANYTHING ABOUT IT.

Not so. You can plan your life so that stress does not overwhelm you. Effective planning involves setting priorities and working on simple problems first, solving them and then going on to more complex difficulties. When stress is mismanaged, it's difficult to prioritise. All your problems seem to be equal and stress seems to be everywhere.

MYTH 4: THE MOST POPULAR TECHNIQUES FOR REDUCING STRESS ARE THE BEST ONES.

Again, not so. No universally effective stress reduction techniques exist. We are all different, our lives are different, our situations are different and our reactions are different. Only a comprehensive program tailored to the individual works.

MYTH 5: NO SYMPTOMS, NO STRESS.

Absence of symptoms does not mean the absence of stress. In fact, camouflaging symptoms with medication may deprive you of the signals you need for reducing the strain on your physiological and psychological systems.

MYTH 6: ONLY MAJOR SYMPTOMS OF STRESS REQUIRE ATTENTION.

This myth assumes that the 'minor' symptoms, such as headaches or stomach acid, may be safely ignored. Minor symptoms of stress are the early warnings that your life is getting out of hand and that you need to do a better job of managing stress.

PHYSICAL EFFECTS OF STRESS

The physical functions of the body are regulated by the nervous, endocrine and immune systems. In humans the nervous system comprises the central and peripheral nervous systems. The central nervous system consists of the brain and spinal cord, the peripheral nervous system and all the other neural structures and pathways in the body. The immune system defends us against infection, including bacteria and viruses, and can protect against some cancers. The endocrine system consists of glands and organs that secrete hormones to regulate metabolism, growth and development. Malfunction in one of these systems will impact on the other systems and cause illness. For example, in a study of 33 anxious and non-anxious women, anxiety was found to be significantly associated with altered and lowered immune functioning (Arranz et al 2007); numerous studies have shown that students' immunity is compromised in the period surrounding exams (Taylor 2012).

PSYCHONEUROIMMUNOLOGY

Psychoneuroimmunology is the multidisciplinary scientific study of the relationship between the nervous system and the immune system. The term

Research focus

Arranz, L., Guayerbas, N., De la Fuente, M., 2007. Impairment of several immune functions in anxious women. Journal of Psychosomatic Research 62, 1–8.

ABSTRACT

Objective

Controversial results concerning immune function changes taking place in anxious subjects have been obtained. The aim of the present work was to study immune function in a group of anxious women.

Methods

Thirty-three anxious and 33 non-anxious age-matched women were included. Anxiety levels were determined by the Beck anxiety inventory. Peripheral blood samples were collected and several leukocyte functions, as well as cytokine release, were studied. Plasma cortisol levels and total antioxidant capacity were also evaluated.

Results

The results showed diminished immunity in anxious women. Plasma cortisol was increased, while total antioxidant capacity was lowered in those subjects.

Conclusions

The findings suggest impaired immune function and cytokine release in anxious women. This might be related to increased cortisol secretion, which would lead to oxidative stress reflected in lowered plasma total antioxidant capacity.

psychoneuroimmunology was coined by George Solomon in 1964, but it would be another decade before research in the field became widespread. This occurred in the 1970s following a finding by Robert Ader, an American psychiatrist, that the immune system of rats could be suppressed through classical conditioning (see Ch 1). Ader published these findings with his colleague, Cohen (Ader & Cohen 1975).

Ader and Cohen's evidence that immune functioning could be affected by the manipulation of psychological processes was a significant milestone in psychoneuroimmunology research. Subsequently, research that investigates the relationship between stress and the immune system has intensified. There is now a substantial body of knowledge to support the hypothesis that immune system alteration precipitated by psychological processes, including stress, can cause physical illness. This applies not only to illnesses that are caused by infection but also to autoimmune and metabolic diseases like multiple sclerosis, asthma and rheumatoid arthritis, and to some cancers (Irwin 2008, Kiecolt-Glasser 2009, 2010).

IMMUNE SYSTEM

The immune system is the body's protection against infection and illness. Its primary function is to detect foreign cells in the body and eradicate them. It consists of organs (such as the spleen) and cells (such as lymphocytes) that detect pathogens like bacteria, viruses and cancer-producing cells, and destroys them. Cells within the immune system have receptors for neuropeptides and hormones enabling them to respond to nervous and neuroendocrine system signals. Nerve fibres connect immune system organs and cells to the autonomic nervous system. Consequently the central nervous system moderates stress through changes in immune cell activity. Because the brain and nervous system are connected to the immune system by neuroanatomic and neuroendocrine pathways, immune functioning can be affected. Figure 10.3 shows the pathway for central nervous system effects on the immune system.

Immunosuppression

Immunosuppression is a consequence of stress that can result from being exposed to both short- and long-term stress. There is an extensive body of research that links stress to immune dysregulation. Effects include: reduced number and function of natural killer cells (whose role is to respond to and reject viral and tumour cells); increased production of proinflammatory cytokines (which are implicated in depression and sleep disorders); and decreased monocytes (which protect the body from foreign substances e.g. infection) (Irwin 2008). The clinical consequence of immunosuppression include chronic low-grade inflammation, delayed wound healing, poor response to vaccines and increased susceptibility to bacterial and viral infections (Gouin 2011, Irwin 2008).

Pathways between the central nervous, endocrine and immune systems travel in two directions. What this means is that not only can the central nervous system affect the endocrine and immune systems but these both have the potential to also affect the central nervous system (see Fig 10.4).

As a consequence of the interrelationship between the three systems not only can cognitions and emotions influence immunity and endocrine function but the immune and endocrine systems can send messages to the brain and influence behaviour. For example, both adrenal corticosteroids and catecholamines can cause immunosuppression that, in turn, can lead to illness behaviour such as tiredness and appetite reduction. Also, in addition to adrenocortical hormones, other hormones including thyroid and growth, can suppress immune function.

In summary, there is now clear evidence that stress-induced immunosuppression can lead to illness. Research that identifies these links provides opportunities for intervention and prevention. Nevertheless, despite the body of research demonstrating the links between stress and illness many questions remain unanswered, namely, how much stress is required to bring about changes to the immune system and how can stress-induced immunosuppression be prevented or mediated?

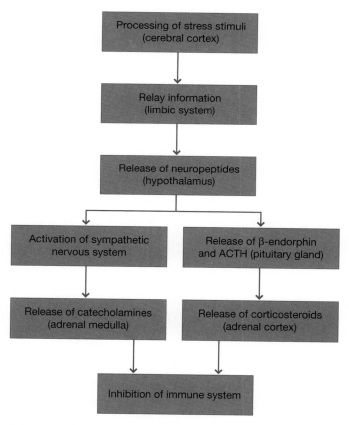

Figure 10.3 Inhibition of immune system

From: Lewis S L, Ruff Dirksen S, McLean Heitkemper M, Bucher L, Camera I N, (eds) 2011 Medical-surgical nursing: assessment and management of clinical problems, 8th edn., Elsevier, St Louis

Psychological effects of stress

The psychological and behavioural health effects of stress also have both short-and long-term consequences. These consequences can include cognitive changes (forgetfulness and obsessional thoughts), affective changes (anxiety and mood alteration) and changes to health behaviours (dietary changes, altered sleep patterns

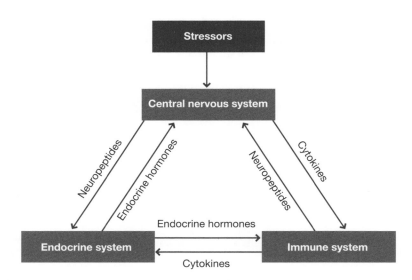

Figure 10.4 Neurochemical links between the nervous, endocrine and immune systems

From: Lewis S L, Ruff Dirksen S, McLean Heitkemper M, Bucher L, Camera I N, (eds) 2011 Medical-surgical nursing: assessment and management of clinical problems, 8th edn., Elsevier, St Louis

and increased tobacco smoking and alcohol/drug use). In the longer term unrelieved stress can have serious lifestyle consequences such as burnout and be a contributing factor in mental illnesses like clinical depression and PTSD.

BURNOUT

Burnout is a psychological syndrome characterised by: emotional exhaustion; depersonalisation and cynicism; and a diminished sense of self-efficacy and personal accomplishment that occurs as a consequence of prolonged chronic workplace stress (Lee & Akhtar 2011, Maslach 2003). According to Maslach (2003) anyone who works with needy people, and particularly healthcare workers, is at risk of burnout. Maslach and Jackson (1981) developed the first tool to identify burnout in human services workers. Their tool measures (1) emotional exhaustion, (2) depersonalisation and (3) reduced personal accomplishment, and has an optional fourth subscale of reduced involvement.

Burnout produces a range of negative outcomes for workers' health and wellbeing including: anxiety and depression; psychosomatic problems such as headaches; and physical health problems such as immunosuppression leading to increased vulnerability to infection (Pipe et al 2009). Other serious consequences of chronic workplace stress include hypertension, coronary heart disease, excessive alcohol use and mental illness (Hurrell & Kelloway 2007). People who work closely with others, such as health professionals, are particularly vulnerable to burnout (Glasberg et al 2007). In a study of burnout among Hong Kong nurses, Lee and Akhtar (2011) found that the 'social context' of nursing work was more significantly associated with burnout than the 'job content'. They defined social context as: lack of professional recognition; professional uncertainty; interpersonal and family conflicts; tensions in work relations; and tensions in nurse–patient relations. Job content, on the other hand, comprised patient care responsibilities, job demands and role conflict. These findings have implications regarding how individual nurses and the organisations they work for address workplace stressors.

Classroom activity

1. In the week preceding the tutorial search the literature for an article about burnout in your intended profession and note:
   - the factors identified as contributing to burnout
   - recommendations and solutions proposed.
2. During the tutorial:
   - Form small groups and present key issues from the article you found to your fellow students.
   - Discuss the implications of the key issues to their intended profession and yourself.

POST-TRAUMATIC STRESS DISORDER

PTSD is a serious, debilitating mental illness that affects some people who experience or witness an extremely traumatic stressful event – one which is outside the realm of usual human experience and involves the threat of death or serious injury. Examples of such events include being the victim of an assault, witnessing a person being run over by a train or the soldier in a war zone who is exposed to gunfire that results in the death and injury of colleagues and bystanders.

Features of PTSD include: insomnia; intrusive thoughts and dreams about the traumatic event; irritability and outbursts of anger; poor concentration; hypervigilance; and an exaggerated startle reflex. People with PTSD may also experience survivor guilt, relationship difficulties, detachment from loved ones, anxiety symptoms and clinical depression (Evans 2012). Furthermore, a study of Vietnam war veterans found that veterans with PTSD also had a 'pattern of physical health outcomes that is consistent with altered inflammatory responsiveness' (O'Toole & Catts 2008 p 33). In other words the stress experienced by these soldiers had not only produced psychological symptoms but also immunosuppression and consequent physical disorders.

While it is clear that experiencing a traumatic stressful event causes PTSD there are still many unanswered questions about this condition. In particular: Why do some people develop PTSD after an extremely traumatic event while others do not? And is stress debriefing beneficial to all victims following a traumatic stress or can this increase psychological distress?

Coping

We will now examine psychological explanations regarding how people cope with excessive stress and stressors. Coping refers to the process of managing demands that challenge or exceed an individual's resources. Its purpose is to enable the person to: tolerate or adjust to stressful events or realities; retain a positive sense of self; and achieve harmonious relationships with others. It includes an evaluation of one's coping resources and the options available to determine if they are sufficient to overcome the threat. Lazarus and Folkman (1984) describe it as the cognitive and behavioural strategies that the individual uses to manage the demands perceived to challenge or exceed their resources.

COPING RESOURCES

The resources one calls on to cope may be internal (within the person), external (within the environment) or both. Internal resources refer to qualities and attributes that the individual possesses and can utilise in response to the stressor. They include the person's cognitive and behavioural responses to stress, personality attributes and disposition. External coping resources are factors external to the person, such as other people and tangible resources they can access that enable them to deal with the stressor. See Table 10.4 for examples of internal and external coping resources.

Table 10.4	
EXAMPLES OF COPING RESOURCES	
Internal	**External**

Health status
Spirituality
Personality attributes
  ■ Optimistic outlook
  ■ Self-efficacy
  ■ Resilience
Communication skills
Problem-solving skills
	Supportive
	  ■ Family
	  ■ Social network
	  ■ Workplace
	Resources
	  ■ Time
	  ■ Financial

Internal coping resources: personality attributes and disposition

Personality refers to the qualities that comprise a person's cognitive, affective and behavioural makeup, and which distinguishes individuals from each other. Personality attributes and disposition are internal resources that can facilitate or hinder coping. Attitudes and disposition identified as influencing coping include: locus of control (Rotter 1966); self-efficacy (Bandura 1977); optimism and pessimism (Seligman 1994, 2011); and resilience (Garmezy 1987). Let us examine the role of personality attributes and disposition in coping.

Locus of control

Locus of control (LOC) is a construct described by the social learning theorist Julian Rotter (1966). It refers to an individual's belief regarding responsibility for reinforcement of a particular behaviour and whether the individual believes that reinforcements (outcomes) are controlled by the self, others or by chance (see also Chs 4 and 9).

People are described as possessing an internal LOC when they believe their behaviour influences outcomes, whereas a person who has an external LOC believes that forces outside the self influence outcomes, that is, chance, fate or other more powerful people. Wallston et al (1978) further refined Rotter's model to propose a 'health LOC' (HLOC) that comprises three attributional constructs, namely, internal, external and powerful others. For example, a person with diabetes who has one of these three attributional constructs would say:

- *internal* – how I manage my diabetes will limit complications
- *external* – no matter what I do my blood sugar levels are always unstable
- *powerful others* – my doctors know more about this than me so I will leave management of my condition to them.

Rotter proposed that a person with an internal attributional style would take more responsibility for their health; however, this only occurs when the reinforcements or outcomes are valued by the individual. For example, Rotter's theory would predict that a person with an internal LOC who valued fitness is more likely to engage in exercise than a person with an internal LOC who did not value fitness.

Furthermore, the model is not predictive of coping when the desired outcome is not exclusively under the control of the individual, for example, a person who has cancer and believes that by adhering to the prescribed treatment they will overcome the disease. While this will initially facilitate coping, should the cancer not be cured, it can have a detrimental impact on the person, who may consequently become depressed. For example, a study that examined HLOC in healthy and cancer patients found that while a high internal HLOC assisted functioning in cancer patients early in the disease, the positive affect was only evident while the patients were sufficiently well enough 'to exert control over their health' (Knappe & Pinquart 2009 p 201).

Self-efficacy

Bandura, too, was a social learning theorist who believed that human behaviour results from the interaction between the individual's perception and thinking and the environment. He proposed the construct of *self-efficacy*, which he described as a personal belief that one is capable of taking action to achieve desired or required outcomes (Bandura 1977, 2001).

According to Bandura's model the thoughts a person has about a particular event or circumstance (their *self-talk*) are predictive of the outcome because the person is cognitively rehearsing the eventual outcome. Self-talk can be either positive or negative. Positive talk increases the likelihood of a positive outcome because the person engages in behaviours that will bring about the desired outcome. For example, a person learning a new skill who tells themselves that 'once I master this I will be right' will engage in behaviours to achieve this, such as practising the skill. Alternatively, the person whose self-talk is negative, for example, 'I will never be able to manage this', is unlikely to practise and therefore less likely to acquire the skill.

Optimism and pessimism

Martin Seligman is a cognitive psychologist who developed the theory of learned helplessness as a cognitive behavioural explanation of depression (Seligman 1974). He later focused his attention on learned optimism, arguing that psychological research has focused excessively on illness with insufficient attention being given to wellness (Seligman 2011). Seligman is attributed as being the founder of the specialist field of *positive psychology*.

A person with an optimistic attribution style believes they can influence the outcomes in certain circumstances. For example, a person with diabetes who has an optimistic attribution style may make the statement, 'Fluctuations in my blood sugar levels are a challenge to be managed'. Whereas a person with a pessimistic style who believes that the outcome has nothing to do with their actions may make the statement, 'Even if I watch my diet my blood sugar levels are high, so I don't bother'.

Rasmussen et al (2009), in a meta-analytic review of optimism and physical health, found that optimism was a significant indicator of physical health, although the exact mechanism of how optimism affects health and disease was not evident. Furthermore, an optimistic outlook is not necessarily the ideal approach in all circumstances and at times may be unrealistic. Segerstrom (2006), for example, found that when an optimist persists in trying to cope with a significant stressor and is unsuccessful they may experience further stress and impaired immune functioning (Segerstrom 2006).

Resilience

As discussed in Chapter 4, resilience refers to the ability to cope with and bounce back from adversity. Research in this area was initiated by Garmezy (1987), who observed that some children coped well despite their adverse family situation. Garmezy identified *protective* factors for these children and explored what facilitated their coping, that is, what enabled some children to be resilient despite living in a challenging family situation.

This and subsequent research has identified that being resilient involves: having caring and supportive relationships within the family and with others; being able to make realistic plans and take steps to carry them out; having a positive view of oneself and belief in one's abilities; good communication and problem-solving skills; and being able to manage strong feelings and impulses. Being resilient, though, doesn't mean that you will never feel stressed, anxious or depressed; it means that you have the requisite internal and external resources to call on in challlenging times (APA 2011).

Garmezy concluded that resilience did not influence vulnerability to stress but, rather, enabled people to cope with challenges and adversity (Garmezy 1991). That is to say that a resilient person is not less vulnerable to stress but that in a stressful situation they are likely to utilise more adaptive coping strategies than those employed by a person who is less resilient. Furthermore, resilience is not a static trait – it can be enhanced. See Box 10.2 from the APA (2011), which outlines strategies for adolescents to build resilience.

COPING STRATEGIES

Coping strategies are the actions people take in response to stress. Lazarus and Folkman (1984) separate coping strategies into two categories: emotion-focused and problem-focused. In using either or both of these coping strategies the person is active not passive and enters a process of engagement with the stressor, which they call a transaction.

Box 10.2 10 ways to build resilience

What are some tips that can help you learn to be resilient? As you use these tips, keep in mind that each person's journey along the road to resilience will be different – what works for you may not work for your friends.

Get together. Talk with your friends and, yes, even with your parents. Understand that your parents may have more life experience than you do, even if it seems they never were your age. They may be afraid for you if you're going through really tough times and it may be harder for them to talk about it than it is for you! Don't be afraid to express your opinion, even if your parent or friend takes the opposite view. Ask questions and listen to the answers. Get connected to your community, whether it's as part of a church group or a high school group.

Cut yourself some slack. When something bad happens in your life, the stresses of whatever you're going through may heighten daily stresses. Your emotions might already be all over the map because of hormones and physical changes; the uncertainty during a tragedy or trauma can make these shifts seem more extreme. Be prepared for this and go a little easy on yourself, and on your friends.

Create a hassle-free zone. Make your room or apartment a 'hassle-free zone' – not that you keep everyone out but home should be a haven free from stress and anxieties. But understand that your parents and siblings may have their own stresses if something serious has just happened in your life and may want to spend a little more time than usual with you.

Stick to the program. Spending time in high school or on a college campus means more choices; so let home be your constant. During a time of major stress, map out a routine and stick to it. You may be doing all kinds of new things, but don't forget the routines that give you comfort, whether it's the things you do before class, going out to lunch, or having a nightly phone call with a friend.

Take care of yourself. Be sure to take of yourself – physically, mentally and spiritually. And get sleep. If you don't, you may be more grouchy and nervous at a time when you have to stay sharp. There's a lot going on, and it's going to be tough to face if you're falling asleep on your feet.

Take control. Even in the midst of tragedy, you can move towards goals one small step at a time. During a really hard time, just getting out of bed and going to school may be all you can handle, but even accomplishing that can help. Bad times make us feel out of control – grab some of that control back by taking decisive action.

Express yourself. Tragedy can bring up a bunch of conflicting emotions, but sometimes, it's just too hard to talk to someone about what you're feeling. If talking isn't working, do something else to capture your emotions like start a journal, or create art.

Cont... ▶

Help somebody. Nothing gets your mind off your own problems like solving someone else's. Try volunteering in your community or at your school, cleaning up around the house or apartment, or helping a friend with his or her homework.

Put things in perspective. The very thing that has you stressed out may be all anyone is talking about now. But eventually, things change and bad times end. If you're worried about whether you've got what it takes to get through this, think back on a time when you faced up to your fears, whether it was asking someone on a date or applying for a job. Learn some relaxation techniques, whether it's thinking of a particular song in times of stress, or just taking a deep breath to calm down. Think about the important things that have stayed the same, even while the outside world is changing. When you talk about bad times, make sure you talk about good times as well.

Turn it off. You want to stay informed – you may even have homework that requires you to watch the news. But sometimes, the news, with its focus on the sensational, can add to the feeling that nothing is going right. Try to limit the amount of news you take in, whether it's from television, newspapers or magazines, or the internet. Watching a news report once informs you; watching it over and over again just adds to the stress and contributes no new knowledge.

Emotion-focused coping uses self-regulation in order to control one's emotional response to a stressor. Stress is moderated when the person engages in strategies that help manage their affective response to the stressor. For example, a person who seeks support from family and friends when given the diagnosis of a terminal illness is using an emotion-focused approach. Problem-focused coping addresses the stressor itself to resolve stress. If the person in the example above had researched the internet to obtain information about the treatments available for their particular illness they would have been using a problem-focused strategy. See Table 10.5 for examples of problem- and emotion-focused coping strategies.

Furthermore, at times both emotion- and problem-focused strategies can be utilised to respond to the same stressor. And while people use both problem- and emotion-focused coping strategies individuals do have a preferred style. In addition a person may use different styles in different situations such as being emotion-focused at home and problem-focused at work (Taylor 2012). Regardless, neither style is preferable – it depends on the context and the demands of the situation.

In summary, while the general intent of coping strategies is to facilitate coping this is not always the outcome. What if, for example, the person who is given the diagnosis of a terminal illness utilises the defence mechanism *denial* (as discussed in Ch 1)? This is an emotion-focused coping strategy that, in the short term, achieves the outcome of minimising the person's anxiety. However, denial is not an effective long-term coping strategy because it does not assist the person and their family to adjust to the reality and consequences of the illness. Furthermore, Hulbert-Williams et al's (2011) study of psychosocial predictors of cancer adjustment found that cognitions and appraisals were more predictive of the outcome than emotions. They concluded that 'the comparative importance of cognitions in outcome prediction suggests that supportive interventions might usefully include theraputic techniques

Table 10.5		
EMOTION- AND PROBLEM-FOCUSED COPING STRATEGIES		
Stressor	**Emotion-focused**	**Problem-focused**
Being diagnosed with diabetes	Joins a diabetes support group	Enrols in a diabetes education class
Made redundant at work	Takes a holiday	Registers with an employment agency
Having recurrent arguments with partner	Goes out with friends	Seeks relationship counselling
Waking up feeling ill on the day of an exam	Rolls over and goes back to sleep	Makes a GP appointment to obtain a medical certificate
A child who is bullied at school	Spends lunchtime in the library to avoid the bullies	Reports the bullying to a teacher

aimed at cognitive re-structuring and/or psychological acceptance of distressing thoughts and feelings' (Hulbert-Williams et al 2011 p 11).

EXTERNAL COPING RESOURCES

In addition to an individual's unique response to stressors, coping is also dependent on the external resources available to the person. These include, but are not limited to, social support (family and friends), education, employment and time. Socioeconomic status (SES) is a significant resource for health, with poverty and disadvantage being predictors of shorter lifespan, poorer health and reduced quality of life (Baum 2008). Conversely people of higher SES generally have more tangible external resources at their disposal to deal with stressors. See Chapter 5 for a more detailed account of the influence of social factors on health.

Social support

Social support refers to the perceived comfort, understanding and help a person receives from others. It was first described as a moderator of stress by Cobb (1976) who defined social support as the perception of being loved and cared for, of feeling esteemed and valued, and of having a social network such as family and friends who could provide resources in times of need. Support may mediate stress either by reducing the impact of stress (buffering effect) or by reducing the likelihood of adverse events (direct effect). Five types of social support that can influence health outcomes are:

- *emotional support* – involves providing empathy and concern for the person, which provides comfort, reassurance and a sense of being loved during difficult times

- *esteem support* – occurs when others express positive regard or encouragement for the person or validate the person's views and feelings that build feelings of self-worth and competence in the person

- *instrumental support* – refers to providing direct assistance like lending the person money or babysitting their children during stressful times, which reduces demand on the person's own resources

- *information support* – involves giving advice and making suggestions to assist decision making or providing feedback on action taken to affirm decisions made, which facilitates self-efficacy

- *network support* – involves being a member of a group of people who share similar values, interests or experiences that provides the person with a sense of belonging, or assists the person to realise that they are not the only person who has experienced the particular stressor.

Evidence that social support also influences health outcomes is abundant (Taylor 2012). A perception that one has adequate social support during illness can moderate the harmful effects of stress and, conversely, having inadequate social support while ill is associated with adverse outcomes. For example, Zhang et al, in a longitudinal study of 1431 elderly people with diabetes, demonstrated a relationship between perceived social support and mortality. Findings were that people who reported a low level of social support had the highest risk of death over the six years of the study. People with moderate social support had 41% less risk of death than people with the lowest reported level of social support. Furthermore, those who reported the highest levels of support were 55% less likely to have died (Zhang et al 2007).

Nevertheless, despite the reported beneficial effects of social support there are some circumstances when it is unhelpful. This can occur when: the help provided is not what the recipient perceives they require; the help is excessive, leading to depletion of the person's coping skills and overdependence on the helper; or harmful coping strategies are encouraged such as excessive alcohol use.

COPING WITH ILLNESS

Being diagnosed with an illness is a stressor that requires a response from the individual. How the person copes is influenced by a number of factors, including: whether the illness is acute, chronic or terminal; whether the person experiences pain, disability or loss; whether stigma is associated with the illness such as mental illness; whether treatment is available; the person's attribution style, such as internal or external LOC; and whether the person has sufficient social support and financial resources to assist coping. Importantly, coping with illness will be influenced by whether the person's quality of life (QoL) is affected. QoL refers to the person's perception of their wellbeing in their physical, functional, psychological/emotional and social/occupational domains (Fallowfield 2009).

Common emotional reactions to illness include denial, anxiety and depression (Taylor 2012). These responses produce additional stressors for the individual, particularly when the illness is chronic. The 'self-regulation model' for coping with chronic illness was proposed by Leventhal et al (1998) to explain how individuals cope with the stress of living with a chronic illness. Self-regulation refers to the individual proactively taking action to manage their health condition and to limit the negative effects of the illness. The stimulus to take action can be either internal, such as a person with diabetes who feels light headed so checks their blood sugar level, or external such as a person with diabetes who keeps a record of their daily blood sugar levels because they know their doctor will want to review them at the next appointment. The self-regulation model is a cognitive one that takes into account a person's view of their physical and social environments, as well as thoughts about themselves. See Chapter 9 for further discussion of chronic illness.

Conclusion

This chapter presented an overview of stress and coping. Stress was defined as the physical and psychological phenomenon experienced when a person perceives an event to threaten, challenge or exceed their available coping resources. While popular opinion views stress as a negative experience and one to be avoided, psychological research demonstrates that stress is a common experience that is a necessary part of everyday life and that stress stimulates an individual to take action in response to life's challenges and threats. Nevertheless, when stress is extreme, prolonged or the person is unable to adapt, negative health consequences can result. This also occurs when the person is overloaded with multiple stresses.

Coping was defined as the processes and strategies that a person adopts as they attempt to accommodate the actual or perceived discrepancies between stressful demands and their coping resources. When coping processes are adaptive they enable the person to respond to and manage the challenge. However, when coping resources are insufficient to manage the threat, physical and psychological illness can result. In summary, this chapter has demonstrated that the process whereby a person perceives and responds to stress is complex and influenced by a range of factors that are both internal and external to that person.

REMEMBER

- Stress and stressors are present in everyday life.
- Essentially people experience stress in the same way, although individuals may respond in different ways to the same stressor.
- Some stress and stressors are beneficial as they stimulate the individual to take action.
- Prolonged and cumulative minor stressors can affect health.
- Traumatic stress can lead to both short- and long-term health consequences.
- How a person copes with stress is influenced by factors that are both internal (within the person) and external (within the environment).

Further resources

Arranz, L., Guayerbas, N., De la Fuente, M., 2007. Impairment of several immune functions in anxious women. Journal of Psychosomatic Research (62), 1–8.

Glasberg, A., Eriksson, S., Norberg, A., 2007. Burnout and 'stress of conscience' among healthcare personnel. Journal of Advanced Nursing 57 (4), 392–403.

Hill Rice, V., 2012. Handbook of stress, coping and health: implications for nursing research, theory and practice, second ed. Sage, Thousand Oaks.

Pipe, T., Bortz, J., Dueck, M., et al., 2009. Nurse leader mindfulness meditation program for stress management: a randomized control trial. The Journal of Nursing Administration 39 (3), 130–137.

Scully, J., Tosi, H., Banning, K., 2000. Life events checklist: revisiting the social readjustment rating scale after 30 years. Educational and Psychological Measurement 60 (6), 864–876.

Weblinks

American Psychological Association

http://www.apa.org/topics/stress/index.aspx

The APA's 'stress' webpage includes tips on stress management and links to publications and research.

Australian Centre for Posttraumatic Mental Health

www.acpmh.unimelb.edu.au

The Australian Centre for Posttraumatic Mental Health undertakes trauma-related research, policy advice, service development and education. This website is a resource for health professionals who work with people who have experienced traumatic events.

Helpguide.org

www.helpguide.org/mental/stress_management_relief_coping.htm

The Helpguide.org website is a resource to help understand, prevent and resolve life's challenges.

Positive Psychology Centre

www.ppc.sas.upenn.edu

This website contains resources, research and publications about positive psychology including the writings of Martin Seligman.

The desk

www.thedesk.org.au

The desk aims to support Australian tertiary students to achieve mental and physical health and wellbeing. Students can access resources to help to improve their wellbeing and be able to study more effectively. The desk offers free access to online modules, tools, quizzes and advice.

References

Ader, R., Cohen, N., 1975. Behaviourally conditioned immunosuppression. Psychosomatic Medicine (37), 333–340.

American Psychological Association, 2012. Six myths about stress. Online. Available: http://www.apa.org/helpcenter/stress-myths.aspx 24 Sep 2012.

American Psychological Association, 2011. Resilience for teens. Online. Available: http://www.apa.org/helpcenter/bounce.aspx 24 Sep 2012.

Armstrong, A., Galligan, R., Critchley, C., 2011. Emotional intelligence and psychological resilience to negative life events. Personality and Individual Differences 51, 331–336.

Arranz, L., Guayerbas, N., De la Fuente, M., 2007. Impairment of several immune functions in anxious women. Journal of Psychosomatic Research 62, 1–8.

Bandura, A., 1977. Self efficacy: towards a unifying theory of behaviour change. Psychological Review 84, 191–215.

Bandura, A., 2001. Social cognitive theory. Annual Review of Psychology 52, 1–26.

Baum, F., 2008. The new public health, third ed. Oxford University Press, Melbourne.

Bosma, H., Marmot, M., Hemingway, H., et al., 1997. Low job control and risk of coronary heart disease in Whitehall II (prospective cohort) study. British Medical Journal 314, 558–565.

Cannon, W., 1932. The wisdom of the body. Norton, New York.

Cobb, S., 1976. Social support as a moderator of life stress. Psychosomatic Medicine 38, 300–314.

Contrada, R., Baum, A., 2010. The handbook of stress science: biology, psychology and health. Springer, New York.

Evans, K., 2012 Anxiety disorders. In: Elder, R., Evans, K., Nizette, D. (Eds.), Psychiatric and mental health nursing, third ed. Elsevier, Sydney.

Fallowfield, L., 2009. What is quality of life? Health economics. Online. Available: http://www.medicine.ox.ac.uk/bandolier/painres/download/whatis/WhatisQOL.pdf 26 Sep 2009.

Garmezy, N., 1987. Stress, competence and development: continuities in the study of schizophrenic adults and the search for stress resistant children. American Journal of Orthopsychiatry 57 (2), 159–174.

Garmezy, N., 1991. Resiliency and vulnerability to adverse developmental outcomes associated with poverty. American Journal of Behavioral Science 34, 416–430.

Glasberg, A., Eriksson, S., Norberg, A., 2007. Burnout and 'stress of conscience' among healthcare personnel. Journal of Advanced Nursing 57 (4), 392–403.

Gouin, J., 2011. Chronic stress, immune dysregulation and health. American Journal of Lifestyle Medicine 5, 476–485.

Holmes, T., Rahe, R., 1967. The social readjustment rating scale. Journal of Psychosomatic Research 11, 213–218.

Hulbert-Williams, N., Neal, R., Morrison, V., et al., 2011. Anxiety, depression and quality of life after cancer diagnosis: what psychosocial variables best predict how patients adjust? Psycho-Oncology 1–11.

Hurrell, J., Kelloway, E., 2007. Psychological job stress. In: Rom, W.N., Markowitz, S.B., (Eds.), Environmental and occupational medicine, fourth ed. Lippincott Williams & Wilkins, New York.

Kiecolt-Glasser, J., 2010. Stress, food and inflammation: psychoneuroimmuniology and nutrition at the cutting edge. Psychosomatic Medicine 72 (4), 365–369.

Irwin, M., 2008. Human psychoimmunology: 20 years of discovery. Brain, Behaviour and Immunity 22, 129–139.

Kiecolt-Glasser, J., 2009. Psychoneuroimmuniology: psychology's gateway to the biomedical future. Perspectives on Psychological Science 4 (3), 367–369.

Kanner, A., Coyne, J., Schaefer, C., et al., 1981. Comparison of two models of stress management: daily hassles and uplifts versus major life events. Journal of Behavioral Medicine 4, 1–39.

Knappe, S., Pinquart, M., 2009. Tracing criteria of successful aging? Health locus of control and well-being in older patients with internal diseases. Psychology Health and Medicine 14 (2), 201–212.

Lazarus, R., 1966. Psychological stress and the coping process. McGraw-Hill, New York.

Lazarus, R., Folkman, S., 1984. Stress, appraisal and coping. Springer, New York.

Lee, J., Akhtar, S., 2011. Effects of the workplace social context and job content on nurse burnout. Human Resources Management 50 (2), 227–245.

Leventhal, H., Leventhal, E., Contrada, R., 1998. Self-regulation, health and behaviour: a perceptual-cognitive approach. Psychology and Health 13, 717–733.

Marmot, M., Kogevinas, M., Elston, M., 1987. Social economic status and disease. Annual Review of Public Health 8, 111–135.

Marmot, M., Bosma, H., Hemingway, H., et al., 1997. Contribution of job control and other risk factors to social variations in coronary heart disease incidence. The Lancet 350, 235–239.

Maslach, C., Jackson, S., 1981. The measurement of experienced burnout. Journal of Occupational Behaviour 2, 99–113.

Maslach, C., 2003. Job burnout: new directions in research and intervention. Current Directions 12, 189–192.

O'Toole, B., Catts, S., 2008. Trauma, PTSD and physical health: an epidemiological study of Australian Vietnam veterans. Journal of Psychosomatic Research 64, 33–40.

Pipe, T., Bortz, J., Dueck, M., et al., 2009. Nurse leader mindfulness meditation peogram for stress management: a randomized control trial. The Journal of Nursing Administration 39 (3), 130–137.

Rasmussen, H., Scheier, M., Greenhouse, J., 2009. Optimism and physical health: a meta-analytic review. Annals of Behavioural Medicine 37, 239–256.

Rotter, J., 1966. Generalized expectancies for internal and external control of reinforcement. Psychological monographs: General and Applied 80, 1–28.

Scully, J., Tosi, H., Banning, K., 2000. Life events checklist: revisiting the social readjustment rating scale after 30 years. Educational and Psychological Measurement 60 (6), 864–876.

Segerstrom, S., 2006. How does optimism suppress immunity: evaluation of three affective pathways. Health Psychology 25, 653–657.

Seligman, M., 1974. Depression and learned helplessness. In: Friedman, J., Katz, M. (Eds.), The psychology of depression: theory and research. Winston-Wiley, Washington.

Seligman, M., 1994. Learned optimism. Random House, Sydney.

Seligman, M., 2011. Flourish: a new understanding of happiness and well-being. Free Press, New York.

Selye, H., 1956. The stress of life. McGraw-Hill, New York.

Taylor, S., 2012. Health psychology, eighth ed. McGraw-Hill, New York.

Wallston, K., Wallston, B., DeVellis, R., 1978. Development of the multidimensional health locus of control (MHLC) scales. Health Education and Behavior 6 (1), 160–170.

Witek-Janusek, L., Barkway, P., 2004. Stress and adaptation. In: Brown, H., Edwards, D. (Eds.), Lewis's medical-surgical nursing, second ed, Australian ed. Elsevier, Sydney.

World Health Organization (WHO), 2008. Closing the gap in a generation: health equity through action on the social determinants of health. WHO Commission on the Social Determinants of Health, Geneva.

Yerkes, R., Dodson, J., 1908. The relation of strength of stimulus to rapidity of habit formation. Journal of Comparative Neurology and Psychology 18, 459–482. Online. Available: http://psychclassics.yorku.ca/Yerkes/Law 24 Sep 2012.

Zhang, X., Norris, S., Gregg, E., et al., 2007. Social support and mortality among older persons with diabetes. Diabetes Educator 33 (2), 273–281.

Chapter 11
Loss

MICHAEL A BULL

Learning objectives

The material in this chapter will help you to:

- understand that loss is a central component of experience of many patients and their families
- identify the wide range of losses patients can experience
- recognise common reactions to loss
- respond appropriately and supportively to grieving patients and their families
- assess when grief may be complicated and requires more advanced support and assistance.

Key terms

- Loss
- Grief
- Disenfranchised grief
- Grief counselling
- Complicated grief

Introduction

Mourning is regularly the reaction to the loss of a loved person, or to the loss of some abstraction which has taken the place of one, such as fatherland, liberty, an ideal and so on ... It is well worth notice that, although grief involves grave departures from the normal attitude to life, it never occurs to us to regard it as a morbid condition and hand the mourner over to medical treatment. We rest assured that after a lapse of time it will be overcome and we look upon any interference with it as inadvisable or even harmful.

(Freud 1917 pp 243–244)

With these words almost a century ago, Freud laid the foundation for understanding the psychological elements of loss, grief and mourning. Indeed, he began to explore the link between grief and healthcare responses. Since then, descriptions of how people grieve and what helps those who experience loss have evolved and expanded. This chapter will explore a range of key theories, models and constructions related to loss, grief, mourning and responses to grief (see Table 11.1), with specific reference to ideas considered relevant to those working in healthcare. Suggestions for helping responses will be discussed. In this chapter, the term 'health professional' or 'helping professional' refers to those from a wide range of disciplines who work in healthcare settings. For simplicity, the term 'patient' is used for those who receive services from and are cared for by health professionals.[1]

Table 11.1	
MODELS OF LOSS, GRIEF AND MOURNING	
Model	Key concepts
Levels of loss (Weenolsen 1988)	Loss is experienced at five levels: ■ primary ■ secondary ■ holistic ■ self-conceptual ■ metaphorical
Ambiguous loss (Boss 2000, 2010)	Some losses are particularly difficult because they are uncertain, unclear or indeterminate; the lost loved one can be: ■ physically absent but psychologically present ■ physically present but psychologically absent
Disenfranchised loss (Doka 2002)	Some losses are not openly acknowledged or socially supported – specific types of relationships, losses, grievers, circumstances and ways of grieving are not socially recognised

Cont... ▶

[1]It is acknowledged that some healthcare settings prefer to use the term 'client' or 'consumer' rather than patient.

Table 11.1 (continued)

MODELS OF LOSS, GRIEF AND MOURNING

Model	Key concepts
Non-finite loss (Bruce & Schultz 2001, Harris & Gorman 2011)	Experiences such as disability, dementia, infertility, involve loss that unfolds throughout the lifespan and involve awareness of the discrepancy between life's events and 'what should have been'
Chronic sorrow (Burke et al 1992, Harris & Gorman 2011, Olshansky 1962)	Some losses, particularly those related to disability, involve intense, pervasive and recurring sadness over a long period of time
Tasks of mourning (Worden 2010)	There are four tasks involved in the process of grieving: ■ to accept the reality of the loss ■ to work through the pain of grief ■ to adjust to an environment without the lost person/thing ■ to emotionally relocate the lost person/thing and move on with life
Continuing bonds (Klass et al 1996)	It is normal and important for grievers to maintain a continuing connection with the person/thing that is lost, rather than having to 'let go'
Dual process model (Stroebe & Schut 1999)	The grief process involves loss-oriented work and restoration-oriented work and the oscillation and interaction between these two aspects of grieving
Complicated grief (Middleton et al 1993, Worden 2010)	Between 10% and 20% of grievers experience ongoing, problematic grief, often associated with factors such as the nature of the relationship with the lost person/thing, lack of preparation for the loss and lack of perceived support
Prolonged grief disorder (Prigerson et al 2008)	This classification of grief is being proposed for the 2013 *Diagnostic and Statistical Manual of Mental Disorders* (DSM-5) and emphasises the griever's intrusive thoughts and persistent, disruptive yearning for the lost person

Defining loss

Loss, in one form or another, will affect all of us – whether we are patients or practitioners. Because loss is a universal experience, defining it may seem unnecessary. However, establishing a common description of loss is probably useful. Loss, write Harvey and Weber (1999 p 320), involves 'a reduction in a person's resources, whether personal, material, or symbolic, to which the person was emotionally attached'. Weenolsen (1988 p 19) succinctly defines loss as 'anything that destroys some aspect, whether macroscopic or microscopic, of life and self'. Loss involves the separation from something – maybe large, maybe small – that has meaning to us and to which we feel strongly connected.

Types of loss

The range of possible losses is almost limitless. How can we attempt to understand the diverse types of losses? Weenolsen (1988) proposes the following classification:

- *Major versus minor loss* – We frequently focus on major losses, such as the death of a family member or the devastation of a bushfire. However, seemingly minor losses can have major significance. Weenolsen describes minor losses as 'the many small deaths of life' (1988 p 21) that can affect us profoundly because they represent larger losses. For example, older people can experience the termination of their driver's licence as the loss of capabilities, mobility and independence, leading to a strong sense of grief.

- *Primary versus secondary loss* – While primary losses usually are identified easily, secondary or derivative losses may not be recognised and can be more painful. A major illness, such as chronic fatigue or heart disease, can lead to secondary losses of unemployment, significant financial loss, family stress and reduced life choices. Healthcare practitioners are challenged to recognise the range of secondary losses experienced by their patients in order to respond holistically to loss-related needs.

- *Actual versus threatened loss* – A loss need not actually occur for a grief response to be generated. Weenolsen notes that a threat to safety, self-identity or health can result in a sense of loss – 'a biopsy may be negative but the self is not the same afterward' (1988 p 22). Threatened loss is similar to Hockley's (1985) description of deprivation loss, where grief is experienced for something the person never had. Couples undergoing in vitro fertilisation treatment can experience a powerful sense of loss each time a treatment is unsuccessful, complicated by the prospect of childlessness that is threatened if a pregnancy never eventuates.

- *Internal versus external loss* – Weenolsen (1988) argues that all losses have an external and internal element. External losses frequently will involve the associated loss of an internalised self-ideal or societal ideal. This type of loss is common after such health-related experiences as mastectomy, amputation, acquired brain injury, burns or chemotherapy-related hair loss. These external losses can challenge the internalised social constructions about appearance, body image, beauty or gender, leading to potentially profound grief reactions.

- *Chosen versus imposed loss* – Losses can result from both chosen and imposed life events. For example, migration as a refugee is imposed by persecution or dislocation, leading to the loss of family connections, freedom and financial security. However, choosing to migrate, while often involving positives such as new opportunities, also can involve associated grief. Those who migrate voluntarily can still experience a sense of loss of homeland, national identity, connections to their past, shared experiences with family 'back home' and continuity of cultural practices. Other life choices, such as to not marry or have children, can result in a strong sense of regret and grief about what 'might have been', even though the loss was chosen.

- *Direct versus indirect loss* – Weenolsen (1988) describes how loss can occur through the experiences of another person. She notes, for example, the grief that parents can experience through the losses affecting their children, such as serious illness, school difficulties, failed relationships or family problems.

LEVELS OF LOSS

Weenolsen also describes five levels of loss, a framework that is particularly useful for understanding the full impact of loss situations:

- *The primary level of loss* – This level of loss is most evident and generally dominates people's perception of a loss situation.

- *The secondary level of loss* – This level is about the derivative, concrete losses that follow directly from, usually with some immediacy after, a primary loss. For example, the primary loss of a diagnosis of childhood leukaemia can lead to such secondary losses as financial pressure due to medical expenses, work time lost due to demands of doctors' appointments, and disruption of school attendance and performance due to treatment side effects.

- *The holistic level of loss* – This level relates to the more abstract losses associated with primary and secondary losses, such as loss of future, dreams, status and security. Childhood leukaemia can result in the loss of hopes for the person's child, loss of safety as the child's life is threatened and loss of family security as the future of a family member becomes uncertain.

- *The self-conceptual level of loss* – A primary loss can lead to changes in how a person sees themselves because part of the self is perceived to be lost. A child with leukaemia may now see herself as 'sick', 'different', 'less competent' in school and a 'burden' on the family's emotional and financial resources.

- *The metaphorical level of loss* – This level recognises the idiosyncratic meaning that a loss has because the person's beliefs are challenged. A significant loss can lead to questioning of values, beliefs and a person's philosophical views. Childhood leukaemia, for example, may challenge assumptions that children will outlive their parents, that parents are able to protect their children from harm or that God will not allow children to suffer.

There are some important implications from Weenolsen's five-level framework. As Weenolsen (1991 p 56) writes, acknowledging the levels 'helps us understand better why loss affects us so deeply'. When we see patients who are grieving, we often witness intense and pervasive reactions. Awareness that they are grieving at several levels can help us make sense of these responses. Second, Weenolsen's model demonstrates how grief 'unfolds' through the levels and is not static or one-dimensional. Third, this framework provides a guide for more comprehensive support and intervention with grieving people. The responses of helping professionals need to consider and address all levels of loss, rather than focus only on the primary loss.

AMBIGUOUS LOSS

Ambiguous loss has been described as the most devastating of all losses in personal relationships due to the uncertain, unclear and indeterminate nature of the loss (Bocknek et al 2009, Boss 2000, 2010). Boss describes two types of ambiguous loss. The first type occurs when a loved one is perceived as physically absent but psychologically present. Such loss relates to situations such as missing soldiers, lost or kidnapped children, family members separated by divorce, and relinquishment through adoption. The second type of ambiguous loss is experienced when a loved one is perceived as physically present but psychologically absent. Health-related conditions such as dementia, addictions, mental illnesses and brain injury involve this type of ambiguous loss. The physically present–psychologically absent dilemma also occurs in palliative care if others treat the dying person as if they are already dead (social death) or if the patient lacks consciousness of existence (psychological death) (Kalish 1966 in Doka 2002, Sudnow 1967). Boss anticipates that, as medical advances keep dying patients alive longer, more families will experience the stress associated with ambiguous loss.

Lack of control makes coping with ambiguous loss so difficult. Five factors can interfere with coping:

- people are confused by the indefinite nature of the loss and become immobilised

- the uncertainty prevents adjustment and results in 'frozen' relationships with the ambiguously lost person

- the ambiguous loss is not recognised by the community, with little validation and no rituals

- ambiguous losses are more confronting, reminding people that life is not always rational or just (this reality can cause potential supports to withdraw)

- because ambiguous loss can be prolonged, those who experience it become physically and emotionally exhausted (Boss 2000, 2010).

To help people deal with ambiguous loss, Boss emphasises sharing information with families, including clinical and technical information. She states that 'clinicians need to realize that by sharing knowledge they are empowering families to take control of their situation even when ambiguity exists' (Boss 2000 p 23). In Bull's (1998) study of families of people with Alzheimer's, respondents listed receiving information as the most helpful thing for dealing with dementia in the family. Information assists in constructing a reality amid the ambiguity. Meeting others who have experienced such a loss further increases a family's information and support base.

Ambiguous loss also can be traumatising, with symptoms similar to post-traumatic stress disorder (PTSD) (Boss 2000, 2010). Like an experience of trauma (Harris & Gorman 2011, Herman 2001), ambiguous loss is outside the realm of usual human experience and often involves a threat to the life or physical safety of a loved one. Trauma often relates to a single traumatising event. However, ambiguous loss usually involves a series of psychological ups and downs, with hopes repeatedly dashed so that continuing to try to cope seems futile and learned helplessness can develop. Boss highlights the importance of allowing those experiencing ambiguous loss to tell their story, to receive validation and to have someone help them make sense of what they are experiencing.

DISENFRANCHISED LOSS AND GRIEF

A concept that has significantly expanded awareness about the nature and impact of loss is disenfranchised grief. Kenneth Doka (2002 p 4) defined disenfranchised grief as 'the grief that persons experience when they incur a loss that is not or cannot be openly acknowledged, publicly mourned, or socially supported! Losses are disenfranchised by the dominant societal norms or 'rules' that define acceptable feeling, thinking and spiritual expression when loss occurs (Doka 2002, Doka & Tucci 2009). Loss experiences that fall outside these rules are not recognised. Doka's work has effectively integrated the psychological and the social elements of loss and grieving by acknowledging that a person's experience of grief is often affected by factors external to the griever.

Doka has proposed the following typology of losses that are disenfranchised:

- *the relationship is not recognised* (e.g. friends, ex-partners, professional helpers, internet relationships, gay partners, companion animals)

- *the loss is not acknowledged* (e.g. abortion, miscarriage, infertility, secondary losses, non-death losses, loss of connection to land)

- *the griever is excluded* (e.g. children, the aged, people with intellectual disabilities)

- *circumstances of the death* (e.g. AIDS-related deaths, suicides, murders)

- *ways people grieve* (e.g. different styles of grieving, cultural differences in grieving).

Health professionals should consider the concept of disenfranchised grief for several reasons. First, we have all been exposed to social norms about 'acceptable' loss and grieving and need to be aware of how these norms may influence our professional thinking and practices, possibly resulting in disenfranchising attitudes and behaviours. Second, as noted in Doka's typology above, there are many health-related losses that are not acknowledged. For example, Corr (2002 p 43) maintains that 'until quite recently and perhaps still today in many segments of society, perinatal deaths, losses associated with elective abortion, or losses of body parts have frequently been disenfranchised!

Third, health professions, by their nature, can sometimes contribute to disenfranchising processes. The primary focus of healthcare is necessarily on treatment, cure, rehabilitation and recovery. Losses may not fit within such a perspective as they may be perceived as healthcare 'failures! Our professional language may be disenfranchising. For example, an amputee rehabilitation setting may describe its work in terms of 'replacement' (through a prosthesis), 'recovery of function' (through physical and occupational therapies), 'adjustment' and 'progress! Such language may limit acknowledgement of the patient's deep sense of bodily impairment, of frustration, of lost possibilities and hopes, and of nothing ever being the same again. Similarly, the focus of health professionals is often on symptomatology. Corr argues that referring to grief *symptoms* disenfranchises grief by failing to recognise the essentially natural and healthy responses to loss found in many grieving behaviours. Speaking about the *signs, manifestations* or *expressions* of grief avoids disenfranchising and even pathologising the wide range of appropriate responses to loss (Corr 2002).

Finally, the grief of health professionals may be disenfranchised (Spidell et al 2011). Such professionals may not be considered as 'legitimate' grievers when, for example, a patient dies. The health professional–patient relationship may not be recognised as one in which the helper's grief is appropriate. Indeed the concept of 'being a professional' often promotes emotional distance between the helper and the patient, resulting in professionals potentially disenfranchising their own grief. For example, after a patient has died nurses are often expected to carry out protocols for managing a dead body and preparing the deceased patient's bed as quickly as possible for the next admission. Frequently little recognition is given by the hospital system, by senior staff and by the nurses themselves to the nurse as a griever.

Classroom activity

1. Using the internet or a community services directory, identify as many services and resources as you can in your local community that are available for grieving people and/or their families. Once you have completed your list, share your findings and ideas with at least one other student in your class.

2. Review Doka's typology of disenfranchised losses on page 257. Under each of the five categories, write down three ways that the healthcare system can disenfranchise the loss and grief of patients and/or families. Then propose strategies by which disenfranchising practices can be avoided or redressed.

NONFINITE LOSS AND CHRONIC SORROW

Another concept of particular relevance to the field of healthcare is nonfinite loss. Bruce and Schultz (2001) developed this term through their clinical and research encounters with families of children with developmental disabilities. They recognised that these parents experienced ongoing loss and grief as the impact of their child's disability unfolded throughout the lifespan. Nonfinite loss is contingent on three elements: lifestage development, passage of time and a lack of synchrony between lived experience and hopes and expectations. The loss is often not identified or named until the person reflects back and realises what did not happen in life in comparison to 'what should have been' (Bruce & Schultz 2001 p 8).

Nonfinite loss has been associated with situations such as: congenital or acquired disabilities; traumatic injury; ongoing or degenerative illnesses such as dementia; adoption; infertility; separation and divorce; and sexual abuse. These experiences can challenge, even shatter, preconceived ideas of what the world should be like, leading to ongoing, nonfinite loss and grief (Bruce & Schultz 2001). Parents of a child with a disability can be repeatedly reminded of what their child has not been able to achieve in comparison to the hopes and dreams they had for that child (Ray & Street 2007). Indeed, Bruce (2000) reported that approximately 20% of mothers experience symptoms of PTSD after the birth of a child with a disability and that their grief is often disenfranchised. Five cycles of nonfinite grief can be experienced, involving themes of shock, protest/demand, defiance, resignation/despair and integration (Bruce & Schultz 2001). The nonfinite nature of the grieving means these cycles recur: 'The cycles are not linear, have no end-point and are prone to recycling again and again' (Bruce & Schultz 2001 p 163).

Similar to nonfinite loss and grief is chronic sorrow. Olshansky (1962) first described chronic sorrow as the intense, pervasive and recurring sadness observed in parents of children with an intellectual disability. Other studies have examined chronic sorrow among parents of children with chronic illness (Bettle & Latimer 2009, Gordon 2009) and female victims of child abuse (Slaughter Smith 2009). Chronic sorrow, while often continuing through a person's life, is considered 'a normal reaction to the significant loss of normality in the affected individual or the caregiver' (Burke et al 1992 p 232). Burke et al, writing from a nursing perspective, argue that it is important to recognise the difference between the normality of chronic sorrow and complicated grief or depression. This caution is an important one for health professionals whose culture characteristically seeks to diagnose and treat pathology. Many patients and families with long-term illnesses will be experiencing nonfinite loss and chronic sorrow (e.g. see Bowes et al's 2009 discussion regarding chronic sorrow in parents of children with type 1 diabetes). By missing or mislabelling their patients' grief, health professionals run the risk of disenfranchising patients' losses or responding inappropriately. Chronic sorrow is best treated through recognition of the family's recurrent experiences of grief and supportive responses to their sadness.

Research focus

Nikcevic, A., Kuczmierczyk, K.A., Nicolaides, K., 2007. The influence of medical and psychological interventions on women's distress after miscarriage. Journal of Psychosomatic Research 63 (3), 283–290.

ABSTRACT

Objective

The aim of this study was to examine the impact of medical and psychological interventions on women's distress after early miscarriage.

Methods

This was a prospective study of women attending for a routine scan at 10–14 weeks of gestation and found to have a missed miscarriage. An intervention group of 66 women had medical investigations to ascertain the cause of miscarriage and at five weeks after the scan, they all had a medical consultation to discuss the results of the investigations. These 66 women were randomly allocated into a group that received further psychological counselling (MPC, n = 33) and a group that received no psychological counselling (MC, n = 33). They were compared with a control group of 61 women who received no specific post-miscarriage counselling. All participants completed pre-intervention and post-intervention measures and four-month follow-up questionnaires.

Results

The scores on the outcome variables decreased significantly with time for all three groups. In group MPC, compared with the control group, there was a significantly greater decrease over time in the levels of grief, self-blame and worry and, compared with group MC, a significantly

Cont... ▶

greater decrease in grief and worry. In group MC, compared with the control group, there was a significantly greater decrease in self-blame. In the MC and MPC groups, those with an identified cause of the miscarriage had significantly lower levels of anxiety and self-blame over time than those with a non-identified cause.

Conclusions

Psychological counselling, in addition to medical investigations and consultation, is beneficial in reducing women's distress after miscarriage. However, absence of an identifiable cause of miscarriage led to the maintenance of the initial anxiety levels, which should have otherwise decreased with time.

Critical thinking

- In relation to the Nikcevic et al (2007) study above, why might having an identified cause of miscarriage assist a woman in her grieving? Consider Worden's first task of mourning and the concepts of disenfranchised grief and ambiguous loss in your thinking.
- Using Table 11.2 on page 266. as a guide, describe grief support activities you would suggest for women who have had a miscarriage. If you are able to access the full article by Nikcevic et al, compare your suggestions with those used in the counselling sessions in the study (see section 'Participants and procedure').

Responses to loss

Since Freud's early writing about grief, health professionals have been trying to understand how people respond to loss. Freud's notion that mourning occurred over a period of time has been accepted and this time element of mourning has been described as the grief process.

THE GRIEF PROCESS

The grief process has been conceptualised in various ways. One approach has been to identify phases or stages in grieving. Erich Lindemann (1944), a pioneer in the study of grief, outlined three phases in the grief process: emancipation from bondage to the deceased, readjustment to the environment without the deceased and the formation of new relationships. Parkes (1972, 1988) and later Bowlby (1980) referred to four phases associated with grieving – numbness, yearning to recover the lost person, disorganisation and despair and reorganisation. Sanders' (1999) model proposed five phases in the mourning process: shock, awareness of loss, conservation-withdrawal, healing and renewal. In her work with terminally ill patients, Kübler-Ross (1969) identified five psychological stages in the dying process. Her staged model of denial, anger, bargaining, depression and acceptance has been used to describe the grieving process. However, Kübler-Ross' work was not intended to describe mourning and has limitations as a grief model (Corr 1993, Worden 2010).

The phase/stage view of grief has been criticised for inferring that the grieving process is essentially passive. Attig (1991 p 386) argues that the phase/stage concept frames 'grieving as yet another thing that happens to bereaved persons, a process into which they are thrust against their will ... (with) little choice of paths through the process'. Attig also cautions against any medical conceptualisations of grief, as these too imply that grief is a kind of illness that happens to people and over which people have no choice once a major bereavement occurs. Instead, Attig sees grieving as an active process through which the griever *relearns* their world.

TASKS OF MOURNING

Psychologist William Worden also argued for a more active view of grieving and developed a widely accepted task model of mourning. Worden (2010) states that a task model fits better with the concept of 'grief work' as described by Freud and Lindemann; that is, grievers need to *act* to move through the grief process. The task model is also seen as consistent with the psychological concept of developmental tasks associated with all human growth. Finally, Worden sees the task model as more useful for practitioners, as 'the approach implies that mourning can be influenced by intervention from the outside' (2010 p 26). Both the griever and the helping professional can approach their grief-related work with a greater sense of agency and mastery. Indeed, this author frequently uses, in his own grief-related practice, the terms 'grieving' (rather than 'grief') and 'work' with clients to communicate the active process in which they are observed to be engaging and to acknowledge the often intense effort (work) that they expend in doing their grieving.

Worden's four tasks of mourning set out specific foci for grievers' actions:

1. *To accept the reality of the loss.* 'The first task of grieving is to come full face with the reality that the person is dead, that the person is gone and will not return' (Worden 2010 p 27). This task addresses the numbness, shock and denial noted in phase models. Denial most often involves the facts of the loss, the meaning of the loss or the irreversibility of the loss. Full denial of a loss may be rare but degrees of denial are not uncommon. As a recognised defence mechanism (Goldstein 1995, Grossberg 2008), denial serves to protect us from the anxiety that may overwhelm us. So we face experiences in smaller parts to deal with what we feel ready to face. Sometimes grievers are described by others as 'being in denial'; health professionals should be aware of not doing this in a way that is dismissive or disenfranchising of patients' or families' grief.

   Funerals and other rituals are useful in providing structure and procedures for gradually facing the reality of a loss. Worden states that both intellectual and emotional acceptance of a loss is necessary; less experienced practitioners can overlook emotional acceptance. This task is more difficult for grievers who have experienced a sudden, unexpected death, especially if the body is not seen. If Weenolsen's levels of loss are also considered, the complexity of this task is further evident. As the levels of loss unfold, the reality of the loss keeps changing, requiring this task to be revisited.

2. *To work through the pain of grief.* Sadness, guilt, anger, loneliness and depressive feelings are often involved in grieving. The intensity of grievers'

emotional pain can go beyond what they have previously experienced and they may wonder if they are 'going crazy'. Because experiencing intense grief pain is so difficult, some people will try to avoid working on this task through stopping painful thoughts, numbing feelings through alcohol or drugs, distracting themselves through work or other activities, or evading painful thoughts and feelings by the 'geographic cure' of moving from place to place (Worden 2010 p 31). Some people are afraid of 'breaking down', stating 'If I allow myself to start feeling (e.g. crying), I'm afraid I will never stop!'. McKissock and McKissock (2012) also describe the 'pharmacological' effects of major loss, as the griever's biochemistry works to numb the immediate emotional reactions. Further emotional distress can be experienced as the numbing wears off in the weeks following the loss. Family and friends do not like to see their loved ones hurting and may feel helpless about how to respond. As a result, they (and helping professionals) can do or say things that give the message 'We don't really want to see your pain'. This is one way that grief responses can be disenfranchised, as discussed above.

3. *To adjust to an environment in which the lost person/thing is missing.* Worden (2010) identifies three types of adjustment: external adjustments, internal adjustments and spiritual adjustments. External adjustments refer to the many functional changes that occur after the death of a loved one. New skills, roles and knowledge – such as cooking meals, driving the family car, parenting without a partner or managing finances – have to be developed. This process can be a challenge both practically and emotionally as many grievers find their energy levels low, their cognitive abilities taxed and their willingness to face more change limited. Internal adjustments relate to changes in the griever's sense of self. These adjustments often will depend on the nature of the relationship and the attachment with the lost person/thing. For example, a relationship that is highly dependent (i.e. one person depends on another to meet their own needs) can lead to significant internal adjustment difficulties. Loss could activate latent self-images (Berzoff 2011, Horowitz et al 1980). Such self-images may be negative, for example, for a woman who experienced childhood sexual abuse before finding some security in the marriage with her now-deceased husband. Alternatively, reactivated self-images may be positive, for example, for a woman who can now pursue career goals that her husband discouraged. Spiritual adjustments involve making sense of or finding meaning in the loss, similar to Weenolsen's idiosyncratic loss discussed above. Basic assumptions such as 'the world is a good place', 'the world makes sense' and 'I am a worthy person' can be replaced by ideas that 'the world sucks!', 'life is not fair!' and 'I must have done something bad for this to happen!' (Janoff-Bulman 1992, Worden 2010).

4. *To emotionally relocate the lost person/thing and move on with life.* This task focuses on the importance of grievers 'finding a place' for the loss in their life while still moving ahead. Worden originally expressed this task as 'withdrawing emotional energy from the deceased and reinvesting it in another relationship' (2010 p 35). However, bereaved people subsequently told Worden that withdrawing was not what they did in their grieving; they tried to stay connected to their loved one. Worden therefore revised this task. Grievers, sometimes with the help of a caring professional, seek to 'find an

appropriate place for the dead in their emotional lives – a place that will enable them to go on living effectively in the world' (Worden 2010 p 36). The importance of *staying connected* is evident in the not uncommon stories grievers tell about how upsetting it is when others do not talk about the deceased person, acting as if the dead person never existed. White (1988) also describes the psychological conflict grievers experience when they feel the need, or are expected, to 'say goodbye'. He proposes that helping grievers to 'say hello' to their dead loved one both releases them from the inappropriate expectation of leaving their loved one behind and empowers them to establish an ongoing connection with the deceased.

CONTINUING BONDS

The importance of 'staying connected' has been reinforced in the work on continuing bonds. Klass et al (1996) present the findings of various theorists and researchers that support the value for grievers in sustaining their relationship with the lost person. They too question the usefulness of grievers having to 'let go':

We propose that it is normative for mourners to maintain a presence and connection with the deceased … We cannot look at bereavement as a psychological state that ends and from which one recovers. The intensity of feelings may lessen and the mourner become more future- rather than past-oriented; however, a concept of closure, requiring a determination of when the bereavement process ends, does not seem compatible with the model suggested by these findings. We propose that rather than emphasizing letting go, the emphasis should be on negotiating and renegotiating the meaning of the loss over time.

(Silverman & Klass 1996 pp 18–19)

The ways in which grievers achieve continuing bonds are creative and fascinating. They reflect the individualised meanings that connecting practices have for the grievers and their families. One family whose daughter died with cancer established a memorial fund at her primary school to cover the costs of their daughter's class cohort for an annual excursion. However, the family realised that this memorial was meaningful primarily to their daughter's classmates and so the funding was maintained only until her class had graduated from their final year of primary school. This memorial provided a continuing bond for both the family and their daughter's school friends.

Marwit and Klass (1996), in their study of 71 university students, identified four ways an important person can play a continuing role after their death. These were:

- *Role model* – someone with whom the student could identify, for example, 'I remember him as the ideal dad; someone I would like to imitate as a parent'.

- *Situation-specific guidance* – situations in which the deceased helps the living with a specific situation, for example, 'I always think about her when I'm trying to make a decision on some big event in my life. I think, *What would she do?*'

- *Values clarification* – choosing for or against a moral position identified with the deceased, for example, 'Rick is sort of a motivation for me to continue being sensitive and patient with people'.

- *Remembrance formation* – remembering the deceased without that person performing any active function, for example, 'Now my dad is someone we enjoy reminiscing about ... We wonder what he would be like 12 years older and what he would be doing' (Marwit & Klass 1996 pp 300–301).

These four ways of continuing bonds can play a significant ongoing function, even when high levels of grief resolution are reported.

THE DUAL PROCESS MODEL

Another perspective on how people respond to loss is presented in the *dual process model*. Stroebe & Schut (1999, 2008) have argued that the concept of 'grief work' does not capture the complexity of activity involved in the process of grieving. They maintain that grief work focuses too much on the need to confront the personal, intrapsychic loss of the loved one without recognising the interpersonal processes that support mourning, the diversity of stressors that grievers need to deal with (in addition to the lost relationship), and the fluctuating nature of grief that can involve swings between the confrontation and avoidance of changes and stressors.

Consequently, the dual process model is constructed around two realms: loss-oriented and restoration-oriented coping (see Fig 11.1). *Loss-orientation* 'refers to the concentration on and dealing with, processing of some aspect of the loss experienced itself, most particularly, with respect to the deceased person' (Stroebe & Schut 1999 p 212). This orientation includes the traditional view of grief work, with its focus on relationship or bonds to the deceased person and the ruminations about the deceased, life together, circumstances surrounding the death and yearning for the deceased. Loss-orientation is usually more evident in early bereavement, although it can dominate the griever's attention periodically over time.

Restoration-orientation addresses the additional stressors associated with a major loss, such as those found in Weenolsen's levels of loss. These stressors include undertaking new tasks, organising one's life without the deceased person, developing

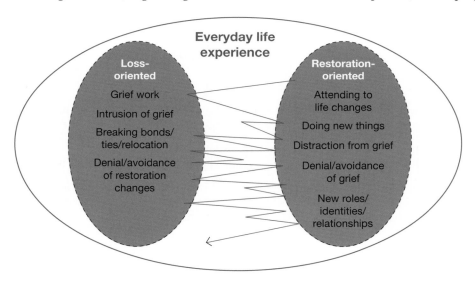

Figure 11.1 The dual process model

Source: Stroebe M, Schut H 1999 The dual process model of coping with bereavement: rationale and description. Death Studies Vol 23, p 197–224

a new identity and constructing some meaning in one's new world. A central element of the dual process model is oscillation: the alternation between loss- and restoration-oriented coping. Stroebe and Schut view oscillation as a dynamic, back-and-forth process that allows the griever to alternatively confront or avoid the loss, depending on various ongoing psychological, social and practical demands. This alternation is seen as having major mental and physical health benefits. The griever may choose to take 'time off' from grieving, to avoid feelings experienced as too painful at a given point and indeed to use denial in a beneficial way. Stroebe and Schut, citing findings about the severe detrimental psychological and physical effects of unremitting avoidance of grief, argue that the dual process model acknowledges the coping value of the oscillation between confrontation and avoidance. The model's flexibility is seen as accommodating such variables as gender, social and cultural differences in grieving styles and methods (Stroebe & Schut 1999, 2008). Overall, the dual process model effectively expresses the unpredictable, vacillating and ongoing complexities of the grief experience.

FOUR ELEMENTS OF GRIEF RESPONSES

Worden (2010) has identified four categories of grief responses – feelings, physical sensations, cognitions and behaviours – that usefully capture the wide range of reactions seen in those experiencing uncomplicated grief.

Feelings

Feelings most commonly include shock, sadness, anger, guilt, anxiety, loneliness, helplessness, yearning, despair, depression, emancipation and relief – sometimes even a lack of feeling (anhedonia) (Stroebe et al 2001, Worden 2010). Particularly difficult to accept and manage can be feelings of anger and guilt. Anger 'is at the root of many problems in the grieving process' (Worden 2010 p 12). Anger can be directed at the person who died, family members, a seemingly insensitive friend, or God/the world. Health professionals can find themselves the target of such anger. It is important to recognise that this anger almost invariably is not intended as a personal attack. It generally comes from the frustration that nothing could prevent the death/loss and the anxiety that results from 'being left' on one's own. Grievers also frequently are able to identify something that should, or should not, have been done in relation to the loss, resulting in feelings of guilt. Anxiety can range from insecurity to anxiety or panic attacks, even phobias in complicated grief reactions. Bereaved people can feel positively about being freed from controlling or abusive relationships or relieved that physical and emotional pain is ended with the death of a suffering loved one.

Physical reactions

Lindemann (1944) is credited with first describing the physical reactions of grief. Such physical sensations as fatigue, hollowness in the stomach, shortness of breath, muscle weakness, oversensitivity to noise and a sense of depersonalisation can exist (Worden 2010). Grievers will sometimes report having the physical symptoms of the person who died (Stroebe et al 2001). Many grievers may not recognise the link between their physical reactions and their grief. It is important therefore for health professionals to be able to identify the physiological elements of grieving and assist grievers in receiving both medical care and grief support.

Cognitive reactions

Cognitive reactions to loss can include disbelief, confusion, problems with memory and concentration, lowered self-esteem, hopelessness, sense of unreality, preoccupation with thoughts of the deceased, sense of presence and hallucinations (Stroebe et al 2001, Worden 2010). It is not unusual for grievers to find their thinking dominated by images and ruminations about the person who died and experiences associated with the death. Some thoughts can be reassuring, such as positive memories about times spent with the deceased loved one, while other thoughts can be distressing. For example, an adult bereaved son reported how the image of his dying father kept appearing over and over again, like a video replaying repeatedly. Thought disturbances are the adjustment required to 're-think' the world in which the lost person or thing is gone.

The cognitive gap or incongruence that results from the absence of a loved one can take some time to be resolved. Preoccupation, sense of presence and hallucinations represent some of the powerful thoughts that occur in grievers' efforts to stay connected to the lost person, while cognitively adjusting to life without that person. Worden (2010) is clear that cognitive processes such as visual and auditory hallucinations belong in a list of normal responses to major loss. Kauffman (2002 p 72) supports this view, stating that 'the hallucinatory power of the image of the deceased functions to mitigate and integrate death loss'. Hallucinations reflect the strong desire to keep alive what is lost because the person is adjusting to the reality of life with that loss. While some grievers may be disconcerted, fearful or ashamed of hallucinatory thoughts, many find them reassuring, with some even seeking them out through those who claim they can make contact with the dead. Kauffman (2002) argues that if such processes as sense of presence or hallucinations are ignored, suppressed or discouraged by self or others, important grief work is disenfranchised and possibly blocked.

Behavioural reactions

Grievers may engage in a range of behavioural reactions. Common behaviours include agitation, crying, social withdrawal, sleep disturbances, appetite changes, absent-minded behaviour, avoiding reminders of the deceased, searching and calling

Table 11.2	
COMMON BEHAVIOURS ASSOCIATED WITH EXPECTED GRIEF	
Life-enhancing behaviours	Life-depleting behaviours

Crying
Talking about the loss
Reaching out for support
Accepting assistance
Taking care of yourself
Exercising
Getting rest/sleep
Seeking out symbolic connection
  with the deceased
	Substance abuse
	High risk-taking behaviours
	Compulsive/excessive behaviours (e.g.
	  eating, shopping, working, gambling)
	Withdrawal and isolation
	Agitated, aggressive and demanding
	  behaviours
	Anxiety-driven behaviours
	Suicidal gestures or attempts

From Pomeroy/Garcia. The Grief Assessment and Intervention Workbook, 1E. © 2009 Wadsworth, a part of Cengage Learning, Inc. Reproduced by permission, www.cengage.com/permissions

out, sighing, restless overactivity and visiting places or carrying objects that remind them of the deceased (Stroebe et al 2001, Worden 2010). Behavioural changes will usually correct themselves over time (Worden 2010) as the griever gradually integrates the impact and meaning of the loss. As behaviours are often the visible expressions of feelings and thoughts, it is important that helping professionals know how to interpret such behaviours. Pomeroy and Garcia (2008 p 52) distinguish between life-depleting and life-enhancing behaviours (see Table 11.2). These authors note that behaviours can be life-enhancing at one point and life-depleting at another. For example, crying can be a life-enhancing expression of sadness but prolonged and excessive crying can lead to exhaustion and disruption to activities of daily living. Similarly, while exercising can enhance the griever's physical health, compulsive exercising may serve to avoid dealing with painful feelings.

CASE STUDY: ELLY

You are doing a practicum as a student health professional at a local teaching hospital. You have been asked to see Elly, a 49-year-old woman who has come for an appointment at the renal outpatient clinic. Your task is to take Elly's medical and social history before she sees the clinician.

After you greet Elly, introduce yourself and explain why you have come to see her, Elly relates the following information:

She was born with cerebral palsy. She currently requires a walker/Zimmer frame to walk, or a wheelchair for longer distances.

Since her childhood, Elly has been hospitalised frequently for numerous surgeries throughout her life, including operations on her legs as a child. Elly states that she wore full leg braces as a child due to her cerebral palsy.

Three years ago Elly was diagnosed with a cancerous lump in her lower back. She had surgery, chemotherapy and radiotherapy for this cancer.

Elly lives in a public housing unit that is specially equipped to assist her with activities of daily living. She lives alone. Her husband of almost 20 years died suddenly eight years ago of a heart attack. Elly's husband was 15 years older than her. Elly has no children. She reports one pregnancy but seems reluctant to discuss this further. She indicates that she had a hysterectomy at age 21.

Elly's family history reveals that both her parents are dead. Her mother died of cancer and her father from a heart attack. She reports that a sister died of suicide, a brother died of drowning and another brother died of cancer.

Elly indicates that over the past six years her sleep has been disrupted. She sleeps for between four and five hours per night, sometimes less. When you ask Elly about particular reasons for this sleep pattern, she states that sometimes she has disturbing dreams from which she wakes suddenly and in a sweat. Elly does not want to talk further about her dreams.

Elly states that she believes her cerebral palsy is worsening. She also notes that she currently sees medical specialists for liver, heart, neurological and cancer problems.

Critical thinking

- While taking Elly's history, you are struck by the number of losses in her life.
- Using Weenolsen's framework of five levels of loss, identify the losses that you think Elly has, or may have, experienced throughout her life.
- Are there any areas of Elly's experience that you believe could be explored further, in terms of her losses and her experience of grief?
- Considering that you have just met Elly and that this may be your only contact with her, can you think of any appropriate, brief comments or responses that you could make to Elly that would acknowledge her losses and demonstrate you understand her losses to some degree? Write out three possible comments/responses.

CULTURAL CONSIDERATIONS

In considering the ideas presented in this chapter, it is worth noting that many of the concepts about loss and grief have come from, and arguably have been dominated by, what might broadly be called Western culture (Allan & Harms 2010, Merritt 2011). Yet, the context of health care is becoming increasingly multicultural. Consequently 'healthcare professionals need to understand the part that may be played by cultural mourning practices in an individual's overall grief experience if they are to provide culturally sensitive care to their patients ... When assessing a person's response to the death of a loved one, clinicians should identify and appreciate what is expected or required by the person's culture' (National Cancer Institute 2012 p 7). The literature on cultural sensitivity emphasises that culture 'creates, influences, shapes, limits, and defines grieving, sometimes profoundly' (Rosenblatt 2008 p 208).

Efforts to understand how a patient or family from any given culture might grieve run the risk of being simplistic and therefore unhelpful (Rosenblatt 2008). However, existing guidelines can make such efforts more productive. The following five questions have been highlighted as particularly important to ask those coping with the death of a loved one:

- What are the culturally prescribed rituals for managing the dying process, the body of the deceased, the disposal of the body, and commemoration of the death?
- What are the family's beliefs about what happens after death?
- What does the family consider an appropriate emotional expression and integration of the loss?
- What does the family consider to be the gender rules for handling the death?
- Do certain deaths carry a stigma (e.g. suicide), or are certain types of death especially traumatic for that cultural group (e.g. death of a child)? (McGoldrick et al 2004, National Cancer Institute 2012).

Although detailed examination of grief-related cultural beliefs and practices is not possible here, examples of cultural beliefs and practices include the following:

- In some cultures, bereaved people 'somaticize grief, so that a grieving person often feels physically ill' (Rosenblatt 2008 p 212).

- Some immigrants to Australia may explain child and maternal death as the result of the life aura of the mother and baby being imbalanced, the mother behaving badly towards her parents, or the mother having an encounter with a malevolent spirit (Rice 2000).

- The Japanese practice of ancestor worship (Kaneko 1990, Klass 1996, Valentine 2009) involves an elaborate set of rituals and enables the living to maintain personal, emotional bonds with relatives who have died over a period of 35–50 years. A focal point for ancestor worship is an altar in the home. Interestingly, in Western societies (that lack the rich memorial/ connecting rituals of other cultures) efforts by grieving families to create spaces for remembering can lead to such disparaging and disenfranchising comments as, 'They have turned that place into a shrine!'

- Australian Aboriginal and Torres Strait Islander people view the loss of land and identity as continuing pervasive losses that influence and interact with their current losses, resulting in what has been described as 'malignant grief' (Merritt 2011).

Health professionals clearly cannot be 'experts' in the various cultures of their patients. However, by making a commitment to cultural sensitivity, they can develop practice that is 'genuinely open, curious, and free of assumptions' (Gunaratnam 1997) and allows them to learn from and work with patients to provide culturally appropriate grief support and care.

Responding to those who are grieving

All health professionals will encounter patients or clients who have experienced significant losses. Most deaths occur in healthcare facilities, particularly hospitals, nursing homes and hospice/palliative care settings. In a Scottish study Stephen et al (2009) found that health professionals were generally the first point of engagement for bereaved individuals and families. It is essential therefore that such professionals are able to recognise their patients' grief and respond in appropriate and helpful ways.

Efforts to determine what kinds of assistance are effective with grievers have identified three levels of intervention. The first level, described as primary preventive intervention (Neimeyer & Currier 2009), would offer assistance to all grievers experiencing uncomplicated grief. Apart from the costs of such a universal approach, there is evidence that primary prevention is not needed by everyone (Worden 2010) and that it generally is not effective (Jordan & Neimeyer 2003, Larson & Hoyt 2007, Neimeyer 2000). Secondary preventive interventions focus on people who are at risk of complications in their grieving and may result in beneficial outcomes, at least in the short term (Schut et al 2001). A third level of intervention involves those who experience complicated grief and research indicates that such intervention reliably achieves positive outcomes for the griever (Boelen et al 2011, Jacobs & Prigerson 2000, Neimeyer 2000).

What works and doesn't work in assisting those who are bereaved remains an area of ongoing debate. The author's clinical experience suggests that grief support and counselling can be beneficial to a wide range of grievers and that we should be cautious about assuming that 'normal' grief does not benefit from supportive intervention. The appreciation that grievers express for the concern, care and support shown by others during times of significant loss clearly indicates there is benefit from such helping actions. For this reason health professionals need to be willing to offer support to grieving patients and families while being respectful of those who do not wish assistance.

The scope of this chapter does not allow a comprehensive discussion of intervention methods. However, Worden (2010 p 52) sets out four useful goals for grief support and counselling, based on his tasks of mourning:

- to increase the reality of the loss
- to help grievers deal with their feelings
- to help the griever overcome obstacles to readjustment after the loss
- to help the griever find a way to remember the deceased/lost object while being prepared to reinvest in life.

Box 11.1 summarises guidelines that health professionals can consider in supporting those who are grieving.

Worden W 2010 Grief counselling and grief therapy: a handbook for the mental health practitioner, 4th edn. Brunner-Routledge, New York – pp 89–104

Box 11.1 How health professionals can support someone who is grieving

HELP THE GRIEVER ACTUALISE THE LOSS

Help grievers express their loss – health professionals can provide a 'fresh' listening ear for the story of loss.

Actively involve grievers in terminal or palliative care situations – this helps make the approaching death more real.

HELP THE GRIEVER IDENTIFY AND EXPERIENCE FEELINGS

Be willing to empathise with the griever's painful feelings.

Responses such as 'It seems like you are really missing _____', or 'I imagine that you must be very lonely since _____ died' help name and express feelings associated with loss.

ASSIST LIVING WITHOUT THE DECEASED

Connect grievers to support groups and services that assist grievers with the adjustments involved after a significant loss.

HELP FIND MEANING IN THE LOSS

Meaning making in grief is highly individual but health professionals can facilitate the process.

Cont... ▶

Ask grievers what their loss has meant to them, share stories of how others have found meaning.

Share own perceptions of meaning – for example, 'It sounds like your life would never have been as happy without your relationship with ____'.

Introduce grievers to meaning-making exercises – for example, Neimeyer (1998, 2007).

FACILITATE EMOTIONAL RELOCATION OF THE DECEASED/LOST OBJECT

Support grievers in remembering and reminiscing about who/what has been lost.

Support grievers regarding concrete efforts to remain connected to the lost person or thing.

Be cautious about grievers' efforts to quickly find a 'replacement'.

PROVIDE TIME TO GRIEVE

Recognise that active grieving can take time, for example, one to two years (or longer).

Avoid giving messages that people should 'be over' their grief.

Remember and support continuing grief at special times, for example, on the anniversary of a death, birthdays or holidays.

Educate the griever's support system (family, friends) that grieving takes time.

INTERPRET NORMAL BEHAVIOUR

Help grievers understand and 'make sense' of their often intense grief responses.

Assure grievers that their reactions are not uncommon, while still acknowledging how the griever might be upset or worried about their reactions.

Connect grievers with those who have had similar experiences, for example, support groups.

ALLOW FOR INDIVIDUAL DIFFERENCES

Recognise the great diversity of grieving responses that can be demonstrated.

Avoid imposing a 'prescription' about how grievers should react.

Educate those around the griever that differences in grieving styles and methods are to be expected.

CONSIDER DEFENCES AND COPING STYLES

Watch for potentially unhelpful grief responses such as excessive use of alcohol or drugs, withdrawal, refusal to be reminded of the loss, 'burying' themselves in work or some other activity.

Cont... ▶

Within a trusting relationship, help the griever explore more useful ways of coping.

IDENTIFY GRIEF COMPLICATIONS AND REFER

Monitor for grief complications (see 'Complicated grief' in this chapter).

In keeping with professional ethics, recognise your own practice limitations.

Refer grievers with complications for more advanced assistance.

Research focus

Carnelley, K., Wortman, C., Bolger, N., et al., 2006. The time course of grief reactions to spousal loss: Evidence from a national probability sample. Journal of Personality and Social Psychology 91 (3), 476–492.

Most studies of widowhood have focused on reactions during the first few years post-loss. The authors investigated whether widowhood had more enduring effects using a nationally representative American sample. Participants were 768 people who had lost their spouse (from a few months to 64 years) prior to data collection. Results indicated that the widowed continued to talk, think and feel emotions about their lost spouse decades later. Twenty years post-loss, the widowed thought about their spouse once every week or two and had a conversation about their spouse once a month on average. About 12.6 years post-loss, the widowed reported only feeling upset sometimes and rarely when they thought about their spouse. These findings add to an understanding of the time course of grief.

Critical thinking

- In view of the findings from Carnelley et al (2006), how do you think that health professionals who work with people in aged care settings (e.g. a nursing home or other residential aged care facility) could support their patients in their long-term grieving for a deceased spouse? For example, how could such settings assist their patients in maintaining continuing bonds with their dead spouses?
- Are there specific things that could be done in terms of the physical environment, staff training or remembering practices?

Complicated grief

Within the loss and grief field, perhaps one of the most enduring and challenging questions has been: 'When is a person's grieving not normal?' The difficulty in understanding 'not-normal' grief is illustrated by the variety of terms that have been used to describe such a phenomenon including absent, abnormal, distorted, morbid, maladaptive, truncated, atypical, pathological, prolonged, unresolved, neurotic, dysfunctional, chronic, exaggerated, masked and delayed grief (Currier et al 2009, Lobb et al 2006, Middleton et al 1993). The preferred term today is complicated grief. It is estimated 10% to 20% of people experience a prolonged, painful grieving process in which the loss is not integrated into their life (Prigerson & Jacobs 2001a, Shear & Shair 2005).

In the first few months after a loss, distinguishing uncomplicated grief from complicated grief is generally difficult due to the intensity of grief in its early acute period. However, after six months, more complicated grief is evident through such indicators as suicidal thoughts and gestures, depressive disorders, post-traumatic reactions and persistent grief reactions (Ray & Prigerson 2006). One of the difficulties in identifying complicated grief has been the lack of valid and reliable measurements of grief. Several grief inventories and questionnaires have been developed; however, the usefulness of many has been questioned (Neimeyer & Hogan 2001). A shortlist of recommended grief measurement instruments includes the Texas Revised Inventory of Grief (TRIG) (Faschingbauer et al 1987), the Grief Experience Inventory (GEI) (Sanders et al 1985) and the Core Bereavement Items (CBI) (Burnett et al 1997), the last developed in Australia. However, such scales are appropriate for identifying complicated grief only if there is a point at which the line between uncomplicated and complicated grief can be determined and more work is needed in this regard.

Another approach has sought to isolate the specific factors and reactions that are particular to complicated grief. Since the 1990s, two groups of researchers have independently been working on a description and measure of complicated grief (Horowitz et al 1997, Prigerson et al 1997). The goal has been to develop criteria for complicated grief that would be accepted within the mental health field, and therefore included in the next *Diagnostic and Statistical Manual of Mental Disorders* (DSM-5), scheduled for publication in May 2013. The DSM is an international reference for diagnosing psychiatric disorders and the current DSM-IV does not categorise complicated grief. The concern was that complicated grief has been inappropriately associated with depressive, anxiety or post-trauma reactions and therefore requires a diagnostic category of its own.

Over time, various diagnostic terms have been suggested by the researchers, including complicated grief disorder (Horowitz et al 1997), traumatic grief (Prigerson et al 1997, Prigerson & Jacobs 2001b) and prolonged grief disorder (Prigerson et al 2008). As a result of this work, the DSM-5 Task Force of the American Psychiatric Association has proposed a new diagnosis, persistent complex bereavement-related disorder, in Section III of DSM-5. The task force acknowledges the significant distress and functional impairment identified in research on the two constructs 'complicated grief' and 'prolonged grief'. However, they see important differences between these constructs and have placed persistent complex bereavement-related disorder in an appendix, with the expectation that further research will occur 'to develop the best empirically-based set of symptoms to characterize individuals with bereavement-related disorders' (APA 2012).

Similar to other disorders in DSM, persistent complex bereavement-related disorder has various criteria (Criterion A to E), all of which must be met for a diagnosis to be made. The death must have occurred at least 12 months before, suggesting that complicated grief is more accurately diagnosed beyond the early months of bereavement. The criteria build on the work of researchers such as Prigerson by including: persistent yearning and preoccupation; difficulty accepting the death; and feelings of anger, isolation and meaningless. Notable is the mention of how criteria should be adapted for bereaved children, and reference to specific factors associated with traumatic bereavement, that is, following a death that occurred in traumatic circumstances, such as by suicide, homicide or in a disaster. The criteria also note the importance of determining whether bereavement reactions are outside accepted religious and cultural norms. Overall, the criteria for persistent complex bereavement-related disorder seek to provide guidelines for determining whether grief reactions are problematic based on their frequency, severity and level of impairment to daily functioning. It will be interesting to see how continuing research on complicated grief influences future classification of this disorder.

Theorists and researchers for some time have explored factors that contribute to complicated grief (Middleton et al 1993). Is it due to the griever's personality, previous life experiences, lack of social support or the nature of the loss? Interestingly, recent work proposes that complicated grief be viewed as an attachment disorder (Prigerson et al 2008, Ray & Prigerson 2006). Previously, Bowlby (1982) conceptualised grief as a response to separation and argued that difficulties grieving as an adult were related to disruptions in a person's childhood attachments with parents or other significant carers. Three pathological attachment patterns were identified:

- An anxious attachment to parents would result in insecure attachments to significant others in adulthood, overdependence and *chronic grief* following a major loss.
- A child who was reluctant to accept care and was highly self-sufficient was described as compulsively self-reliant and therefore likely to deny loss and experience *delayed grief*.
- Chronic grief also was likely to be experienced by a compulsive caregiver, someone whose role as a child was one of giver rather that receiver of care.

Prigerson's research group (Ray & Prigerson 2006) suggests that attachment-related risk factors for complicated grief include:

- the closeness of the relationship with the deceased
- dependent, confiding, close relationships – these lead to poorest bereavement adjustment, whereas conflicted relationships result in lower rates of bereavement disorders
- weak parental bonding
- damaged sense of security due to childhood abuse or severe neglect
- childhood separation anxiety
- people who are generally averse to change of any kind.

Two other risk factors are the griever's perception of being unsupported and lack of preparation for the death. This latter factor, among others, makes suicide deaths particularly difficult to deal with. Loss through suicide has been identified as a specific risk factor for complicated grief (as noted above in relation to traumatic bereavement in DSM-5). For further information about helping those bereaved through suicide see Clark and Goldney (2002), Hawton and Simkin (2008) or Maple et al (2010).

Significant negative health outcomes have been associated with complicated grief, including cancer risk, hypertension, suicidal ideation, hospitalisations, alcohol/ cigarette consumption and depressive symptoms (Buckley et al 2009, Ray & Prigerson 2006). For example, people experiencing complicated grief at six months post-loss are 16 times more likely to have changes in smoking at 13 months post-loss, seven times more likely to experience changes in eating, and almost three times more likely to experience depression (Zhang et al 2006 p 1195).

The proposed DSM-5 model arguably is current best practice in distinguishing between normal and complicated grief and is expected to play a key role in establishing a 'gold standard' for reliably identifying complicated grief as a specific disorder. The benefits of such a consensus about complicated grief include: more accurate assessment/diagnosis of complicated grief; increased consistency of practice within the loss and grief field; and greater access to appropriate services by those experiencing complicated grief. Establishing complicated grief as a specific disorder could, for example, enable grievers to more readily access mental health services under Medicare funding. On the other hand, including complicated grief in the DSM potentially stigmatises grievers, as can happen to others with mental health problems. A possible response to this argument is that complicated grief is currently disenfranchised by not being accurately recognised by practitioners and health policymakers and that situating complicated grief among depressive and post-trauma reactions is already stigmatising.

Conclusion

This chapter highlights the importance that experiences of loss and grief reactions can play in the lives of those with whom we work as health professionals. Losses and grief reactions need to be incorporated into health assessments and appropriate supportive responses included in healthcare plans. If this does not happen we run the risk of further disenfranchising the grief of our patients and missing opportunities to assist them in their grief work. Health professionals from all disciplines are positioned to play a key role in the identification, assessment and support of grief reactions. It is hoped that readers of this chapter will consider how they can take up this challenge in their practice.

REMEMBER

- Most patients with whom health professionals work have experienced significant loss or losses that can affect physical, social, emotional and psychological wellbeing.
- While a major factor in grief is loss of a loved one through death, there also are many non-death losses experienced by patients and their families.

Cont... ▶

- The loss and grief of patients is often unrecognised, leading to the disenfranchisement of their loss experiences.
- Grief is expressed through a diverse range of feelings, thoughts, behaviours and physical reactions that health professionals can learn to identify.
- Health professionals can play a vital role in identifying and supporting the grief of patients and their families.
- Some grief can become more complicated and can be assessed by health professionals so that appropriate assistance can be provided.

Further resources

Dickenson, D., Johnson, M., Katz, J. (Eds.), 2000. Death, dying and bereavement. Sage, London.

Doka, K. (Ed.), 2002. Disenfranchised grief: new directions, challenges and strategies for practice. Research Press, Champaign.

McKissock, M., McKissock, D., 2012. Coping with grief, fourth ed. ABC Books, Sydney.

Stroebe, M., Schut, H., Stroebe, W., 2007. Health outcomes of bereavement. The Lancet 370, 1960–1973.

Worden, W., 2010. Grief counselling and grief therapy: a handbook for the mental health practitioner, fourth ed. Springer, New York.

Weblinks

Australian Centre for Grief and Bereavement

www.grief.org.au

This website for the Australian Centre for Grief and Bereavement (Melbourne) links to an extensive list of related websites, provides information on the peer-reviewed journal *Grief Matters: The Journal of Grief and Bereavement* and describes continuing education events. Look under 'Resources' for weblinks and podcasts of conference presentations.

Australian Child & Adolescent Trauma, Loss & Grief Network

www.earlytraumagrief.anu.edu.au

Affiliated with the Australian National University, this network brings together evidence-based resources and research to make them more accessible to those working with, or interested in, children and young people who have been affected by trauma and grief. Check the section on 'Grief & loss' for a range of resources.

Bereavement Care Centre

www.bereavementcare.com.au

This website for the Bereavement Care Centre in Sydney includes a useful section on 'Resources'. In particular, look at the *Health Care Report* under 'Articles' (in the 'Resources' section) for a discussion debunking some myths about bereavement and grief.

British Medical Journal

www.bmj.com

This website of the *British Medical Journal* includes many articles and news items about grief associated with healthcare-related experiences. Click on the 'Search' window and use 'grief' or 'loss' as key words.

Grief Link

www.grieflink.asn.au

This South Australian website provides information on many aspects of death-related grief for the general community and professionals in contact with people who are grieving.

References

Allan, J., Harms, L., 2010. 'Power and prejudice': thinking differently about grief. Grief Matters 13 (3), 72–75.

Attig, T., 1991. The importance of conceiving of grief as an active process. Death Studies 15, 385–393.

Berzoff, J., 2011. The transformative nature of grief. Clinical Social Work Journal 39, 262–269.

Bettle, A., Latimer, M., 2009. Maternal coping and adaptation: a case study examination of chronic sorrow in caring for an adolescent with a progressive neurodegenerative disease. Canadian Journal of Neuroscience Nursing 31 (4), 15–21.

Bocknek, E., Sanderson, J., Broitner, P., 2009. Ambiguous loss and posttraumatic stress in school-aged children of prisoners. Journal of Child Family Studies 18, 323–333.

Boelen, P., deKeijser, J., van den Hout, A., et al., 2011. Factors associated with outcomes of cognitive-behavioural therapy for complicated grief: a preliminary study. Clinical Psychology and Psychotherapy 18, 284–291.

Boss, P., 2000. Ambiguous loss: learning to live with unresolved grief. Harvard University Press, Cambridge.

Boss, P., 2010. The trauma and complicated grief of ambiguous loss. Pastoral Psychology 59, 137–145.

Bowes, S., Lowes, L., Warner, J., et al., 2009. Chronic sorrow in parents of children with type 1 diabetes. Journal of Advanced Nursing 65 (5), 992–1000.

Bowlby, J., 1980. Loss: sadness and depression, Vol 3: Attachment and loss. Penguin Press, London.

Bowlby, J., 1982. Attachment and loss: retrospect and prospect. American Journal of Orthopsychiatry 52, 664–678.

Bruce, E., 2000. Grief, trauma and parenting children with disability: cycles of disenfranchisement. Grief Matters 3 (2), 27–31.

Bruce, E., Schultz, C., 2001. Nonfinite loss and grief: a psychoeducational approach. Paul H Brookes, Baltimore.

Buckley, T., Bartrop, R., McKinley, S., et al., 2009. Prospective study of early bereavement on psychological and behavioural cardiac risk. Internal Medicine Journal 39, 370–378.

Bull, M.A., 1998. Losses in families affected by dementia: strategies and service issues. Journal of Family Studies 4, 187–199.

Burke, M., Hainsworth, M., Eakes, G., et al., 1992. Current knowledge and research on chronic sorrow: a foundation for inquiry. Death Studies 16, 231–245.

Burnett, P., Middleton, W., Raphael, B., et al., 1997. Measuring core bereavement phenomena. Psychological Medicine 27, 49–57.

Carnelley, K., Wortman, C., Bolger, N., et al., 2006. The time course of grief reactions to spousal loss: Evidence from a national probability sample. Journal of Personality and Social Psychology 91 (3), 476–492.

Clark, S., Goldney, R., 2002. The impact of suicide on relatives and friends. In: Hawton, K., van Heeringen, K. (Eds.), The international handbook of suicide and attempted suicide. Wiley, Chichester.

Corr, C., 1993. Coping with dying: lessons that we should and should not learn from the work of Elisabeth Kübler-Ross. Death Studies 17, 69–83.

Corr, C., 2002. Revisiting the concept of disenfranchised grief. In: Doka, K. (Ed.), Disenfranchised grief: new directions, challenges and strategies for practice. Research Press, Champaign.

Currier, J., Holland, J., Neimeyer, R., 2009. Assumptive worldviews and problematic reactions to bereavement. Journal of Loss and Trauma: International Perspectives on Stress and Coping 14 (3), 181–195.

Doka, K., Tucci, A., 2009. Living with grief: diversity and end of life care. Hospice Foundation of America, Washington.

Doka, K. (Ed.), 2002. Disenfranchised grief: new directions, challenges and strategies for practice. Research Press, Champaign.

Faschingbauer, T., Zisook, S., DeVaul, R., 1987. The Texas revised inventory of grief. In: Zisook, S. (Ed.), Biopsychosocial aspects of bereavement. American Psychiatric Press, Washington DC.

Freud, S. 1917. Mourning and melancholia. The standard edition of the complete psychological works of Sigmund Freud, volume XIV (1914–1916): on the history of the psycho-analytic movement. Papers on metapsychology and other works, 237–258.

Goldstein, E., 1995. Ego psychology and social work practice, second ed. Free Press, New York.

Gordon, J., 2009. An evidence-based approach for supporting parents experiencing chronic sorrow. Paediatric Nursing 35 (2), 115–119.

Grossberg, R., 2008. Psychoanalytic contributions to the care of medically fragile children. Journal of Psychiatric Practice 14 (5), 307–311.

Gunaratnam, Y., 1997. Culture is not enough: a critique of multi-culturalism in palliative care. In: Field, D., Hockey, J.L., Small, N. (Eds.), Death, gender, and ethnicity. Routledge, London.

Harvey, J., Weber, A., 1999. Why there must be a psychology of loss. In: Harvey, J. (Ed.), 1999. Perspectives on loss: a sourcebook. Bruner/Mazel, Philadelphia.

Harris, E., Gorman, D., 2011. Grief from a broader perspective: non finite loss, ambiguous loss and chronic sorrow, Ch 1 in D. Harris Reflecting on change loss and transitions in everyday life. Routledge, New York.

Hawton, K., Simkin, S., 2008. Help is at hand: a resource for people bereaved by suicide and other sudden, traumatic death. The Centre for Suicide Research, University of Oxford. Online. Available: http://cebmh.warne.ox.ac.uk/csr/linksbereaved.html 10 Sep 2012.

Herman, J., 2001. Trauma and recovery: from domestic abuse to political terror. Pandora, London.

Hockley, R., 1985. The precipitants of grief. In: National Association for Loss and Grief, The family and grief, Proceedings of the Fourth National Conference. National Association for Loss and Grief, Sydney, pp. 45–56.

Horowitz, M.J., Siegel, B., Holen, A., et al., 1997. Diagnostic criteria for complicated grief disorder. The American Journal of Psychiatry 154, 904–910.

Horowitz, M.J., Wilner, N., Marmar, C., et al., 1980. Pathological grief and the activation of latent self images. American Journal of Psychiatry 137 (10), 1157–1162.

Jacobs, S., Prigerson, H., 2000. Psychotherapy of traumatic grief: a review of evidence for psychotherapeutic treatments. Death Studies 24, 479–495.

Janoff-Bulman, R., 1992. Shattered assumptions: towards a new psychology of trauma. Free Press, New York.

Jordan, J., Neimeyer, R., 2003. Does grief counselling work? Death Studies 27, 765–786.

Kalish, R., 1966. A continuum of subjectively perceived death. The Gerontologist 6, 73–76.

Kaneko, S., 1990. Dimensions of religiosity among believers in Japanese folk religion. Journal of the Scientific Study of Religion 29 (1), 1–18.

Kauffman, J., 2002. The psychology of disenfranchised grief: liberation, shame and self-disenfranchisement. In: Doka, K. (Ed.), Disenfranchised grief: new directions, challenges and strategies for practice. Research Press, Champaign.

Klass, D., 1996. Grief in an Eastern culture: Japanese ancestor worship. In: Klass, D., Silverman, P., Nickman, S. (Eds.), Continuing bonds: new understandings of grief. Taylor and Francis, Philadelphia.

Klass, D., Silverman, P., Nickman, S. (Eds.), 1996. Continuing bonds: new understandings of grief. Taylor and Francis, Philadelphia.

Kübler-Ross, E., 1969. On death and dying. Macmillan, New York.

Larson, D., Hoyt, W., 2007. What has become of grief counselling? An evaluation of the empirical foundations of the new pessimism. Professional Psychology: Research and Practice 38 (7), 347–355.

Lindemann, E., 1944. Symptomatology and management of acute grief. American Journal of Psychiatry 101, 141–148.

Lobb, E., Kristjanson, L., Auon, S., et al., 2006. An overview of complicated grief terminology and diagnostic criteria. Grief Matters 9 (2), 28–32.

Maple, M., Edwards, H., Plummer, D., et al., 2010. Silenced voices: hearing the stories of parents bereaved through the suicide death of a young adult child. Health and Social Care in the Community 18 (3), 241–248.

Marwit, S., Klass, D., 1996. Grief and the role of the inner presentation of the deceased. In: Klass, D., Silverman, P., Nickman, S. (Eds.), Continuing bonds: new understandings of grief. Taylor and Francis, Philadelphia.

McGoldrick, M., Schlesinger, J., Lee, E., et al. (Eds.), 2004. Living beyond loss: death in the family. WW Norton, New York.

McKissock, M., McKissock, D., 2012. Coping with grief, fourth ed. ABC Books, Sydney.

Merritt, S., 2011. First Nations Australians – surviving through adversities and malignant grief. Grief Matters 14 (3), 74–77.

Middleton, W., Raphael, B., Martinek, N., et al., 1993. Pathological grief reactions. In: Stroebe, M., Stroebe, W., Hanssen, R. (Eds.), Handbook of bereavement: theory, research and intervention. Cambridge University Press, Cambridge.

National Cancer Institute, 2012. Cross-cultural responses to grief and mourning. Online. Available: http://www.cancer.gov/cancertopics/pdq/supportive-care/bereavement/HealthProfessional/page7 10 Sep 2012.

Neimeyer, R., 1998. Lessons of loss: a guide to coping. McGraw-Hill, New York.

Neimeyer, R., 2000. Searching for the meaning of meaning: grief therapy and the process of reconstruction. Death Studies 24, 531–558.

Neimeyer, R., 2007. Meaning reconstruction and the experience of loss. American Psychological Association, Washington DC.

Neimeyer, R., Currier, J., 2009. Grief therapy: evidence of efficacy and emerging directions. Current Directions in Psychological Science 18 (6), 352–356.

Neimeyer, R., Hogan, N., 2001. Quantitative or qualitative? Measurement issues in the study of grief. In: Stroebe, M., Hansson, R., Stroebe, W., et al. (Eds.), Handbook of bereavement research: consequences, coping and care. American Psychological Association, Washington DC.

Nikcevic, A., Kuczmierczyk, A., Nicolaides, K., 2007. The influence of medical and psychological interventions on women's distress after miscarriage. Journal of Psychosomatic Research 63 (3), 283–290.

Olshansky, S., 1962. Chronic sorrow: a response to having a mentally defective child. Social Casework 43, 191–193.

Parkes, C.M., 1972. Bereavement: studies of grief in adult life. Tavistock, London.

Parkes, C.M., 1988. Bereavement as a psychosocial transition: process of adaptation to change. Journal of Social Issues 44, 53–65.

Pomeroy, E., Garcia, R., 2008. The grief assessment and intervention workbook: a strengths perspective. Brooks/Cole, Belmont.

Prigerson, H.G., Bierhals, A.J., Kasl, S.V., et al., 1997. Traumatic grief as a risk factor for mental and physical morbidity. The American Journal of Psychiatry 154, 616–623.

Prigerson, H., Jacobs, S., 2001a. Caring for bereaved patients: all the doctors just suddenly go. The Journal of the American Medical Association 286, 1369–1376.

Prigerson, H.G., Jacobs, S.C., 2001b. Diagnostic criteria for traumatic grief: a rationale, consensus criteria, and preliminary empirical test. American Psychological Association, Washington DC.

Prigerson, H., Vanderwerker, L., Maciejewski, P., 2008. A case for inclusion of prolonged grief disorder in DSM-V. In: Stroebe, M., Hansson, R., Schut, H., et al. (Eds.), Handbook of bereavement research and practice: advances in theory and intervention. American Psychological Association, Washington DC.

Ray, R., Street, A., 2007. Non-finite loss and emotional labour: family caregivers' experiences of living with motor neurone disease. Journal of Clinical Nursing 16 (3a), 35–43.

Ray, A., Prigerson, H., 2006. Complicated grief: an attachment disorder worthy of inclusion in DSM-V. Grief Matters 9 (2), 33–38.

Rice, P.L., 2000. Death in birth: the cultural construction of stillbirth, neonatal death, and maternal death among Hmong women in Australia. Omega: The Journal of Death and Dying 41, 39–57.

Rosenblatt, P., 2008. Grief across cultures: a review and research agenda. In: Stroebe, M., Hansson, R., Schut, H., et al. (Eds.), Handbook of bereavement research and practice: Advances in theory and intervention. American Psychological Association, Washington DC.

Sanders, C.M., Mauger, P., Strong, P., 1985. A manual for the grief experience inventory. Consulting Psychologists Press, Palo Alto.

Sanders, C.M., 1999. Grief the mourning after: dealing with and bereavement, second ed. Wiley, New York.

Schut, H., Stroebe, M., van den Bout, J., et al., 2001. The efficacy of bereavement interventions: determining who benefits. In: Stroebe, M., Hansson, R., Stroebe, W., et al. (Eds.), Handbook of bereavement research: consequences, coping and care. American Psychological Association, Washington DC.

Shear, K., Shair, H., 2005. Attachment, loss and complicated grief. Developmental Psychobiology 47, 253–276.

Silverman, P., Klass, D., 1996. Introduction: What's the problem? In: Klass, D., Silverman, P., Nickman, S. (Eds.), Continuing bonds: new understandings of grief. Taylor and Francis, Philadelphia.

Slaughter Smith, C., 2009. Substance abuse, chronic sorrow, and mothering loss: relapse triggers among female victims of child abuse. Paediatric Nursing 24 (5), 401–412.

Spidell, S., Wallace, A., Carmack, C., et al., 2011. Grief in healthcare: an investigation of the presence of disenfranchised grief. Journal of Health Care Chaplaincy 17, 750–786.

Stephen, A., Wimpenny, P., Unwin, R., et al., 2009. Bereavement and bereavement care in health and social care: provision and practice in Scotland. Death Studies 33, 239–261.

Stroebe, M., Schut, H., 1999. The dual process model of coping with bereavement: rationale and description. Death Studies 23, 197–224.

Stroebe, M., Schut, H., 2008. The dual process model of coping with bereavement: overview and update. Grief Matters 11 (1), 4–10.

Stroebe, M., Hansson, R., Stroebe, W., et al., 2001. Introduction: concepts and issues in contemporary research on bereavement. In: Stroebe, M., Hannson, R., Stroebe, W., et al. (Eds.), Handbook of bereavement research: consequences, coping and care. American Psychological Association, Washington DC.

Sudnow, D., 1967. Passing on: The social organisation of dying. Prentice Hall, Englewood Cliffs.

Valentine, C., 2009. Continuing bonds after bereavement: a cross-cultural perspective. Bereavement Care 28 (2), 6–11.

Weenolsen, P., 1988. Transcendence of loss over the life span. Hemisphere, New York.

Weenolsen, P., 1991. Transcending the many deaths of life: clinical implications for cure versus healing. Death Studies 15, 59–80.

White, M., 1988. Saying hullo again: the incorporation of the lost relationship in the resolution of grief. Dulwich Centre Newsletter, Spring, pp 7–11.

Worden, W., 2010. Grief counselling and grief therapy: a handbook for the mental health practitioner, fourth ed. Springer, New York.

Zhang, B., El-Jawahri, A., Prigerson, H., 2006. Update on bereavement research: evidence-based guidelines for the diagnosis and treatment of complicated bereavement. Journal of Palliative Medicine 9 (5), 1188–1203.

Chapter 12
Pain

SARAH OVERTON & MARIA DE SOUSA

Learning objectives

The material in this chapter will help you to:

- explain what pain is
- describe a biopsychosocial model of pain
- explain the difference between nociceptive and neuropathic pain and the role of central sensitisation
- explain the roles of beliefs, fear avoidance, distress, pain behaviour, coping strategies, learning and environment in a chronic pain presentation
- explain the difference between acute and chronic pain and describe some of the factors that can contribute to the transition from acute to chronic
- list the main biomedical interventions for pain and describe the components of a cognitive-behavioural approach to managing pain
- understand that in the case of chronic pain the treatment goal shifts from trying to reduce or eliminate the pain to learning to live with the pain and return to normal activities and function despite the pain.

Key terms

- Nociception
- Neuropathy
- Central sensitisation
- Acute versus chronic pain
- Fear avoidance
- Pain behaviour
- Cognitive-behavioural pain management program

Introduction

Pain is an important issue for all health professionals to be aware of. It accompanies most health presentations and is commonly understood to be a warning system signifying the need for immediate attention. Our response to it as health professionals can have a significant impact on outcome in terms of gaining the trust and cooperation of our patients, and making the appropriate decisions for management.

Pain is a multifactorial experience with sensory and emotional aspects and it is best understood within a biopsychosocial framework. Although we now have a much better understanding of the neurobiological basis of pain, the lack of direct correlation between actual injury or pathology and reported pain and pain behaviour can only be understood when all aspects of the presentation are taken into account. Psychological and environmental factors can play a particularly important role in the transition from acute to chronic pain and its ongoing maintenance. Given that approximately one in five adults may suffer from chronic pain (Blyth et al 2001) and that biomedical interventions have limitations, understanding and managing all aspects of such a presentation is essential.

What is pain?

Most of us think we know exactly what pain is through our own experience and most of us would assume that pain is clearly linked to injury. Moreover, many of us would further believe that the intensity of pain is somehow proportional to the severity of the injury that has occurred. In fact, these seemingly obvious assumptions are not simply incorrect but misleading in terms of allowing health professionals to best assist patients in assessing and managing pain.

A comprehensive overview of the history of pain concepts and treatments can be found in Cope (2010). Here you will see that pain in different eras and different cultures has been viewed both as a sensation and therefore tied to the stimulus (or injury) and as an experience with strong emotional features (e.g. a quality or passion of the soul or a form of punishment). The former view is more consistent with commonly held contemporary views of pain, especially in the Western world. However, for researchers and health professionals working in the area of pain, it has become increasingly obvious that pain is not adequately explained by linking it to a noxious stimulus. A brief paper by Wall and McMahon (1986) clearly outlines that the evidence of a relationship between perceived pain and the firing of specific types of nerve fibres, or nociception, is not simply variable but sometimes nonexistent. Melzack and Wall (1982) provide an excellent overview of the variability of this relationship, discussing a range of phenomena, for example, congenital analgesia (people who are born without the ability to feel pain and therefore have no automatic warning system of injury), episodic analgesia (the inability to feel pain in certain situations such as when trying to survive on the battlefield), phantom limb pain (the experience of pain in a limb that does not exist) and, most commonly of all for many people in our society, the persistence of pain long after the healing of whatever injury was associated with its onset.

The important points to note from the above are that pain is not nociception. Nociception is simply activity in the nervous system generated by a noxious stimulus and it is quite possible for this to take place without any conscious awareness, such as when one is under anaesthetic. Pain, on the other hand, is a conscious, subjective experience with a number of dimensions.

This more complex understanding of what pain is has led to the following definition of pain from the International Association for the Study of Pain (IASP) Task Force on Taxonomy (1994), that it is 'an unpleasant sensory and emotional experience associated with actual or potential tissue damage, or described in terms of such damage.'

The following notes provided by the task force clearly emphasise the understanding that pain has a strong subjective, emotional component and that tissue damage can only be a poor guide to what the person may or may not be experiencing.

Pain is always subjective. Each individual learns the application of the word through experiences related to injury in early life ... It is unquestionably a sensation in a part or parts of the body but it is also always unpleasant and therefore also an emotional experience.

Many people report pain in the absence of tissue damage or any likely pathophysiological cause; usually this happens for psychological reasons. There is usually no way to distinguish their experience from that due to tissue damage if we take the subjective report. If they regard their experience as pain and if they report it in the same ways as pain caused by tissue damage, it should be accepted as pain. This definition avoids tying pain to the stimulus. Activity induced in the nociceptor and nociceptive pathways by a noxious stimulus is not pain, which is always a psychological state, even though we may well appreciate that pain most often has a proximate physical cause.

(IASP 1994 p 210)

The biopsychosocial model of pain

The biopsychosocial model was discussed in Chapter 4. There it was pointed out that health or illness is influenced by a complex interplay of biological, psychological and social factors. In terms of understanding and providing a formulation of the experience of pain, the biopsychosocial model has been widely accepted by health professionals as providing the best possible template to assess and manage the presentation of pain. Given the IASP definition cited above that describes pain as an unpleasant sensory and emotional experience, this of course makes perfect sense.

The biopsychosocial model originally delineated by Engel (1977) has been applied to pain by a number of important researchers in the field, including Fordyce (1976), Loeser (1982) and Waddell et al (1984).The broad components of the model are essentially the same in all versions and are elaborated in Figure 12.1. These components will be discussed in turn below but it is important to note that at all levels every component can impact on another level, in both directions. Therefore changes at the physiological level initiated by trauma may have impact at the psychological and behavioural levels in terms of distress and/or avoidance of activity but equally changes at the psychological or behavioural level can, in turn, have an impact at the physiological level, such as physical deconditioning (Turk & Monarch 2002).

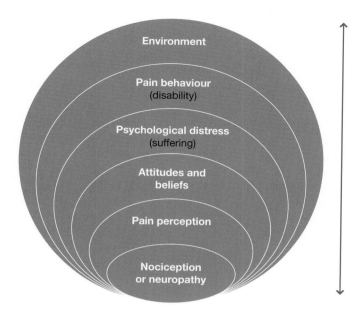

Figure 12.1 Biopsychosocial model of pain

Source: Drawn from Fordyce 1976, Loeser 1982 and Waddell et al 1984

NOCICEPTION OR NEUROPATHY

When considering the biological contributors to the experience of pain, we can divide pain into two types – nociceptive and neuropathic – depending on the structures and mechanisms involved. Pain can further be classified clinically as acute or chronic. These distinctions are important because different types of pain, with different characteristics and underlying mechanisms, have different responses to treatment.

Nociceptive pain

According to the IASP, nociceptive pain refers to pain arising from actual or threatened damage to non-neural structures and is due to the activation of nociceptors (Turk & Okifuji 2010). Nociceptive pain is generally described as aching or dull and, in the case of musculoskeletal pain, usually related to activity or posture. For example, soft tissue sprains and strains, bone fractures and appendicitis may give rise to nociceptive pain.

Neuropathic pain

Neuropathic pain refers to pain arising as a direct consequence of a lesion or disease of the somatosensory system (Turk & Okifuji 2010). Neuropathic pain is confined to a region of sensory disturbance that is consistent with the distribution of the affected peripheral nerve, root or central pathway, and is often described by patients as burning or shock-like (Haanpää et al 2011). Episodes of neuropathic pain can occur spontaneously or as an exaggerated response to minor stimulation. An exaggerated response to a non-painful stimulus, such as light touch, is called allodynia. An exaggerated response to a painful stimulus is called hyperalgesia. Patients with neuropathic pain may also describe dysaesthesias, which are unpleasant and strange sensations in the skin such as ants crawling, water running, tingling, and pins and needles (Freynhagen & Bennett 2009). Neuropathic pain may occur following traumatic nerve injury, multiple sclerosis or spinal cord injury (Haanpää & Treede 2010). Postherpetic neuralgia and diabetic polyneuropathy may also give rise to neuropathic pain (Haanpää et al 2011). Depending on the site of the lesion, other symptoms may occur, such as muscle cramps, autonomic nerve damage symptoms and motor weakness (Haanpää & Treede 2010).

This current definition distinguishes neuropathic pain from pain arising as a consequence of neuroplastic changes, as in central sensitisation (see section below on pain processing), which occur in response to strong nociceptive stimulation (Haanpää et al 2011). For example, in a patient who presents with deep aching pain in the hypothenar region of the hand, intermittent stabbing pain without obvious triggers, and the fact that this pain initiated after an injury to the area, is suggestive of an ulnar nerve lesion (Geber et al 2009). A clinical examination that finds sensory disturbance consisting of negative (hypoaesthesia or reduced sensation) and/or positive sensory signs (hyperalgesia and allodynia) would confirm a diagnosis of neuropathic pain (Geber et al 2009). Alternatively, a patient presenting with depression and widespread pain that could not be apportioned to an anatomically defined nervous system lesion, and who had a normal sensory examination with no suggestion of neurologic disease or neural damage, is unlikely to be experiencing neuropathic pain but might fulfill the criteria for fibromyalgia (Geber et al 2009).

Mixed pain

It is worth noting that, in many patients, neuropathic and nociceptive pains coexist and it is therefore important that clinicians identify these different components and treat them according to the best available evidence (Haanpää & Treede 2010) (see Table 12.1). For example, a patient presenting with low back and leg pain may have referred pain from a degenerative facet joint and/or sciatica from irritation or compression of a lumbar nerve root. A diagnosis of definite neuropathic pain would depend on a history of pain radiating along the leg, a positive MRI scan and an altered somatosensory examination (i.e. hypoaesthesia, hyperalgesia and allodynia) within the distribution of the affected nerve root.

Pain processing in the peripheral and central nervous systems

Understanding the nature of pain has consumed humankind throughout the ages. During the 19th and 20th centuries, advances in the study of anatomy, physiology and histology prompted the formulation of several physiologic theories of pain. Of these, the gate control theory (Melzack & Wall 1965) was the most influential and the first attempt to combine neurophysiological mechanisms with psychological processes such as cognitions and emotions. In this model, pain was viewed as an end product of a number of interacting processes in which the central nervous system played an active role in determining the nature and degree of pain following harmful stimulation in the periphery. Although we now know that this theory is overly simplistic, it nevertheless provides us with an understanding of the types of mechanisms involved in the processing and modulation of the experience of pain.

A simple explanation of the nervous system changes that occur in response to pain is that injury, disease or inflammation in tissues activates local nociceptor terminals to transmit information about physical damage to the dorsal horn of the

Table 12.1		
DIFFERENTIATING NOCICEPTIVE PAIN FROM NEUROPATHIC PAIN		
	Nociceptive pain	Neuropathic pain
Biological basis	Damage and/or disease in somatic and visceral structures such as bone fractures, ligament sprains, appendicitis	Damage and/or disease in peripheral or central neural structures such as peripheral nerve injury, postherpetic neuralgia (shingles), spinal cord injury
Symptoms	Dull, aching pain In the case of musculoskeletal pain, worse with movement or certain postures	▪ Burning, shock-like or electric spontaneous pain, unrelated to activity ▪ Associated with numbness, pins and needles or dysaesthesias
Signs	Tenderness on palpation Restriction of movement	Sensory and motor disturbance Altered reflexes Autonomic changes such as changes in temperature, sweating, skin colour, hair and nail growth, and oedema

spinal cord. These nociceptors become sensitised by the release of chemicals from the damaged tissue and by the release of neurotransmitters from sensory nerve endings. This process is called peripheral sensitisation and is responsible for primary hyperalgesia or increased sensitivity to mechanical and thermal stimulation at the site of injury or pain. Once noxious information reaches the spinal cord, it is modulated by cells within the spinal cord and by the activation of descending pathways from the brain, which might be either inhibitory or excitatory. Continued transmission of noxious information from the periphery leads to a cascade of events within the central nervous system (spinal cord and brain) that contribute to an increase in responsiveness of central neurons. This is known as central sensitisation.

In the case of neuropathic pain following peripheral nerve injury, the peripheral processes of nociceptors can become traumatised and undergo numerous changes that lead to increased activation of peripheral and central pain circuits that sometimes become chronic and debilitating. As noted above, allodynia, hyperalgesia, dysaesthesias and spontaneous pain are common features of neuropathic pain and are mediated by central sensitisation.

Under normal conditions central sensitisation resolves following recovery. In some cases, however, central changes persist and symptoms associated with these changes are seen in pathological pain states such as complex regional pain syndrome (CRPS), failed back surgery syndrome and phantom limb pain.

From the spinal cord, noxious signals reach the brain via a number of ascending tracts that terminate in many structures throughout the brainstem, thalamus and cortex (Woolf 2011). The thalamus acts as a major relay station in the transmission of noxious signals. As these signals reach the brain, many other regions are also activated, including those that control a number of autonomic and homeostatic mechanisms such as blood pressure regulation and respiration (Woolf 2011). In addition, there are descending mechanisms mediated by a variety of neurotransmitters, acting at subcortical and spinal cord levels, modulating ascending information (Randich & Ness 2010).

The higher brain centres used in pain processing can be divided into those involved in the sensory-discriminative component of pain perception (somatosensory cortex) and the affective component of pain perception (such as the cingulate cortex). However, this may be an oversimplification. Functional imaging studies have now identified a widely distributed network of cortical and subcortical areas that are activated by noxious stimuli (Apkarian et al 2011). These include sensory, limbic, associative and motor areas. Functional imaging studies have also shown significant differences in brain activation between people with no pain, acute pain and chronic pain (Apkarian et al 2011). Figure 12.2 shows the mechanisms of pain.

PAIN PERCEPTION

Pain does not occur in isolation but, rather, within a context that has a direct bearing on the person's perception of pain and on their response to pain. A person's subjective perception of pain may be viewed as the net result of transduction (the conversion of energy from the initiating stimulus into an electric signal), transmission (the propagation of action potentials from the peripheral nerve terminal to the central terminal) and modulation of sensory information (Turk et al 2010). Some modulatory

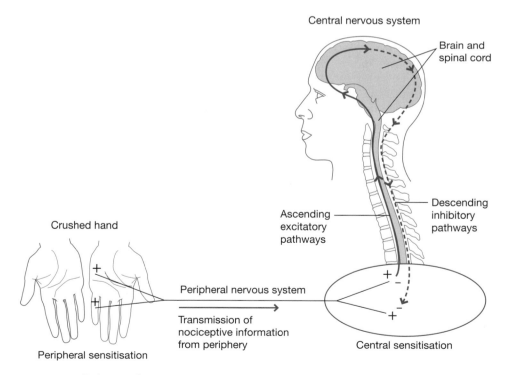

Figure 12.2 Pain mechanisms

effects are predictable and reliable, while others are less predictable, being dependent on psychological/cognitive processes that may involve learning, motivation and emotional status (Randich & Ness 2010). Pain can be extremely variable; it can attain intolerable intensity, persist beyond tissue healing or disappear on the battlefield. The way we interact with our environment is significantly altered by pain and our behaviour changes over time as pain continues. Therefore, in order to fully understand a person's perception and response to pain, a biopsychosocial approach is required, with consideration given to the interrelationships between the biological changes, psychological status and the sociocultural context in which pain occurs (Turk et al 2010).

Given that pain is an experience that is modulated by a complex set of emotional, environmental and psychophysiological variables, one would expect pain to influence brain processing on many levels (Apkarian et al 2011). Consideration of the neural representations of pain processing should therefore also include the neural representations of the mechanisms involved in pain modulation (including the role of learning, meaning, attention, anticipation and avoidance). A number of research techniques have been used to study these representations:

- injection of dyes or markers into nerves or supraspinal structures to allow researchers to trace their pathways

- immunohistochemical techniques to study changes in gene expression in neurons following noxious stimulation

- functional neuroimaging techniques such as positron emission tomography (PET) and functional magnetic resonance imaging (fMRI) to detect changes in regional blood flow or changes in local blood oxygen levels that coincide with changes in local functional brain activity in pain versus non-pain states (e.g. Apkarian et al 2011)

- anatomical imaging using voxel-based morphometry (VBM) to study the anatomical changes that occur in the brain of patients with chronic pain (e.g. Ruscheweyh et al 2011).

In recent years, human functional brain imaging has added significantly to our knowledge of where and how pain is processed in the brain (Apkarian et al 2011). As pointed out earlier, the processing of pain can no longer be viewed as a simple 'hard-wired' system with a strong relationship between stimulus and response (Cope 2010). We now have a better understanding of the neuroplastic changes that occur within the central nervous system in the presence of pain and hence the changes that should be addressed as part of an integrative approach to pain management (Tracey & Bushnell 2009).

ATTITUDES AND BELIEFS

What the pain means to a particular person at a particular time will have a clear influence on how that person subsequently responds. For example, if a person wakes in the night with stomach pain, he or she may think 'I should not have eaten so much', groan, roll over and eventually fall back to sleep. However, if they think that the pain may be an indicator of stomach cancer, perhaps because they saw a program on television about stomach cancer the previous evening or because they have a close relative with that disease, they are then likely to begin monitoring the pain, become worried and distressed, be unable to fall back to sleep and so on. Pain can sometimes be accepted as a necessary accompaniment to another valued goal such as in childbirth or in the pursuit of sporting success. It can even be pursued for pleasure as in certain sexual practices. Chapman and Okifuji (2004) discuss three main cognitive factors that will influence the pain experience:

- The degree of *attention* paid to the pain modulates the pain experience such that a person is likely to experience less pain if their attention is actively engaged elsewhere. People who report greater attention to pain have been shown in a number of studies to also report higher pain intensity, emotional distress, psychosocial disability, and pain-related healthcare utilisation (e.g. McCracken 1997).

- *Expectations* about pain – a number of studies have demonstrated that when expectations about pain are manipulated the level of pain changes. Expectations in this context can refer to 'response expectancies' or the response a person predicts they will have to a certain stimulus, for example, a pain medication or an activity. Response expectancies have a significant impact on actual pain experience. For example, Whalley et al (2008) showed that placebo effects were significantly associated with response expectancy.

- Expectations can also refer to 'efficacy expectancies' (e.g. self-efficacy) or a person's confidence that they have the ability to cope with pain or an activity. Self-efficacy has been shown to predict pain behaviour and avoidance (Asghari & Nicholas 2001), even when controlling for 'catastrophising'. Catastrophising is discussed below.

- *Appraisals* – what the person assumes the pain means; at the extreme level this can lead to 'catastrophising' about the pain which, in turn, can lead to high levels of distress and disability. A number of studies have shown that the meaning ascribed to the pain, particularly as it relates to tissue damage, can influence the experienced intensity (e.g. Arntz & Claassens 2004). Other studies have shown that pain patients with a high level of pain-related fear can have a bias to interpret innocuous or pain-related stimuli in a threatening way (e.g. Vancleef et al 2009).

Catastrophising

Catastrophising has been identified as a robust psychological predictor of pain-related outcomes. It refers to the tendency to exaggerate the negative consequences of actual or anticipated pain to an extreme level and comprises elements of rumination about the pain, magnification of its effects and helplessness (Sullivan & Martel 2012). A large number of studies have attested to the link between catastrophising about pain and increases in disability, distress and pain intensity. For example, Hanley et al (2008) found that changes in catastrophising and belief in one's ability to control pain were each significantly associated with greater pain interference and poorer psychological functioning, while changes in social support and specific coping strategies were not.

Fear avoidance

People in pain can evidence a high level of 'fear avoidance', such that they become fearful of engaging in physical activity due to the risk of increased pain and/or (re) injury and therefore avoid the activity (see Fig 12.3) (Vlaeyen et al 1995, Vlaeyen &

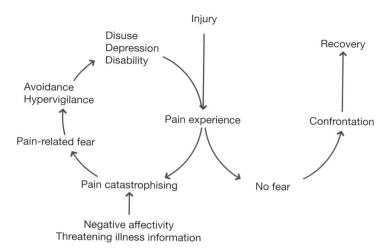

Figure 12.3 The fear-avoidance model

Figure 2 from Vlaeyen Johan WS and Linton Steven J. Fear-avoidance and its consequences in chronic musculoskeletal pain: a state of the art. PAIN® 2000 April 85(3); 317–332. This figure has been reproduced with permission of the International Association for the Study of Pain® (IASP). The figure may NOT be reproduced for any other purpose without permission.

Linton 2000). Over time this can result in significantly reduced activity levels, increased disability, deconditioning and depression or distress. Fear avoidance provides an excellent example of the interaction of three separate levels of the biopsychosocial model. Beliefs or appraisals of pain at one level result in anxiety or fear at the next level that, in turn, results in disability or pain behaviours at the next. The latter then further entrench the negative aspects of the pain experience and therefore fear avoidance becomes established. Leeuw et al (2007) recently published a comprehensive review of the current evidence for the fear-avoidance model and concluded that there is accumulating support for its various components.

PSYCHOLOGICAL DISTRESS (SUFFERING)

For many people pain, by definition, entails suffering. Nevertheless the degree of suffering is clearly variable and likely to be influenced by a range of factors. For example, the duration, severity, frequency and number of sites of pain (Fishbain et al 1997) may impact on the level of suffering. The contributors to distress and suffering for a person with pain can be widespread and significant (Turk et al 2010, Williams 1998). They may experience a wide range of losses both material and intangible, covering everything from employment and finances, to changes in relationships, being able to maintain independence, issues of self-worth and so on. They also often experience symptoms such as fatigue, difficulty concentrating, muscle tension, disturbed sleep, side effects of medication and deconditioning. In addition they may have to deal with a range of health professionals, with possible disbelief and lack of understanding from some and undergo a variety of tests and interventions. They may have numerous fears or worries, including fear about the cause of the pain or that the doctors have missed something, fear of re-injury, worries about the future, financial concerns and so on.

An important point to note here, in terms of the biopsychosocial model, is the way in which each of these factors has the potential to impact on every other factor.

For example, a person may avoid certain activities as a result of pain, experience weight gain, deconditioning and loss of social contact as a result, followed by a drop in mood. Then, due to low mood, they have great difficulty in being motivated to become active again and therefore the low mood and deconditioning become further entrenched.

There is often considerable overlap between the symptoms of mood disturbance and those caused by the pain or factors related to it such as inactivity and the side effects of medications. For example, disrupted sleep, low energy, poor concentration, sexual dysfunction and weight changes can be the result of any of these.

Given all the issues faced by people with persistent pain it is not surprising that a large proportion may be diagnosed as having depression or an anxiety disorder (Turk et al 2010). Although issues of measurement and definition make establishing prevalence difficult (Williams 1998), few would dispute that it is a major issue for a large number of such people. Studies in the area of depression suggest a wide range of prevalence ranging from 10% to as high as 100% but with the majority reporting it in over 50% of cases (Sullivan 2001).

There has been much debate about the relationship between depression and chronic pain, particularly regarding the question of whether pain causes depression or depression leads to pain (Turk et al 2010). A comprehensive review of the literature on the pain–depression association by Fishbain et al (1997) found little evidence for the hypothesis that depression leads to pain, while all studies relating to the hypothesis that pain can lead to depression had results consistent with that hypothesis. In addition, increased pain led to increased depression rather than the other way around. Having said that, it would of course always be important to establish if there is any history of depression or other psychiatric illness.

In addition to anxiety and depression, anger is a very common feature of a persistent pain presentation (Turk et al 2010). There are many possible sources of anger including inability of the medical profession to help, repeated treatment failures, frustration at not being able to do things, anger with people who do not appear to understand or believe the pain is real, difficulties in dealing with insurers or employers, and so on.

Post-traumatic stress disorder (PTSD) and chronic pain can share a specific relationship in that very often the accident or trauma that occasioned the ongoing pain has also caused post-traumatic stress symptoms (see Sharp & Harvey 2001). For example, as a result of a motor vehicle accident, a person may experience pain from physical injuries and post-traumatic stress symptoms relating to the accident. A study by Tsui et al (2010) suggested that hyperarousal (a symptom of PTSD) can be a significant predictor of pain-related disability and decreased acceptance. Not surprisingly, as with depression, having PTSD and chronic pain means an additional load and likely interactions for the patient. This means both must be addressed.

PAIN BEHAVIOUR (DISABILITY)

As pointed out by Fordyce (1976), the only way in which we can know that a person is in pain is by their display of pain behaviour, by observing what they do or do not do and what they tell us. There is no objective measure of pain available to us other than this. Moreover, as pointed out earlier in the chapter, there is often no correlation between what we observe in this regard and identifiable tissue damage. Pain behaviours can take many forms from grunting, moaning and groaning, to limping, distorted posture and being hunched over. People may tell you that they are in pain but equally their lack of social engagement may be an indicator of discomfort. They may take medication, attend numerous medical appointments or treatments and they may take time off work, lie down or cease activities. Equally they may rate their pain as being very high on questionnaires or in response to questions about their pain. It is important to note in relation to pain behaviours that, because pain is a completely subjective experience and because there are no objective measures, health professionals can only go by the person's report. A *change* in such behaviours and reports can at least indicate that, for that person, at that time, there has been a change in their experience of the pain. Note also, suggesting to a person that they are not in pain may only serve to increase the display of pain behaviour. The important point here is that if pain is viewed as an experience, the distinction between real, exaggerated or fabricated pain becomes irrelevant. For health professionals the targets of treatment become not the pain itself but the associated suffering or disability (Fordyce 1988).

ENVIRONMENT

The environment or context in which pain occurs can have a significant impact on a person's experience of that pain. Environment or context can refer to a range of factors including: the situation in which the pain occurred, for example, while playing sport, during an argument or slipping on a step; the response of others such as family or health professionals to the pain; and legal or compensation matters.

The role of learning

Fordyce (1976) proposed that operant learning plays an important role in the development and maintenance of pain behaviour. Operant conditioning (see Chs 1 and 7) refers to the reinforcement or rewarding of a behaviour, such that it is more likely to occur in the future. In the case of pain, for example, reinforcement of behaviours, like groaning and grimacing by encouraging the person to rest and take medication, is likely to lead to increased groaning and grimacing in the future, especially if it allows the person to avoid aversive tasks. On the other hand, reinforcing activity and normal function, while at the same time extinguishing pain behaviours through lack of reinforcement, can be an effective intervention for pain (Eccleston et al 2009, Guzman et al 2001). Research in the area has shown that reinforcement contingencies cannot only modify pain behaviours but also influence the development and maintenance of these behaviours (Jolliffe & Nicholas 2004, see *Research focus*).

Classical conditioning (see Chs 1 and 7) can also play a role in maintaining pain behaviour. Linton et al (1985) proposed that pain can act as an unconditioned stimulus (UCS), eliciting physiological responses that may become conditioned to other stimuli (CS) present at the same time as the painful stimulation. For example, stimuli associated with painful experiences such as needles when having an injection or the sound of a drill when at the dentist can become conditioned (through pairings

Research focus

Jolliffe, C.D., Nicholas, M.K., 2004. Verbally reinforcing pain reports: an experimental test of the operant model of chronic pain. Pain 107, 167–175.

ABSTRACT

This study demonstrates that pain responses can be conditioned (controlled by reinforcement contingencies), independently of the noxious stimulus. The pain reports from a blood pressure cuff on the arm were measured over two sets of 15 trials in 46 healthy undergraduates. In one set of trials the pressure from the cuff remained stable; in the other set the pressure reduced over time. The students were split into two groups with one group being 'praised' or reinforced for higher pain ratings across trials and 'punished' for lower pain ratings. The experimenter expressed praise with comments like 'that's good' and punishment with comments like 'that's a bit odd'. The other group (the control group) received no verbal feedback. After the 15 trials the average pain reports of the reinforced group were significantly higher than those of the control group, in both sets of trials.

Critical thinking

- Consider the study described in the *Research focus* on the conditioning or reinforcement of pain reports.
- What do you think might have happened if the pressure in the cuff had increased rather than decreased over time?
- Do you think there could be a limit to the power of conditioning pain reports?
- This study cites an average pain report across each group but some participants will not have responded in the direction of the average. How might you explain the responses of these participants?
- How might you explain what happened in this study in terms of 'pain processing'?
- Consider your own experience in this area – can you think of examples where your response to a stimulus has been conditioned by factors other than the actual stimulus?

with pain) to elicit fear and physiological changes, such as muscle tension, even in the absence of pain. Recent literature has pointed out that interoceptive stimuli (internal bodily sensations) can also become predictors of pain (De Peuter et al 2011) through a process of classical conditioning. For example, stiff joints or muscle twitches can elicit a defensive or conditioned response and pain patients may try to avoid such sensations by minimising activity. This in turn can lead, through a process of operant conditioning, to a vicious circle whereby the reduced activity is reinforced by a reduction in fear or the non-occurrence of pain.

Partner or significant other

An important source of reinforcement contingencies is a person's partner and/or family. A number of studies have shown that these can play an important role in developing or maintaining pain behaviour (Cano & Leong 2012). While social support may be an important factor in helping a person to cope with pain, such support can become 'solicitous' and there is clear evidence that solicitous partners can maintain and even increase disability and pain behaviour. 'Solicitous' in this context refers to behaviours by others such as sympathy, taking over tasks, and assistance, which serve to reinforce or reward pain behaviours. Note that the dynamics can be complex, with a number of other factors influencing outcome such as the person's level of depression, their satisfaction with the marriage or relationship, and the context in which the interaction takes place, for example, in front of mates as opposed to in the hospital (Newton-John 2002). Contrary to what might be expected, punishing responses to pain behaviour from a partner can also serve to increase that behaviour, possibly by contributing to levels of depression (Cano & Leong 2012). Importantly it is the *perception* on the part of the pain patient of the partner's response that matters.

Gender and cultural factors

Gender appears to have an influence on pain, with a number of studies clearly demonstrating that women report more pain, both acute and chronic, than men (Fillingim 2010). The reasons for this are not clear but studies have suggested that gender differences in nociceptive processing and hormonal influences may play a role. Stereotypic gender roles appear to account for some differences, especially in the reporting of pain in experimental pain responses (Fillingim 2010), with both men and women reporting that women are more comfortable than men to report pain.

In the case of cultural factors, the research is again not conclusive, partly because culture is itself not a clear construct and can be influenced by a number of factors, including ethnicity, gender, education and religion. The information available suggests that cultural factors, particularly those influenced by ethnic background, can be important in the expression and conceptualisation of pain. For example, studies have shown that certain ethnic groups may report higher levels of pain, be more disabled and display a higher level of pain behaviour (Otis et al 2004). Although ethnicity may affect pain, this appears to be primarily through sociocultural influences rather than through genetics (Morris 2010). People's attitudes and responses to pain are shaped by social norms within particular social contexts and can change over generations. This is most clearly illustrated by differences in response to health issues between immigrants and their acculturated offspring (Morris 2010). Moreover, it is likely that there are as many differences between people of a certain cultural background as there are similarities. Therefore, in the clinical context, although it is important to be culturally sensitive to a person's background, it is equally important to avoid stereotyping (Ng et al 1996).

A number of studies in the United States have shown that health professionals are not immune to practising discrimination, whether they are aware of it or not (Morris 2010). For example, studies by Todd et al (1993) and Todd (1996) have shown that people from a Hispanic background presenting at an emergency department with fractures were twice as likely as similar Caucasian patients to go without pain medication. Other studies have shown that African-American patients with sickle cell disease seeking pain relief have been suspected of drug seeking (Wailoo 2001). Studies of pain treatment in cancer patients have also suggested that people from minority groups experience inadequate pain relief (Cleeland et al 1997). The reasons for this may be complex including language difficulties and/or socioeconomic status, but such findings also suggest the possibility of stereotyping.

The healthcare system and healthcare providers

The information and treatments provided to a person in pain can have a strong impact on both their expectations and understanding of the pain and consequent self-management. Information given to the patient such as advising a person to let pain be their guide can contribute to a sense of helplessness and increased disability (Kouyanou et al 1997). Facial expressions and the language health professionals use can inadvertently encourage catastrophising in patients (Vlaeyen & Linton 2006); for example, the term 'degeneration' of the spine can lead a patient to think that their spine is crumbling away and they must be very careful. This is despite the fact that an x-ray of anyone's spine over the age of 30 will show some signs of degeneration.

In the case of chronic pain, ongoing recommendations for biomedical investigations, interventions and passive treatments implies to the patient that there is indeed something wrong and that it needs to be fixed before they can resume normal life activities. This is despite the fact that, at present, there is little evidence that commonly practised medical treatments for chronic pain make any difference in terms of increasing function and returning people to work (Hansson & Hansson 2000).

A number of studies have suggested a clear link between higher fear-avoidance beliefs in healthcare practitioners and increased recommendations for rest, and less advice to maintain physical activities and higher fear-avoidance beliefs in patients (Coudeyre et al 2006, Linton et al 2002, Poiraudeau et al 2006). This may represent confusion between acute and chronic pain states, but even in acute and subacute back pain, the available evidence and a range of guidelines clearly recommend reassurance by the clinician and encouragement for resumption of activity (e.g. Van Tulder et al 2005).

Research focus

Linton, S.J., Vlaeyen, J., Ostelo, R., 2002. The back pain beliefs of healthcare providers: are we fear avoidant? Journal of Occupational Rehabilitation 12 (4), 223–232.

The beliefs of health professionals regarding the management of pain are passed on to their patients and can be detrimental in terms of promoting fear avoidance and increased disability. In this study 71 physiotherapists and 60 general practitioners (GPs) were given a questionnaire measuring fear-avoidance beliefs and related management of their patients. More than two-thirds reported that they would recommend patients avoid movements that cause pain, more than one-third believed that pain must reduce before returning to work and 25% believed that taking time off work is a good treatment for back pain. Importantly these beliefs are not consistent with the current evidence for the optimal management of back pain.

Critical thinking

Consider the study described in the *Research focus* on the pain beliefs of healthcare providers and examine your own beliefs and behaviours in relation to pain.

- How do you respond to pain? Rest? Take medications? Go to the doctor? 'Soldier on'?
- How would your response differ depending on the type of pain or the situation?
- What do you advise others to do?
- Would your advice change if the pain continued over time?
- Do you think pain is a sign of damage or injury?
- Have you ever ignored pain? What was the context?
- Do you sometimes think that other people exaggerate or pretend to have pain? How would you know? Why do you think they would do that?

The workplace and the compensation system

A number of factors relating to the workplace have been identified as impacting on outcome in terms of return to work (Shaw et al 2012). Work-related risk factors include physical work demands such as lack of modified duties and heavy or fast work; social factors such as lack of support or having little control; perceptions about work especially job dissatisfaction; and workplace disability management (Shaw et al 2012).

People with compensation claims are often regarded as having a motive for exaggerating their pain or disability, but in fact research in the area suggests that there are no important differences between compensated and non-compensated patients and the vast majority of workers do recover and get back to work (Robinson & Loeser 2012). However, a systematic review by Harris et al (2005) of a large number of postoperative cases in many countries did find that having a compensation claim was strongly associated with poorer health outcomes. Likewise an Australian study looking at people injured in motor vehicle accidents found that a compensation claim was associated with poorer health outcomes (Gabbe et al 2007).

The reasons for these poorer outcomes are unclear, but proposed contributing factors include the possibility of secondary gains such as financial compensation, avoidance of unpleasant tasks and attention from others. Note claimants may not be consciously aware of the pursuit of these gains and most also experience a wide range of secondary losses (Robinson & Loeser 2012). Other proposed contributing factors include a difficult claims and settlement process, inability to move on with life during this process, extreme dislike of medicolegal assessments, necessity of legal representation and a perceived lack of trust about having to prove an injury or disability (Murgatroyd et al 2011). Of notable importance is that people in the compensation system are required, by the system itself, to constantly report and demonstrate their symptoms in order to be compensated, which, in turn, encourages focusing on disability rather than rehabilitation (Nicholas 2002).

Acute versus chronic pain

Acute pain is short-lived; it can last from a few seconds to a few hours but generally less than three months and is associated with injury, disease or inflammation of somatic, visceral or nervous system structures. Acute pain is generally thought to have a protective biological function, for example, when a person touches a hot stove, pain alerts them to immediately withdraw their hand. Likewise, following a fracture, pain imposes significant limitation of function that is useful in preventing further damage (Hurley et al 2010). However, in some instances, the warning (pain) comes too late to avoid injury. Sunburn is such an example.

As noted above, the distinction between acute and chronic pain has traditionally relied on a measure of time; however, using time to distinguish between acute and chronic pain is subjective and can be ambiguous (Turk & Okifuji 2010). For example, pain that persists for extended periods of time in the presence of ongoing pathology might be viewed by some as acute, whereas others would classify it as chronic (Turk & Okifuji 2010). Moreover, pain can be considered chronic if it extends beyond tissue healing, even when this is only a relatively short period of time. This ambiguity has led Turk and Okifuji (2010) to propose a two-dimensional conceptualisation of acute and chronic pain, one that is based on time and physical pathology. From this two-dimensional perspective, pain of short duration or associated with high physical pathology is acute, whereas pain associated with low physical pathology or of long duration is chronic (Turk & Okifuji 2010).

The nervous system changes that occur in response to injury or disease were discussed earlier in this chapter. Acute pain may be associated with anxiety and fear, particularly if it is unexpected and severe and can have deleterious effects if left unchecked (Hurley et al 2010). The emphasis in managing acute pain therefore, should be to identify the cause and provide pain relief until healing occurs. Adequate analgesia is necessary, particularly in the case of severe trauma and postoperative pain, to reduce the risk of acute pain persisting (Hurley et al 2010). Under normal conditions, following recovery, the pain and associated nervous system responses usually disappear within days or weeks.

Chronic pain, on the other hand, results in numerous pathophysiological peripheral and central nervous system changes and is only rarely amenable to effective biomedical treatment (Turk & Okifuji 2010). It may represent a low level of underlying pathology (e.g. as in osteoarthritis), but usually such pathology fails to explain the presence and/or extent of pain. While chronic pain may have been initiated by an injury or disease, the factors that maintain it are more than likely both physically and pathogenetically removed from the originating cause (Turk & Okifuji 2010).

Persistent pain can have a strong impact on psychological function and can have significant functional consequences. People report mood and sleep disturbance, irritability, distress, helplessness and depression. They may lose confidence in their ability to perform tasks and become fear avoidant. There may be other consequences such as loss of status, relationship breakdown and loss of employment. Therefore, in order to successfully manage chronic pain, it is necessary to assess the relative contribution of physical, psychological and environmental factors, and to address the consequences of pain.

In some cases, it may be possible to address the initial pathology resulting in significant reduction or resolution of pain and its associated consequences. For example, pain and secondary changes such as central sensitisation, mood disturbance and disability will generally disappear following a procedure (e.g. hip replacement surgery) that successfully resolves the initial pathology, regardless of chronicity (e.g. Rodriguez-Raecke et al 2009). However, in other cases, it may be impossible to identify or adequately treat the initial pathology. In these cases, the focus should be on dealing with the initial pathology if possible, but of equal importance is to identify and address the functional consequences of pain, such as depression, sleep disturbance, loss of meaning in personal relationships and work, fear avoidance of activities and postural changes. Persisting with the search for a cause or a cure of their chronic pain can prevent a person from accepting and dealing with their pain and can prolong or exacerbate their suffering and disability (McCarberg 2010).

TRANSITION FROM ACUTE TO CHRONIC PAIN AND DISABILITY

Many people with chronic pain continue to lead active lives despite ongoing pain. An epidemiological study by Blyth et al (2001) established that in Australia just over 17% of male adults and 20% of adult females report having chronic pain. Nearly half of those reported that it was having little impact on their lives, while the other half reported varying levels of interference, some to a significant degree. A more recent population study conducted in South Australia confirmed the overall prevalence of chronic pain and noted that the degree to which pain interfered 'extremely' with activity was 5% (Currow et al 2010).

For those who do experience this level of interference, one might assume that this is because of the severity of the injury and pain. In fact, research in this area has made it increasingly clear that many factors unrelated to the physical injury can have a significant impact on a person's recovery and return to normal function (Nicholas et al 2011). Importantly, after three to six months, the likelihood of a person recovering and returning to normal activities becomes increasingly less likely, despite ongoing consumption of healthcare resources (Cohen et al 2000).

This means, of course, that it would be very useful to be able to predict who might be at risk of developing chronic pain and a high level of disability, and provide appropriate interventions at an early stage. There has been extensive research into which factors might be relevant in the development of chronic pain and a range of psychological, social and environmental risk factors have been identified. Table 12.2 outlines some of these factors, differentiating psychological factors from work and biomedical factors according to a system of coloured flags. Some of these factors were discussed earlier in the section on the workplace and the compensation system. A number of screening tools have been developed to help health professionals identify people at risk for persisting pain and disability (Nicholas et al 2011).

Interventions and management for pain

BIOMEDICAL INTERVENTIONS

A discussion of the interventions used to manage pain should be prefaced by a discussion of the nonspecific effects of treatment. One could argue that a positive

Table 12.2

RISK FACTORS FOR TRANSITION OF PAIN FROM ACUTE TO CHRONIC, ACCORDING TO THE COLOURED FLAG SYSTEM

Flag	Type	Examples
Red	Signs of serious pathology	Tumour; infection; cauda equina syndrome; fracture; neurological signs
Orange	Psychiatric issues	Major depression; schizophrenia
Yellow	Psychological factors	High levels of distress or anxiety; beliefs about pain (e.g. increased pain means further damage); expectation of need for resolution of pain; over-reliance on passive treatments; avoidance of activity due to fear of pain and/or damage
Blue	Perceptions about workplace and health	Job dissatisfaction; belief that there is a lack of support at work; belief that the job is too demanding physically and/or mentally; attribution of pain condition to work
Black	System factors – occupational and legal	Availability of modified duties; lack of support from the workplace; limitations imposed by legislation or the return to work system; conflict with the insurer or workplace

Source: Nicholas MK, Linton SJ, Watson PJ, Main CJ, the 'Decade of the Flags' Working Group. Early identification and management of psychological risk factors ('yellow flags') in patients with low back pain: a reappraisal. Phys Ther. 2011;91:737–753. © 2011 American Physical Therapy Association

Research focus

Buchbinder, R., Jolley, D., Wyatt, M., 2001. Effects of a media campaign on back pain beliefs and its potential influence on management of low back pain in general practice. Spine 26 (23), 2535–2542.

ABSTRACT

This study looks at the effects of a statewide public health intervention to alter beliefs about back pain and influence its medical management and reduce disability and workers' compensation-related costs. In 1997 a multimedia campaign was begun in Victoria, Australia that positively advised people with back pain to remain active, exercise, minimise resting and stay at work. The influence of that campaign was measured by comparing beliefs before and after the campaign, in the general population and in GPs, with demographically identical groups in New South Wales (NSW), where there had been no such campaign. A total of 4730 people were contacted by telephone and 2556 GPs completed mailed surveys regarding their approaches to treatment of back pain. The results showed a significant improvement in back pain beliefs over time in Victoria but not in NSW. Likewise, GPs in Victoria reported significant improvements over time in their beliefs about back pain management, compared with GPs in NSW.

Critical thinking

- Consider the study described in the *Research focus* on the effects of a media campaign on back pain beliefs.
- How else could people's beliefs be changed over time?
- What methods would be most effective and be long lasting?
- Why do you think GPs might change their beliefs due to a media campaign as opposed to, for example, reading the current literature on back pain?
- What other areas of healthcare and management have been or might be addressed by a campaign such as this?
- Have you changed your views on any areas of health as a result of media campaigns?

response following treatment may come about in three ways: the specific effects of the treatment; natural history or regression to the mean; and nonspecific effects, such as attention from healthcare providers, a desire to improve, a reduction in anxiety and improved coping (Jamison 2011). In other words, the overall response to an active treatment can be viewed as the sum of the treatment itself and the context in which treatment is given (Finniss et al 2010). There is growing evidence from the placebo literature that these nonspecific or placebo effects are genuine psychobiological phenomena attributable to the therapeutic context, including individual patient and clinician factors, and the interaction between the clinician, the patient and the therapeutic environment (Finniss et al 2010). For example, in a series of large trials comparing traditional acupuncture, sham acupuncture and either no treatment or usual clinical care, patients' expectation of pain relief was the most powerful predictor of treatment benefit, regardless of group allocation to traditional or sham acupuncture (Linde et al 2007).

The emphasis in managing acute pain is to identify and treat the cause or to provide pain relief until healing occurs. Acute musculoskeletal pain can respond well to a short course of a variety of medications. Simple analgesics such as paracetamol and NSAIDs (non-steroidal anti-inflammatory drugs) are mostly used for mild pain, compound analgesics (e.g. paracetamol plus codeine) and weak opioids (e.g. tramadol) are used for moderate pain and strong opioids (e.g. morphine, oxycodone) are used for severe pain. The choice of medication should be individualised and should include a discussion with the patient of the potential benefits and risks of therapy (Chou 2010).

In the past 20 years there has been a swing to increased use of strong opioids for treating chronic pain. However, the use of these drugs has been linked with nausea, constipation, drowsiness, mood change, poor concentration, drug tolerance and dependence. Long-acting formulations and transdermal patches are able to provide more stable levels of analgesia but a large number of people on strong opioid medication still report ongoing pain and minimal functional gain (Nicholas et al 2006).

Neuropathic pain, on the other hand, generally does not respond well to NSAIDs, and opioids should only be considered as second- or third-line options in noncancer neuropathic pain treatment due to the risks associated with long-term use such as opioid-induced hyperalgesia (Attal & Finnerup 2010). However, tricyclic antidepressants (TCAs), in lower doses than would normally be used for treating depression, can be effective in treating neuropathic pain and may also help with sleeplessness and comorbid depression. Side effects include weight gain, constipation, blurred vision, drowsiness, poor concentration and clouded thinking. Anticonvulsants generally reduce the abnormal firing of sensory nerves that occurs with neuropathic pain. The newer anticonvulsants, such as gabapentin and pregabalin, have fewer side effects but are nevertheless associated with a number of adverse reactions and are more expensive. Side effects include impaired memory and reduced concentration. Additionally, the newer serotonin-noradrenaline reuptake inhibitor (SNRI) antidepressants (e.g. duloxetine and venlafaxine) have established efficacy in the treatment of neuropathic pain and are recommended as first-line treatments, along with TCAs, gabapentin and pregabalin (Attal & Finnerup 2010).

Surgery

Surgery has a major role to play in managing some pain conditions, such as where a lesion or abnormality is able to be identified and resected, repaired, reconstructed, reinforced or replaced, but outcomes are not as good if the main reason for surgery is pain relief (Ghabrial & Bogduk 2010). For example, outcome studies have concluded that although surgery can be indicated for patients with specific spinal conditions, such as cauda equina syndrome, there is little advantage of surgery over conservative treatment at 12–24 months for patients with low back pain and sciatica (Koes et al 2007). There is also the possibility that surgery may make the pain worse.

A number of techniques are available to cut nerves in an attempt to eliminate pain. These procedures are mostly used for severe cancer pain in terminally ill patients and are not recommended for treating chronic pain. An exception is radiofrequency (RF) lesioning of the small nerves that supply the facet joints in the spine. This procedure can relieve pain by stopping nociceptive inputs from reaching the spinal cord and brain (Dreyfuss et al 2000). However, it is only suitable for a very small group of people with a specific form of spinal pain and the pain can return when the nerves re-grow.

Injections

Different types of injections can be used to treat pain; these include local anaesthetic blocks and steroid injections. Local anaesthetic blocks may be useful as a diagnostic procedure and can assist in temporarily reducing chronic pain. Steroid injections can be helpful in reducing inflammation in some acute conditions but they cannot be repeated very often and are associated with a number of side effects.

Stimulation techniques

A variety of stimulation techniques have also been used for treating pain with varying levels of success. These include acupuncture, transcutaneous electrical nerve stimulation (TENS), spinal cord stimulation and deep brain stimulation. Acupuncture has been demonstrated to be useful for some types of acute and chronic pain but the effects are short lived and, in the case of chronic pain, treatment needs to be repeated at regular intervals. The other stimulation techniques mentioned above are thought to act on inhibitory mechanisms at the level of the spinal cord and brain and can be particularly useful for treating certain types of neuropathic pain.

Physical therapies and exercise

A number of physical and manual therapies are used in the treatment of both acute and chronic musculoskeletal pain, although there is continuing debate about the effectiveness of such treatments in the long term. Passive modalities include massage, manipulation, ultrasound, hot packs and cold packs. These can be helpful in relieving acute musculoskeletal pain but, as the effects are short lived, they are less useful in managing chronic pain and in returning people to normal activities. A greater understanding of the biopsychosocial model of pain calls for a novel approach to physical therapy, termed 'psychologically informed practice', whereby treatment of patients anywhere along the pain continuum incorporates systematic attention to the psychosocial factors that are associated with poorer treatment outcomes (Main & George 2011).

Research into the treatment of patients with subacute low back pain has demonstrated that physiotherapist-directed exercise and advice have beneficial effects on pain and function at six weeks, when compared with placebo (Pengel et al 2007). In the case of ongoing pain, the focus of treatment shifts from pain relief to a gradual resumption of normal activities despite the presence of pain. Exercise can be beneficial in reversing some of the secondary changes that occur such as decreased mobility and strength and reduced fitness. Exercise programs typically include stretching, strengthening, aerobic and functional components and should focus on encouraging a return to normal function. Exercise should be progressed gradually to minimise over-stimulation of a sensitised nervous system and should be based on the individual's functional goals. A recent systematic review of physical conditioning programs with a stated relationship to the workplace and a focus on job demands by Schaafsma and colleagues (2010) concluded that intensive physical conditioning programs improved long-term return to work outcomes for patients with chronic low back pain compared with routine clinical care. It is important to note that for patients with chronic pain, exercise is not an end in itself but a means of exposure to feared or avoided activities and forms a series of stepping stones towards achieving functional goals.

PSYCHOLOGICAL APPROACHES

A range of psychological strategies can be used to help people manage both acute and chronic pain. In the case of acute pain, information and education about what is going to happen in a proposed treatment and what to expect in terms of pain can be helpful in terms of allaying fears and reducing distress, for example, prior to a surgical procedure. Training a patient in ways to calm themselves, such as by relaxation, forms of meditation and self-hypnosis, can also be beneficial. Attentional techniques such as distraction can be useful. However, studies on the effectiveness of all these techniques suggest they have variable rates of success (Macintyre et al 2010). Repeated practise by the patient appears to be important as does structure, specific (written) instructions, and an understanding that the primary goal is to reduce distress rather than pain. In the case of education and information it is important to check what the beliefs and concerns of the patient actually are. Simply providing education and information will not necessarily remove fear.

In the case of chronic pain the above techniques can also be of benefit but the emphasis shifts to long-term management of the pain, rather than simply dealing with the current episode of pain. In practice this means learning to live with the pain and returning to normal activities and function despite pain. The patient can sometimes interpret this as 'a last resort' or as an indication that they are being told their pain is 'all in their head'. Therefore it is essential to clarify the rationale and benefits of psychological management strategies when introducing them. Education regarding the physiological mechanisms causing persisting pain can play an important role in reassuring patients that persisting pain is not necessarily a sign of further damage and that it is safe to upgrade activity levels. Psychological strategies can be introduced at the same time as biomedical interventions, or in a planned sequence. In the case of chronic pain it can sometimes be useful to introduce them when biomedical interventions have been completed because of the different goal: improved self-management and adjustment to the pain as opposed to pain reduction.

CASE STUDY: PENELOPE

Penelope is a married 30-year-old mother of two children aged four and two. Apart from several months off work for the birth of each child, she had worked part time as a legal secretary for seven years. A year ago she slipped and fell while getting heavy files down from a shelf in her workplace. She experienced an immediate onset of pain in her lower back and left leg and was advised by her GP to take two weeks off work and rest. Her pain did not resolve and a subsequent MRI scan identified a postero-lateral disc bulge at L4/5, mildly abutting the thecal sac, without disc protrusion or nerve root compromise. She was prescribed analgesic medication and referred for physiotherapy treatment.

After three months, the pain had not resolved and she was referred to an orthopaedic surgeon for review but surgery was not recommended. Instead she was advised to try to increase her activity levels but to stop if the pain increased. She was also prescribed stronger analgesics. Now, a year later, she has not returned to work, she is doing little housework and her two children are being cared for during the day by relatives. Penelope reports feeling depressed and hopeless and her GP has started her on antidepressants. She describes herself as previously having been a very active cheerful person and is frustrated by her current inability to do things. She reports difficulty with remembering things and poor concentration, which she thinks may be a side effect of the pain medication she is on. She is anxious that her pain has not resolved and is concerned that increases in pain are a sign of further damage. She believes that overall her pain is getting worse. She worries that the doctors may have missed something and both she and her husband believe that her pain would have to resolve before she could become more active.

As well as physiotherapy, Penelope has tried acupuncture and has weekly massages. She has tried to do the exercises given to her by her physiotherapist but then usually takes extra medication to cope with the increased pain and spends the following day resting to recover. Recently she has stopped doing the exercises altogether. Her sleep is disrupted and she frequently naps during the day. Penelope's husband is working extra shifts to meet their financial commitments and has taken over her chores at home. He has apparently tried to be supportive but they are now arguing more and sleep in separate rooms.

Cont... ▶

Penelope notes that when she is very distressed or upset her pain is worse. The family no longer has any social activities and Penelope rarely attends her children's activities. Penelope's job still remains open for her but she says she could not sit for long enough to do her previous work and is concerned about her poor concentration and memory.

Classroom activity

1. Refer back to the case of Penelope. Think about the way her case has been managed to date by the various health professionals involved and how each of them may or may not have contributed to her current presentation.
   » What decisions were made?
   » What advice was she given?
   » What decisions or advice might have been more helpful?
2. Formulate a plan for management of her current presentation.
   » What would be the components of the plan?
   » What health professionals would need to be involved?
   » How could the plan best be delivered (individual sessions, a group format)?
   » Who else would it be important to include in formulating and implementing the plan and how (husband, family, GP, workplace, insurance company and so on)?
3. Using the biopsychosocial model of pain, identify all the relevant components of Penelope's case. Think carefully about how each component of the model impacts on every other component. Use the specific facts of Penelope's case to show these links. It may be helpful to construct this as a diagram on a whiteboard, similar to the diagram used in Figure 12.4.

COGNITIVE-BEHAVIOURAL APPROACHES

There is good evidence that cognitive behavioural therapy (CBT) to help people manage pain, particularly chronic pain, is effective for the targeted outcomes (e.g. increased function, improved mood, reduced use of medications and return to work) (Eccleston et al 2009, Guzman et al 2001, Nicholas et al 2012). It can be delivered in individual sessions with different health professionals, for example, a physiotherapist and a psychologist, but the evidence available suggests that it is more effective when delivered as part of a structured intensive program, particularly for those who are more disabled and distressed (Haldorsen et al 2002). It is of course important that all health professionals working with a patient deliver a consistent message and work within the same biopsychosocial framework.

For patients who have had chronic pain for some time and who have not managed to return to normal function, the impact on many areas of their lives can be

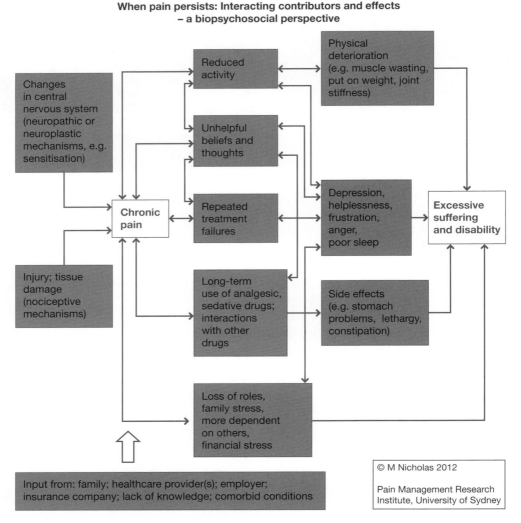

Figure 12.4 When chronic pain becomes a problem

Adapted with permission from MK Nicholas

significant and seem insurmountable. They often report feeling that they have tried everything and there is now little hope for improvement. The diagram in Figure 12.4, based on the biopsychosocial model of pain, outlines the typical experience for a chronic pain patient.

In cases such as these, a comprehensive and intensive cognitive-behavioural program can be used to target and improve all aspects of the presentation. Such a program is usually delivered by a physiotherapist and psychologist, specially trained in the area of chronic pain management, who work together as an integrated team. Other health professionals involved may include a doctor (to rationalise and/or reduce medication), a nurse and a work rehabilitation adviser. The typical components of such a program include education about pain, setting functional goals, upgrading activity levels in a paced manner so as to progress towards those goals, programmed exercises and stretches, applied relaxation training, desensitisation to the pain, identifying and changing unhelpful beliefs and thought patterns, learning effective problem-solving techniques, reduction of medication use and other passive strategies such as resting or avoidance of activities and, where relevant, formulating a plan to return to work. Some of these components are illustrated in Tables 12.3 and 12.4 and Figure 12.5. Note that pain reduction itself is not specifically targeted as this can lead to constant monitoring of the pain along with unhelpful attempts to avoid and reduce it. However, there is increasing evidence that

Table 12.3

SETTING FUNCTIONAL GOALS

Long-term goal	Short-term goals	Physical abilities
Return to work	Sit longer Stand longer Walk further Lift up to 10 kg occasionally	Identify and improve sitting, standing and walking tolerances Train technique and improve lifting tolerance Improve back and leg mobility Improve abdominal and back extensor strength Improve arm and leg strength
Surfing	Lying on stomach Paddling Balance	Identify and improve prone lying tolerance Improve back and shoulder mobility Improve scapular muscle and upper limb strength Identify and improve paddling tolerance Improve abdominal and back extensor strength Improve hip and lower limb strength Improve balance

Table 12.4

IDENTIFYING AND CHANGING UNHELPFUL BELIEFS

Situation	Thoughts	Feelings/behaviours	Alternative/helpful thoughts	Outcome
Increase in pain	The doctors must have missed something	Worried, visit more specialists	I have had many tests already and nothing serious was found	Calmer, continue with activity
	My life is ruined; I can't do anything	Depressed, do nothing	If I pace myself I can gradually build up my activities	More motivated, continue with activity
	I need to stop and rest	Frustrated, lie down	I know that pain does not mean more damage	Reassured, continue with activity

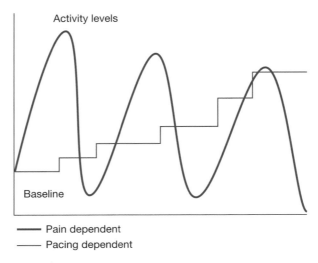

Figure 12.5 Using pacing to structure activity levels

once people are managing their pain better and are more engaged in life, they often report reduced pain (e.g. Nicholas et al 2012).

Conclusion

This chapter gives an overview of the current understanding of the experience of pain. It explains the neurobiological basis of pain, including the difference between nociceptive and neuropathic pain, the role of central sensitisation and the distinction between acute and chronic pain. It further explains that despite this neurobiological basis, the presentation of pain can only be usefully explained and understood when all relevant psychological and environmental factors are taken into account. This is particularly important in the case of chronic pain where biomedical interventions have only limited effectiveness and the emphasis shifts from pain relief to pain management and specifically to more adaptive management of relevant psychosocial factors.

REMEMBER

- Pain is an unpleasant sensory and emotional experience that is not adequately explained by simply linking it to a noxious stimulus.
- There are two main types of pain: nociceptive, which is pain arising from injury or pathology in somatic or visceral structures where it activates nociceptors in the affected tissues; and neuropathic, which is pain arising as a direct consequence of damage or disease affecting the somatosensory system.
- Pain is best understood within a biopsychosocial model with factors at all levels impacting on the experience: nociception or neuropathy; pain perception; attitudes and beliefs; psychological distress (suffering); pain behaviour (disability); and environment interactions.

Cont... ▶

- Pain can also be divided into acute pain (less than three months) and chronic pain (three months or more). Chronic pain can also be thought of as 'pain that extends beyond the expected period of healing'.
- In the acute phase biomedical interventions can be effective in reducing pain and increasing function; in chronic pain such interventions become increasingly less effective and the emphasis often shifts from pain relief to pain management.

Further resources

Fishman, S.M., Ballantyne, J.C., Rathmell, J.P. (Eds.), 2010. Bonica's management of pain, fourth ed. Lippincott Williams & Wilkins, Philadelphia.

Hasenbring, M.I., Rusu, A.C., Turk, D.C. (Eds.), 2012. From acute to chronic back pain: risk factors, mechanisms, and clinical implications. Oxford University Press, New York.

International Association for the Study of Pain (IASP) Task Force on Taxonomy, 1994. Classification of chronic pain. Descriptions of chronic pain syndromes and definitions of pain terms, second ed. IASP, Washington DC.

Melzack, R., Wall, P.D., 1982. The challenge of pain. Basic Books, New York.

Turk, D.C., Monarch, E.S., 2002. Biopsychosocial perspective on chronic pain. In: Turk, D.C., Gatchel, R.J. (Eds.), Psychological approaches to pain management. A practitioner's handbook, second ed. Guilford Press, New York, pp. 3–29.

Vlaeyen, J.W.S., Linton, S.J., 2000. Fear-avoidance and its consequences in chronic musculoskeletal pain: a state of the art. Pain 85 (3), 317–332.

Weblinks

International Association for the Study of Pain (IASP)

www.iasp-pain.org

The IASP was founded in 1973 and is the world's largest multidisciplinary organisation focused specifically on pain research and treatment. It brings together scientists, health professionals, healthcare providers and policymakers to stimulate and support the study of pain. The website gives details of all its activities, publications, events and meetings and also provides links to many other useful websites.

PAIN – the official journal of IASP

www.sciencedirect.com/pain

PAIN is the official journal of the International Association for the Study of Pain. The IASP publishes 18 issues per year of original research on the nature, mechanisms and treatment of pain. This peer-reviewed journal provides a forum for the dissemination of research in the basic and clinical sciences of multidisciplinary care.

Pain Management Research Institute, Royal North Shore Hospital

www.pmri.med.usyd.edu.au

The Pain Management Research Institute (PMRI) is a joint initiative between the University of Sydney and Royal North Shore Hospital. It conducts basic and clinical research programs and also operates a national and international educational program leading to a master's qualification in pain management. The PMRI works in close collaboration with the Pain Management and Research Centre (PMRC), which treats patients with acute pain, cancer pain and chronic non-cancer pain. The website gives details of all these activities and provides links to a wide range of other useful websites.

The Australian Pain Society

www.apsoc.org.au

APSOC was formed in 1979 as the Australian chapter of the International Association for the Study of Pain.

The New Zealand Pain Society

www.nzps.org.nz

NZPS was formed in 1984 as the New Zealand chapter of the International Association for the Study of Pain.

References

Apkarian, A.V., Hashmi, J.A., Baliki, M.N., 2011. Pain and the brain: specificity and plasticity of the brain in clinical chronic pain. Pain 152 (Suppl 3), S49–S64.

Arntz, A., Claassens, L., 2004. The meaning of pain influences its experienced intensity. Pain 109, 20–25.

Asghari, A., Nicholas, M.K., 2001. Pain self-efficacy beliefs and pain behavior: a prospective study. Pain 94, 85–100.

Attal, N., Finnerup, N.B., 2010. Pharmacological management of neuropathic pain. IASP Pain Clinical Updates 18 (9), 1–8.

Blyth, F.M., March, L.M., Brnabic, A.J.M., et al., 2001. Chronic pain in Australia: a prevalence study. Pain 89, 127–134.

Buchbinder, R., Jolley, D., Wyatt, M., 2001. Effects of a media campaign on back pain beliefs and its potential influence on management of low back pain in general practice. Spine 26 (23), 2535–2542.

Cano, A., Leong, L., 2012. Significant others in the chronicity of pain and disability. In: Hasenbring, M.I., Rusu, A.C., Turk, D.C. (Eds.), From acute to chronic back pain: risk factors, mechanisms, and clinical implications. Oxford University Press, New York.

Chapman, C.R., Okifuji, A., 2004. Pain mechanisms and conscious experience. In: Dworkin, R.H., Breitbart, W.S. (Eds.), Psychosocial aspects of pain: a handbook for health care providers. Progress in Pain Research and Management. Vol. 27. IASP Press, Seattle.

Chou, R., 2010. Pharmacological management of low back pain. Drugs 70 (4), 387–402.

Cleeland, C., Gonin, R., Baez, L., et al., 1997. Pain and treatment of pain in minority patients with cancer: the Eastern Cooperative Oncology Group Minority Outpatient Pain Study. Annals of Internal Medicine, 127, 813–816.

Cohen, M., Nicholas, M., Blanch, A., 2000. Medical assessment and management of work-related low back pain or neck/arm pain. Journal of Occupational Health and Safety – Australia NZ 16, 307–317.

Cope, D.K., 2010. Intellectual milestones in our understanding and treatment of pain. In: Fishman, S.M., Ballantyne, J.C., Rathmell, J.P. (Eds.), Bonica's management of pain (online), fourth ed. Lippincott Williams & Wilkins, Philadelphia.

Coudeyre, E., Rannou, F., Tuback, F., et al., 2006. General practitioners' fear-avoidance beliefs influence their management of patients with low back pain. Pain 124, 330–337.

Currow, D.C., Agar, M., Plummer, J.L., et al., 2010. Chronic pain in South Australia – population levels that interfere extremely with activities of daily living. Australian and New Zealand Journal of Public Health 34 (3), 232–239.

De Peuter, S., Van Diest, I., Vansteenwegen, D., et al., 2011. Understanding fear of pain in chronic pain: interoceptive fear conditioning as a novel approach. European Journal of Pain 15, 889–894.

Dreyfuss, P., Halbrook, B., Pauza, K., et al., 2000. Efficacy and validity of radiofrequency neurotomy for chronic lumbar zygapophysial joint pain. Spine 25 (10), 1270–1277.

Eccleston, C., Williams, A.C.D.C., Morley, S., 2009. Psychological therapies for the management of chronic pain (excluding headache) in adults. Cochrane Database of Systematic Reviews Issue 2. Art. No.: CD007407. DOI: 10.1002/14651858.CD007407. pub2.

Engel, G.L., 1977. The need for a new medical model: a challenge for biomedicine. Science 196, 129–136.

Fillingim, R.B., 2010. Individual differences in pain: the roles of gender, ethnicity, and genetics. In: Fishman, S.M., et al. (Eds.), Bonica's management of pain, fourth ed. Lippincott Williams & Wilkins, Philadelphia.

Finniss, D.G., Kaptchuk, T.J., Miller, F., 2010. Biological, clinical, and ethical advances of placebo effects. The Lancet 375 (9715), 686–695.

Fishbain, D.A., Cutler, R., Rosomoff, H.L., et al., 1997. Chronic pain-associated depression: antecedent or consequence of chronic pain? A review. Clinical Journal of Pain 13 (2), 116–137.

Fordyce, W.E., 1976. Behavioural methods for chronic pain and illness. Mosby, St Louis.

Fordyce, W.E., 1988. Pain and suffering: a reappraisal. American Psychologist 43, 276–283.

Freynhagen, R., Bennett, M.I., 2009. Diagnosis and management of neuropathic pain. British Medical Journal 339, 391–395.

Gabbe, B.J., Cameron, P.A., Williamson, O.D., et al., 2007. The relationship between compensable status and long-term patient outcomes following orthopaedic trauma. Medical Journal of Australia 187, 14–17.

Geber, C., Baumgärtner, U., Schwab, R., et al., 2009. Revised definition of neuropathic pain and its grading system: an open case series illustrating its use in clinical practice. The American Journal of Medicine 122 (10A), S3–S12.

Ghabrial, Y., Bogduk, N., 2010. Surgery for low back pain. In: Fishman, S.M., Ballantyne, J.C., Rathmell, J.P. (Eds.), Bonica's management of pain (online), fourth ed. Lippincott Williams & Wilkins, Philadelphia.

Guzman, J., Esmail, R., Karjaleinan, K., et al., 2001. Multidisciplinary rehabilitation for chronic low back pain: systematic review. British Medical Journal 322, 1511–1516.

Haanpää, M., Attal, N., Backonja, M., et al., 2011. NeuPSIG guidelines on neuropathic pain assessment. Pain 152 (1), 14–27.

Haanpää, M., Treede, R.D., 2010. Diagnosis and classification of neuropathic pain. IASP Pain Clinical Updates 18 (7), 18–27.

Haldorsen, E.M.H., Grasdal, A.L., Skouen, J.S., et al., 2002. Is there a right treatment for a particular patient group? Comparison of ordinary treatment, light multidisciplinary treatment, and extensive multidisciplinary treatment for long-term sick-listed employees with musculoskeletal pain. Pain 95, 49–63.

Hanley, M.A., Raichle, K., Jensen, M., et al., 2008. Pain catastrophising and beliefs predict changes in pain interference and psychological functioning in persons with spinal cord injury. The Journal of Pain 9, 863–871.

Hansson, T.H., HanSson, E.K., 2000. The effects of common medical interventions on pain, back function and work resumption in patients with chronic low back pain. Spine 25, 3055–3064.

Harris, I., Mulford, J., Solomon, M., et al., 2005. Association between compensation status and outcome after surgery. Journal of the American Medical Association 293 (13), 1644–1652.

Hurley, R.W., Cohen, S.P., Wu, C.L., 2010. Acute pain in adults. In: Fishman, S.M., Ballantyne, J.C., Rathmell, J.P. (Eds.), Bonica's management of pain (online), fourth ed. Lippincott Williams & Wilkins, Philadelphia.

International Association for the Study of Pain (IASP) Task Force on Taxonomy, 1994. Classification of chronic pain. Descriptions of chronic pain syndromes and definitions of pain terms, second ed. IASP, Washington DC.

Jamison, R.N., 2011. Nonspecific treatment effects in pain medicine. IASP Pain Clinical Updates 19 (2).

Jolliffe, C.D., Nicholas, M.K., 2004. Verbally reinforcing pain reports: an experimental test of the operant model of chronic pain. Pain 107, 167–175.

Koes, B.W., van Tulder, M.W., Peul, W.C., 2007. Diagnosis and treatment of sciatica. British Medical Journal 334 (7607), 1313–1317.

Kouyanou, K., Pither, C.E., Wesley, S., 1997. Iatrogenic factors and chronic pain. Psychosomatic Medicine 59, 597–604.

Leeuw, M., Goossens, M.E.J.B., Linton, S.J., et al., 2007. The fear-avoidance model of musculoskeletal pain: current state of scientific evidence. Journal of Behavioural Medicine 30 (1), 77–94.

Linde, K., Witt, C.M., Streng, A., et al., 2007. The impact of patient expectations on outcomes in four randomized controlled trials of acupuncture in patients with chronic pain. Pain 128 (3), 264–271.

Linton, S.J., Melin, L., Stjernlof, K., 1985. The effects of applied relaxation and operant activity training on chronic pain. Behavioural Psychotherapy 13, 87–100.

Linton, S.J., Vlaeyen, J., Ostelo, R., 2002. The back pain beliefs of healthcare providers: are we fear-avoidant? Journal of Occupational Rehabilitation 12 (4), 223–232.

Loeser, J.D., 1982. Concepts of pain. In: Stanton-Hicks, M., Boas, R. (Eds.), Chronic low back pain. Raven Press, New York, pp. 145–148.

Macintyre, P.E., Schug, S.A., Scott, D.A., et al.; APM:SE Working group of the Australian and New Zealand College of Anaesthetists and Faculty of Pain Medicine, 2010. Acute pain management: Scientific evidence, third ed. ANZCA & FPM, Melbourne.

Main, C.J., George, S.Z., 2011. Psychologically informed practice for management of low back pain: future directions in practice and research. Physical Therapy 91 (5), 820–824.

McCarberg, B., 2010. Pain management in primary care. In: Fishman, S.M., Ballantyne, J.C., Rathmell, J.P. (Eds.), Bonica's management of pain (online), fourth ed. Lippincott Williams & Wilkins, Philadelphia.

McCracken, L.M., 1997. 'Attention' to pain in persons with chronic pain: a behavioral approach. Behavior Therapy 28, 271–284.

Melzack, R., Wall, P.D., 1965. Pain mechanisms: a new theory. Science 150 (3699), 971–978.

Melzack, R., Wall, P.D., 1982. The challenge of pain. Basic Books, New York.

Morris, D.B., 2010. Sociocultural dimensions of pain management. In Fishman, S.M., et al. (Eds.), Bonica's management of pain, fourth ed. Lippincott Williams & Wilkins, Philadelphia.

Murgatroyd, D.F., Cameron, I.D., Harris, I.A., 2011. Understanding the effect of compensation on recovery from severe motor vehicle crash injuries: a qualitative study. Injury Prevention 17, 222–227.

Newton-John, T.R.O., 2002. Solicitousness and chronic pain: a critical review. Pain Reviews 9, 7–27.

Ng, B., Dimsdale, J.E., Rollnick, J.D., 1996. The effect of ethnicity on prescriptions for patient-controlled analgesia for post-operative pain. Pain 66, 9–12.

Nicholas, M.K., 2002. Reducing disability in injured workers: the importance of collaborative management. In: Linton, S.J. (Ed.), New avenues for the prevention of chronic musculoskeletal pain and disability. Pain Research and Clinical Management. Vol. 12. Elsevier Science BV, pp. 33–46.

Nicholas, M.K., Asghari, A., Corbett, M., et al., 2012. Is adherence to pain self-management strategies associated with improved pain, depression and disability in those with disabling chronic pain? European Journal of Pain 16, 93–104.

Nicholas, M.K., Linton, S.J., Watson, P.J., et al., 2011. Early identification and management of psychological risk factors ('yellow flags') in patients with low back pain: a reappraisal. Physical Therapy 91, 737–753.

Nicholas, M.K., Linton, S.J., Watson, P.J., et al, the "Decade of the Flags" Working Group, 2011. Early identification and management of psychological risk factors ('yellow flags') in patients with low back pain: a reappraisal. Physical Therapy 91, 737–753. © 2011 American Physical Therapy Association.

Nicholas, M.K., Molloy, A.R., Brooker, C., 2006. Using opioids with persisting noncancer pain: a biopsychosocial perspective. Clinical Journal of Pain 22 (2), 137–146.

Otis, J.D., Cardella, L.A., Kerns, R.D., 2004. The influence of family and culture on pain. In: Dworkin, R.H., Breitbart, W.S. (Eds.), Psychosocial aspects of pain: a handbook for health care providers. Progress in Pain Research and Management. Vol. 27. IASP Press, Seattle, pp. 29–45.

Pengel, L.H.M., Refshauge, K.M., Maher, C.G., et al., 2007. Physiotherapist-directed exercise, advice, or both for subacute low back pain: a randomized trial. Annals of Internal Medicine 146 (11), 787–796.

Poiraudeau, S., Rannou, F., Baron, G., et al., 2006. Fear-avoidance beliefs about back pain in patients with subacute low back pain. Pain 124, 305–311.

Randich, A., Ness, T., 2010. Modulation of spinal nociceptive processing. In: Fishman, S.M., Ballantyne, J.C., Rathmell, J.P. (Eds.), Bonica's management of pain (online), fourth ed. Lippincott Williams & Wilkins, Philadelphia.

Robinson, J.P., Loeser, J.D., 2012. Effects of workers' compensation systems on recovery from disabling injuries. In: Hasenbring, M.I., Rusu, A.C., Turk, D.C. (Eds.), From acute to chronic back pain: risk factors, mechanisms, and clinical implications. Oxford University Press, New York.

Rodriguez-Raecke, R., Niemeier, A., Ihle, K., et al., 2009. Brain gray matter decrease in chronic pain is the consequence and not the cause of pain. The Journal of Neuroscience 29 (44), 13746–13750.

Ruscheweyh, R., Deppe, M., Lohmann, H., et al., 2011. Pain is associated with regional grey matter reduction in the general population. Pain 152 (4), 904–911.

Schaafsma, F., Schonstein, E., Whelan, K.M., et al., 2010. Physical conditioning programs for improving work outcomes in workers with back pain. The Cochrane Database of Systematic Reviews Issue 1.

Sharp, T.J., Harvey, A.G., 2001. Chronic pain and posttraumatic stress disorder: mutual maintenance? Clinical Psychology Review 21 (6), 857–877.

Shaw, W.S., Pransky, G.S., Main, C.J., 2012. Work-related risk factors for transition to chronic back pain and disability. In Hasenbring, M.I., Rusu, A.C., Turk, D.C. (Eds.), From acute to chronic back pain: risk factors, mechanisms, and clinical implications. Oxford University Press, New York.

Sullivan, M.D., 2001. Assessment of psychiatric disorders. In: Turk, D.C., Melzack, R. (Eds.), Handbook of Pain Assessment, second ed. Guilford Press, New York, pp. 275–291.

Sullivan, M.J.L., Martel, M.O., 2012. Processes underlying the relation between catastrophising and chronic pain: Implications for intervention. In: Hasenbring, M.I., Rusu, A.C., Turk, D.C. (Eds.), From acute to chronic back pain: risk factors, mechanisms, and clinical implications. Oxford University Press, New York.

Todd, K.H., 1996. Pain assessment and ethnicity. Annals of Emergency Medicine 27, 421–423.

Todd, K.H., Samaroo, N., Hoffman, J., 1993. Ethnicity as a risk factor for inadequate emergency department analgesia. The Journal of the American Medical Association 269, 1537–1539.

Tracey, I., Bushnell, M.C., 2009. How neuroimaging studies have challenged us to rethink: Is chronic pain a disease? The Journal of Pain 10 (11), 1113–1120.

Tsui, P., Stein, T., Sonty, N., 2010. The relationship among PTSD symptoms, chronic pain acceptance and disability. The Journal of Pain 11, S58.

Turk, D.C., Monarch, E.S., 2002. Biopsychosocial perspective on chronic pain. In Turk, D.C., Gatchel, R.J. (Eds.), Psychological approaches to pain management: a practitioner's handbook, second ed. Guilford Press, New York, pp. 3–29.

Turk, D.C., Okifuji, A., 2010. Pain terms and taxonomies of pain. In: Fishman, S.M., Ballantyne, J.C., Rathmell, J.P. (Eds.), Bonica's management of pain (online), fourth ed. Lippincott Williams & Wilkins, Philadelphia.

Turk, D.C., Swanson, K.S., Wilson, H.D., 2010. Psychological aspects of pain. In: Fishman, S.M., Ballantyne, J.C., Rathmell, J.P. (Eds.), Bonica's management of pain (online), fourth ed. Lippincott Williams & Wilkins, Philadelphia.

Van Tulder, M., Becker, A., Bekkering, T., et al., 2005. on behalf of the COST B23 Working Group on Guidelines for the Management of Acute Low Back Pain in Primary Care. Online. Available: www.backpaineurope.org 10 Sep 2012.

Vancleef, L.M.G., Peters, M.L., De Jong, P.J., 2009. Interpreting ambiguous health and bodily threat: are individual differences in pain-related vulnerability constructs associated with an on-line negative bias? Journal of Behavior Therapy and Experimental Psychiatry 40, 59–69.

Vlaeyen, J.W.S., Kole-Snijders, A.M.J., Boeren, R.G.B., et al., 1995. Fear of movement/(re) injury in chronic low back pain and its relation to behavioral performance. Pain 62 (3), 363–372.

Vlaeyen, J.W.S., Linton, S.J., 2000. Fear-avoidance and its consequences in chronic musculoskeletal pain: a state of the art. Pain 85 (3), 317–332.

Vlaeyen, J., Linton, S.J., 2006. Are we fear-avoidant? Pain 124, 240–241.

Waddell, G., Bircher, M., Finlayson, D., et al., 1984. Symptoms and signs: physical disease or illness behaviour? British Medical Journal 289, 739–741.

Wailoo, K., 2001. Dying in the city of the blues: sickle cell anemia and the politics of race and health. University of North Carolina Press, Chapel Hill.

Wall, P.D., McMahon, S.B., 1986. The relationship of perceived pain to afferent nerve impulses. Trends in Neuroscience 9 (6), 254–255.

Whalley, B., Hyland, M.E., Kirsch, I., 2008. Consistency of the placebo effect. Journal of Psychosomatic Research 64 (5), 537–541.

Williams, A.C.D.C., 1998. Depression in chronic pain: mistaken models, missed opportunities. Scandinavian Journal of Behaviour Therapy 27 (2), 61–80.

Woolf, C.J., 2011. Central sensitization: implications for the diagnosis and treatment of pain. Pain 152 (Suppl 3), S2–S15.

Chapter 13
Health promotion

PATRICIA BARKWAY

Introduction

Health promotion consists of a set of activities and programs that aim to facilitate wellness, prevent illness and foster recovery for individuals, communities and wider society. It is a relatively new endeavour in the health field and draws on 'the knowledge and methods of diverse disciplines and being informed by new evidence about health needs and their underlying determinants' (Smith et al 2006 p 340). Health promotion is not only informed by research evidence, it is also underpinned by ethical and social justice principles (Carter et al 2011). This chapter will examine the development of the health promotion movement from its emergence in the 1970s as a specific intervention to change individual health and lifestyle behaviours through to its evolution to a social determinants approach in the 21st century.

Initially, health promotion programs in the 1970s sought to improve health by encouraging individuals, through health education and counselling, to make behavioural and lifestyle changes. Through the 1980s health professionals became aware that broader social, political and economic forces also played a role in health outcomes, and health promotion activities expanded to reflect this. Consequently, contemporary health promotion has evolved to include population-focused models that utilise interdisciplinary, intersectoral and partnership approaches.

What is health promotion?

Health promotion consists of a range of strategies and activities that are designed to facilitate health and wellbeing and to prevent illness. Definitions of health promotion range from those that focus more on the individual and their personal responsibility for their health outcomes (O'Donnell 2008) to definitions that take account of the wider social, political and economic forces that influence the health of individuals, communities and wider society (World Health Organization (WHO) 1998). The editor of the *American Journal of Health Promotion*, for example, defines health promotion as:

... the science and art of helping people change their lifestyle to move towards a state of optimal health. Optimal health is the process of striving for a dynamic balance of physical, emotional, social, spiritual and intellectual health and discovering the synergies between core passions and each of those dimensions. Lifestyle change can be facilitated through a combination of efforts to enhance awareness, increase motivation, build skills and most importantly, to provide opportunities for positive health practices.

(Michael P. O'Donnell, PhD, MBA, MPH)

WHO, however, defines health promotion more broadly as:

A comprehensive social and political process [that] not only embraces actions directed at strengthening the skills and capabilities of individuals, but also action directed towards changing social, environmental and economic conditions so as to alleviate their impact on public and individual health. Health promotion is the process of enabling people to increase control over the *determinants of health* and thereby improve their *health*.

(WHO 1998 pp 1–2)

While seemingly disparate the two explanations are both valid because they offer definitions that are applicable in different contexts. O'Donnell's definition can be applied to health promotion for specific people with a specific purpose, for example, diabetes education for a newly diagnosed person with diabetes or antenatal classes for prospective parents. The WHO definition, on the other hand, applies to population approaches to health promotion in which the social determinants of health, like housing, employment and education, are addressed in order to improve the health of individuals and communities.

Health promotion, therefore, is a term that can be broadly interpreted and applied to a variety of healthcare practices and research activities that range from promoting wellbeing and preventing illness through to rehabilitation and recovery from illness. Also in this chapter health promotion will be presented as distinct from illness prevention. Health promotion is defined here as being concerned with fostering *protective* factors for health, while illness prevention is concerned with identifying, reducing and responding to the *risk* factors for illness.

PROTECTIVE AND RISK FACTORS

Rickwood (2006), in distinguishing protective and risk factors for mental health and illness, states that protective factors reduce the likelihood of a mental disorder developing by reducing the *exposure* to risk, and by reducing the *effect* of risk factors for people exposed to risk. Protective factors also foster resilience in the face of adversity and moderate against the effects of stress. Risk factors, however, increase the likelihood that a mental disorder will develop, exacerbate the burden of an existing disorder and can indicate a person's vulnerability. Both protective and risk factors comprise individual characteristics and social influences including biological, behavioural, sociocultural and demographic conditions. Individual attributes include genetics, disposition and intelligence, while external drivers comprise the social determinants of health related to social, economic, political and environmental factors including the availability of opportunities in life and access to health services (Provencher & Keyes 2011).

Protective factors assist people to maintain physical, emotional and social wellbeing, and to cope with life experiences including adversity. They can provide a buffer against stress as well as being a set of resources to draw upon to deal with stress. Factors that have been identified as protective for healthy development in children include, for example: easy temperament, family harmony, positive social networks (e.g. peers, teachers, neighbours); access to positive opportunities (e.g. education); and religious faith (Commonwealth of Australia 2009).

Risk factors increase vulnerability to illness and injury and work against recovery from the illness or injury. Developmental risk factors in children have been identified as: 'low birth weight, prematurity, birth injury; delayed development; poverty; low parental education; family conflict; family breakdown; parental alcoholism; and parental mental illness' (Commonwealth of Australia 2009).

It cannot be assumed, though, that identifying protective and risk factors can lead to accurately predicting who will or will not be healthy. Demographic data, epidemiological data and research findings merely indicate levels of risk and vulnerability in certain populations, or the increased likelihood of some people for particular illnesses – and their interaction is complex. The significant contribution made by health promotion research findings is that it provides evidence for health professionals and policymakers about opportunities for intervention to promote health and wellbeing, and to prevent illness for individuals and populations.

Classroom activity

1. In small groups identify risk and protective factors for the following health issues:
   » HIV/AIDS
   » depression
   » cardiovascular disease
   » unplanned parenthood
   » obesity.
2. If funding were available for a health promotion initiative to address **one** of these issues which one would you pick? And why?
3. Pair up with another student who selected a different issue to you and explain the reasons for your choice to each other.
4. In small groups identify and discuss the challenges faced by health planners when allocating funding for health promotion initiatives.

History of health promotion

Health promotion commenced in the 1970s following the identification of lifestyle as being a major contributor to health and illness (Baum 2008) and the development of psychological models for understanding and changing health behaviours. The health belief model (see also Ch 7) was especially influential in early health promotion campaigns and was viewed as the way forward in changing unhealthy lifestyle practices, particularly in relation to diet, physical activity, tobacco smoking and alcohol consumption. Health promotion initiatives, at this time, mainly consisted of: health education and counselling of individuals regarding lifestyle; illness prevention strategies like mass vaccination and screening initiatives; and lifestyle education programs such as stress management.

PSYCHOLOGY AND HEALTH PROMOTION

Contributions to the field of health promotion by the discipline of psychology have been significant since the 1970s when psychological theories like the health belief model, transtheoretical model and health action process approach were first used in health education and counselling to bring about targeted individual behaviour and lifestyle changes. In later years, with the rise in the prevalence and burden of chronic illnesses in Western countries, the focus of health promotion efforts shifted from reducing mortality to reducing morbidity or the burden of disease (Taylor 2012). Additionally, psychological research that had initially focused on identifying risk factors shifted to understanding and facilitating 'protective' factors for health like resilience (Garmezy 1991).

In contemporary health promotion, psychological theory contributes to an interdisciplinary approach across the range of activities at all levels of intervention from that of the individual to that of the wider population. Motivational interviewing, for example, is a psychologically based counselling intervention aimed at changing unhealthy behaviours. It utilises a client-centred, semi-directed approach and focuses on reasons for and against the change to motivate the person to change to a healthier lifestyle (see also Ch 7). In larger scale health promotion interventions behavioural and cognitive principles that are derived from psychological theory are incorporated in mass media health education campaigns, particularly those targeting lifestyle.

PRIMARY HEALTH CARE MOVEMENT AND HEALTH PROMOTION

During the 1980s it became apparent that health education and counselling approaches, on their own, were insufficient to bring about the required changes in many instances because people's behaviour is also shaped by the social, political and economic environments in which they live (Braveman et al 2011, Marmot et al 2008). It was at this time that WHO (1986) released its seminal document, the *Ottawa Charter for Health Promotion* (see Ch 4), which subsequently became the cornerstone of the health promotion movement. The Charter shifted the emphasis of health promotion from the individual and called on governments and health services to address the wider social, political and economic drivers of health. As a consequence health promotion became located in, and was central to, the emerging primary health care movement.

The shift from an individual to a societal and population focus precipitated a change in perceptions of responsibility for health away from the individual to wider society and the environments in which people live. While both individual and population-focused approaches have a role to play in contemporary health promotion practice, a population approach that addresses the social determinants of health offers greater opportunity to influence health outcomes for a greater number of people. Nevertheless, individual approaches do continue to play a role in assisting people to engage in healthy lifestyle practices and can facilitate the utilisation of strategies of the Ottawa Charter in healthcare practice, for example, the development of personal skills through health education and counselling. Despite originating in the 1980s the Ottawa Charter remains relevant in the 21st century as a framework for health promotion, as evidenced by its frequent citing in the literature and its widespread utilisation in healthcare practice and programs (McQueen 2008).

Levels of intervention

Theories and models for health promotion offer opportunities for intervention at three levels, namely, the level of the individual, the community and at a population level. These are also referred to as downstream (individual), midstream (community) and upstream (population) levels.

The upstream/midstream/downstream distinction is best illustrated by the allegory popularised by John McKinlay, a medical sociologist in the 1970s. McKinlay's tale tells of a physician who was standing by a swiftly flowing river when a drowning man floated past. The physician jumped in the water and rescued the man. However, no sooner had the physician rescued the man when another drowning person came by. Repeatedly, the physician rescued and resuscitated drowning people as they floated past. In fact the physician was so busy rescuing the drowning people that he did not have time to go upstream to see who was pushing them in (McKinlay 1974). This frequently repeated scenario is now an enduring primary health care metaphor that illustrates that while downstream interventions are effective in responding to a health problem they do nothing to address the actual upstream cause of the problem.

The medical model operates primarily as a downstream approach in which people with health problems seek assistance from their general practitioner (GP) or the healthcare system. An exception is mass immunisation programs, which are a biomedical intervention with an illness prevention focus. Downstream approaches also occur mainly at the individual level. Downstream approaches are generally limited to disease-specific interventions such as dietary advice to lower cholesterol. Midstream interventions operate at a local community level and utilise education and intervention strategies to prevent illness. Upstream interventions operate at a societal level whereby social policy and planning is utilised to address the social determinants of health and to re-dress social inequities. Psychosocial models, including primary health care, operate at all three levels. Table 13.1 summarises intervention levels in health promotion and Table 13.2 cites examples of upstream, midstream and downstream approaches to addressing poor nutrition to promote heart health as outlined by Raine (2010).

Classroom activity

In small groups identify upstream, midstream and downstream interventions for the following health issues:

- tobacco smoking
- cancer
- type 2 diabetes mellitus
- not having a child immunised
- unsuitable housing
- polluted waterways.

Primary, secondary and tertiary interventions

The terms primary, secondary and tertiary prevention are used to distinguish between levels of intervention that foster wellness, treat illness and restore function following illness (recovery) (McMurray 2011). According to Kaplan (2000) primary prevention is distinct from healthcare service delivery, which is the provision of treatment for health problems. At each level of intervention the goal of health promotion is to ensure that public policy is healthy, environments are supportive of health, community action is strengthened, personal skills are developed and that health services are reoriented. In other words, that the strategies for health promotion as articulated in the Ottawa Charter (WHO 1986) are implemented.

Table 13.1

LEVELS OF INTERVENTION

Health promotion: intervention levels

Upstream	Midstream		Downstream	
Primary	**Primary**		**Secondary**	**Tertiary**
Services/programs for: • health • social • welfare • environment	Services/programs to: • prevent illness • eradicate health risks in at-risk groups	Services/programs to: • prevent illness • eradicate health risks for at-risk individuals	Services/programs for illness: • diagnosis • treatment • management	Services/programs for: • recovery • rehabilitation • management
Enduring social, political change and policy about: • health • social • welfare • environment				
Outcomes	**Outcomes**		**Outcomes**	
Healthy society and members Individual behaviour change Sustainable environments for health Health promotion	Healthy community and individuals Individual behaviour change Environmental change Illness prevention		Healthy individuals Individual behaviour change Illness management Recovery	

Table 13.2		
ADDRESSING POOR NUTRITION TO PROMOTE HEART HEALTH		
Upstream	Midstream	Downstream
Policy change to improve nutritional value of food (similar to tobacco legislation)	Workplace weight-reduction programs and education	Dietary education to assist individuals to eat healthy food
Tax unhealthy foods	Improve access to healthy foods by offering healthy options in workplaces and school canteens	Shopping advice regarding choosing healthy food

PRIMARY PREVENTION

Primary prevention aims to foster wellbeing and prevent the occurrence of illness. It includes both midstream and upstream strategies. Midstream strategies focus on 'at-risk individuals' and 'at-risk groups', with the goal of changing the individual's risky behaviour, like ceasing tobacco smoking or reducing risk in the community (by improving access to healthcare services for people who live in regional areas, for example). Further examples of population-focused primary prevention include mass vaccination programs, legislation to protect vulnerable members of the society such as anti-discrimination laws, social inclusion policy and economic policies to fund health screening and public housing.

SECONDARY PREVENTION

Secondary prevention refers to interventions that are, in the main, delivered downstream when symptoms, injury or illness are identified and treated as early as possible to restore health. It includes the range of health services that the general public will be most familiar with, for example, attending an emergency department when injured or visiting a GP when symptoms are present.

In addition to treating illness and health problems a further goal of secondary prevention is early intervention. Hence, some interventions will occur midstream, such as health screening like mammograms, or hearing tests for infants. In this instance the purpose of early intervention is to identify and address health issues before they become a problem or to minimise the impact of an illness or disability on the individual. An example of the effectiveness of early intervention was demonstrated by Hakama et al (2008) whose research found that the incidence and mortality rates of cervical cancer was significantly reduced through population screening by undertaking cytological smears.

TERTIARY PREVENTION

Tertiary prevention is also a downstream approach and is implemented when the disease cannot be cured or the illness process is prolonged. Its aim is to assist individuals (and their family and carers) to cope with a change in their health status, to limit disability from the health problem and to promote health and quality of life (recovery). Interventions include: treatment programs for chronic illnesses like emphysema and irritable bowel syndrome; rehabilitation and recovery programs for conditions like mental illness, post-coronary heart disease and post-stroke; and palliative care for terminal illnesses like cancer and dementia.

Recovery, which is a goal of tertiary prevention, is a concept that evolved as part of the reform of mental health services that has occurred in Western countries over recent decades. A recovery approach has subsequently become an integral component of mental health clinical practice (Slade 2009). Recovery for the client refers to living well with a chronic illness or disability. It may include learning about the condition and what triggers episodes, and making lifestyle changes. For health professionals it means not only working with clients to manage the symptoms of care problems, but also to work in collaboration with clients to manage a life lived well despite illness or disability. The approach acknowledges that lifestyle and the social context of people's lives can positively or negatively influence the course of the ongoing illness. Hence, a recovery approach encompasses more than merely treating or managing the symptoms of the illness. It also includes recognition of and attention to social, economic and political aspects of people's lives. In a recovery-focused model of care health professionals and clients work together in partnership to maximise the quality of life for the person living with the ongoing illness (see also Ch 9).

While, to date, the recovery model has mainly focused on minimising the disability from mental illness and to enable people with mental illness to live a fulfilling life despite their condition, the approach does have wider applicability for people who live with other chronic illnesses and for those health professionals who work with people living with a chronic illness or disability. An example of a recovery-focused tertiary intervention that has a broad application is the 'Flinders Program™' of chronic disease self-management developed by health professionals and researchers at Flinders University, Adelaide. The model is underpinned by cognitive behavioural therapy (CBT) principles. It utilises a partnership approach in which health professionals and clients collaborate on problem identification, goal setting and developing an individualised care plan. The model has proved to be effective in facilitating self-management among people with chronic health conditions and improves health-related behaviour and health outcomes (Harvey et al 2008).

In summary, health promotion can be implemented at primary, secondary or tertiary levels to target individual, community or population health needs. Secondary and tertiary approaches are effective in diagnosing, treating and managing illness. However, as McKinlay's (1974) primary health care metaphor tells us, responding to health problems with a treatment response will deal with the symptoms but not necessarily the cause of the health problem. Therefore, in order to address the cause of a health problem, it is evident that primary intervention, alongside treatment and recovery models, is required. See Table 13.2, which summarises the health promotion levels of intervention.

Classroom activity

Programs and activities to promote mental health and prevent mental illness are less prolific than health promotion initiatives in the physical health arena. One of the explanations given for this is that the stigma attached to mental illness marginalises the field making it a less popular area in which to work as a health professional or in which to conduct research.

In small groups identify and discuss health promotion initiatives that could address the stigma of mental illness.

Evidence for health promotion

There is now a growing and convincing body of evidence that shows that the health of individuals, communities and populations are influenced by a broad range of factors, many of which are outside the health sector. Research findings also demonstrate that social and economic factors have more influence on health outcomes than lifestyle or healthcare (Keleher & MacDougall 2011, WHO 2008). The challenge though is to undertake research that demonstrates that health promotion interventions make a difference to the health of individuals and communities. Difficulties in delivering evidence include the multifactorial nature of many health problems and the length of time (often decades) that elapses before outcomes are seen. Nevertheless, evidence is available to support the effectiveness of specific health promotion interventions for some health issues. One of these specific interventions – reduction of tobacco smoking – will now be examined.

EVIDENCE FOR HEALTH PROMOTION: TOBACCO SMOKING

According to the Australian Institute of Health and Welfare (AIHW) tobacco smoking is 'the single most preventable cause of ill health and death in Australia' (AIHW 2012 p 221). It is responsible for more admissions to hospital and deaths than illicit drug use and alcohol combined, and accounts for 9.6% of the disease burden in men and 5.8% in women (7.8% overall). Illnesses for which smoking is a major risk factor include coronary heart disease, peripheral vascular disease, stroke and cancer (AIHW 2010 pp 67, 86).

Since the 1980s public health programs with a whole-of-population focus have targeted tobacco smoking cessation and successfully reduced smoking rates in developed countries. In Australia the daily smoking rate, which is now among the lowest for OECD countries, dropped from one in three adults in 1985 to less than one in five in 2010 and the level continues to fall (AIHW 2012). Health promotion initiatives since the 1980s have successfully reduced smoking from 33% in 1985 for men to 18% in 2010, and from 26% in 1985 for women to 15% in 2010 (see Fig 13.1).

This outcome has been achieved by not just one strategy but by several interventions interacting together to achieve the reduction in the percentage of the population who smoke tobacco. Health promotion strategies to reduce tobacco smoking have included a range of activities such as: increased taxation; restriction of advertising; health education in schools; social marketing in the mass media that

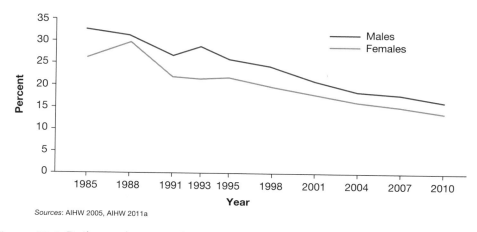

Figure 13.1 Daily smokers aged 14 years and over, 1985–2010

Source: Australian Institute of Health and Welfare. Australia's health 2012, Cat. no. AUS 156 p. 223

utilises both education and fear appeal principles (graphic images on tobacco products); legislation (the banning of smoking in public places); and access to QUIT programs and other supports for smokers who wish to give it up. In summary, several Ottawa Charter strategies have been used concurrently to reduce smoking.

Health promotion approaches

Health promotion is delivered through interdisciplinary and intersectoral activities that are influenced and driven by the underlying values, theories and research findings of the relevant discipline. Interventions, therefore, vary enormously depending on the disciplinary approach and whether the interventions target individuals, communities or whole populations. Biomedical approaches, for example, identify causative factors within the individual and their environment to prevent illness (e.g. provision of clean water supply and immunisation) or early identification and intervention (health screening). Psychological theories of behaviour change, as discussed in Chapter 7, are utilised in health education and counselling approaches to assist people to engage in behaviours that contribute to a healthy lifestyle. A social determinants approach incorporates primary health care values and practices, is underpinned by social justice principles and aims to reduce health inequities and thereby improve the health of a population and its members. Each lends itself to different approaches to health promotion, which will now be examined. These are health education, social determinants/health inequities, settings for health promotion and population-focused approaches.

HEALTH EDUCATION

Health education is a health promotion strategy that generally refers to a process of enabling people to make behaviour and lifestyle changes (Baum 2008). It can be delivered in a one-on-one situation (such as health counselling) in the form of dietary advice from a nutritionist, in a group setting, for example, parenting classes, or through population-focused interventions such as social marketing media campaigns like television media advertisements to discourage drink driving or gambling. In the main these interventions utilise cognitive and behavioural strategies derived from psychological theory.

While health education is a common approach to health promotion it is also one of the most problematic because educating people about what they should do does not address the social and economic environments in which they live and that shape their behaviour (Keleher & MacDougall 2011). This critique applies particularly to early health education approaches that were delivered in the traditional biomedical model. This model was concerned with compliance and positioned the client in a dependent role with the health professional *expert*. Subsequent client-centred models, like the Flinders Program™ for chronic condition self-management, engage the client in a partnership regarding decision making about management of the health issue.

Health education can also be undertaken by adopting a population approach that targets whole communities through strategies such as social marketing. This approach uses marketing principles and theory from the disciplines of psychology, sociology and communications to identify solutions to social and health problems, and to encourage individuals and populations to lead healthy lifestyles. Successful social marketing campaigns have been undertaken, for example, to promote wearing seatbelts in cars, bicycle helmets while cycling and using sun protection. Campaigns are generally carried out through the media, which is the primary source of health information for most Australians (Janda et al 2007).

HEALTH EDUCATION: A POPULATION APPROACH

Australia has the highest rate of skin cancer in the world, mostly caused by over exposure to ultraviolet (UV) radiation. Around 380,000 people are treated for skin cancer and 1600 people die from the disease every year (SunSmart Victoria 2012). In 1981, in response to this alarming statistic, Australia introduced a social marketing health campaign titled 'Slip-Slop-Slap', which was led by a seagull named Sid. Australians were encouraged to 'slip on a shirt, slop on sunscreen and slap on a hat' before venturing outdoors to prevent sunburn and skin cancer. The campaign included print and television media advertisements, a jingle, education resources for school teachers and visits by the mascot, Sid Seagull, to schools and public events. A similar campaign was undertaken in New Zealand where the mascot was a lobster (SunSmart NZ 2012). In subsequent years seeking shade and wearing sunglasses were added to the health message and people are now encouraged to 'slip, slop, slap, seek (shade) and slide (on sunglasses)'.

Following this public health campaign the incidence of basal cell carcinoma (BCC) and squamous cell carcinoma (SCC), the most common forms of skin cancer, were reduced. However, the incidence of melanoma, which is the most fatal form of skin cancer, was not affected. This is most likely because the use of sunscreen does not prevent the development of melanoma, whereas sunscreen prevents BCCs and SCCs by preventing sunburn (Planta 2011). It is therefore a false confidence for a person to believe that applying sunscreen will provide protection against all forms of skin cancer.

Furthermore, despite the overall decrease in skin cancer rates, another health issue has arisen as a consequence of reduced sun exposure. Vitamin D deficiency, which predisposes people to increased risk of bone fractures, particularly in later life, has been observed in some sections of the population, especially the elderly, people with dark skin, and people who cover their body in clothing for religious or cultural reasons (Hedges & Scriven 2008, Henry et al 2007). Vitamin D deficiency is linked to insufficient sun exposure, and sunlight is the major source of vitamin D for Australians and New Zealanders. It seems that the prevention of one health problem may predispose a person to another.

These findings highlight the importance of evaluating health promotion interventions to ascertain that the intervention has the required outcome, and that other unwanted effects do not occur. Even interventions that have intuitive appeal and can demonstrate positive health outcomes (e.g. the SunSmart campaign) may not be effective for all people or all forms of skin cancer. And for some population groups, like the elderly, the intervention may have other unwanted side effects (e.g. reducing uptake of vitamin D).

Finally, while psychological behaviour change models and psychosocial principles are used in health education approaches, the social determinants of health as identified by WHO (2008) are not necessarily addressed in behaviour change programs and these may be more influential in determining lifestyle choices, as was found in the Whitehall study (see Ch 10) (Marmot et al 1997, WHO 2008). Finally, considering the inconclusive results from health education initiatives to promote health, Keleher suggests that in order for health education to be effective it must move beyond the advice giving – knowledge transfer – symptom-control model to one of empowerment (Keleher & MacDougall 2011) that is inherent in a social determinants approach.

Classroom activity

1. In small groups make a list of common health education messages such as quit smoking, and slip, slop, slap, seek, slide.
2. Discuss in pairs:
   » What impact do such messages have on you?
   » Have you ever changed a health behaviour in response to a health education message?
3. In small groups discuss whether you think such messages influence people in general. Why or why not?
4. What are some of the underlying assumptions of health education?
5. In what circumstances might health education have a negative impact?

SOCIAL DETERMINANTS/HEALTH INEQUITIES APPROACH

Social determinants refer to the 'wide range of social (including economic and political) conditions that are strong influences on health, such as wealth and educational attainment of the family into which one is born, neighbourhood social conditions, and the social policies which determine these conditions' (Schrecker et al 2010 p 33). A social determinants approach to health promotion addresses health inequities and is, therefore, underpinned by the principles and values of social justice, equity and respect for the rights of others. There is recognition that drivers outside the health arena influence health outcomes and a commitment to working in partnership with individuals and communities. In this approach health – not medicine – is the focus (Braveman et al 2011). The WHO Commission on the Social Determinants of Health report (WHO 2008) advocates strongly for a social justice approach to health that includes recognising and addressing health inequities.

Given the range of social determinants that impact on health, it is evident that at a government level the health portfolio alone cannot sufficiently redress these. This was reinforced in the recommendations made to the South Australian Government by the 2010 South Australian Thinker in Residence, Ilona Kickbusch, which stated that a whole-of-government approach was required including input from the portfolios of justice, transport, education, employment, housing and welfare (Kickbusch & Buckett 2010a, 2010b). In conclusion, health promotion that utilises a social determinants approach to address health inequities 'is the process of enabling people to increase control over their health, resulting from the synergy of healthy policy in all sectors of society and health education for all' (Mittelmark et al 2008 p 225).

HEALTH INEQUITIES

Health is essential to wellbeing and quality of life, therefore, health inequities further disadvantage groups of people who are already socially disadvantaged due to poverty, gender or being a member of a disenfranchised racial, ethnic or religious group. Furthermore, equity is a social justice principle and closely related to human rights (Braveman 2010). The Victorian Health Promotion Foundation (2011) defines health inequity as the 'unfair and avoidable differences in health status between different populations of people that are 'evident through a range of measures, including illness and death rates, and self-reported health status'. Three dimensions of inequality are identified by the foundation, all of which need to be addressed to overcome health inequalities. They are:

1. *Inequality of access* – as a result of barriers to support services required for health and wellbeing. This can result from costs of the service, lack of transport to the service, services that are inaccessible for people with special needs and services that are culturally inappropriate for some population groups.

2. *Inequality of opportunity* – as a result of social, geographic or economic resources for health including education, employment and suitable housing.

3. *Inequality of impacts and outcomes* – differences in health outcomes between groups and populations such as mortality and morbidity rates or self-reported health rates (Victorian Health Promotion Foundation 2011).

Redressing health inequities for Indigenous people

Indigenous Australians and New Zealand Māori experience poorer health outcomes than the non-Indigenous people of these two countries. In addition to health inequities, many Indigenous people also experience disadvantage regarding education, employment status, economic status, housing and lack of appropriate environmental infrastructure (Baum 2008). Therefore, when planning and implementing health promotion with Indigenous people it is essential that social justice and human rights be incorporated because social conditions, health equity and human rights are interrelated (Braveman 2010).

VicHealth, in collaboration with Aboriginal Affairs Victoria, conducts an Indigenous leadership health promotion program to support the development of young Indigenous leaders in order to promote the emotional and spiritual wellbeing of Indigenous communities in Victoria. The goal of the program is to build leadership potential among young people and to enable young Indigenous people to develop the skills required to combat experiences of discrimination, and to enable positive futures for the participants. The program is conducted in metropolitan and rural areas across Victoria and provides a range of personal development projects based in leadership training, mentoring by senior community members, support and providing resources to develop leadership skills and access to participation in a range of community and professional activities (VicHealth 2005).

In New Zealand health promotion practice takes account of the 1840 *Treaty of Waitangi*, which is the country's founding contract between Māori and the Crown and the 1986 *Ottawa Charter for Health Promotion*. Māori health is understood as a holistic concept in which health is recognised as being dependent on a balance of factors that influence wellbeing. These contributing factors include spiritual (wairua), mental (hinengaro), physical (tinana), language (te reo rangatira) and family (whanau), which interact to enable wellbeing, as does the environment (te ao turoa). Therefore, in understanding Māori health, it is evident that the social, economic and cultural position of Māori must be taken into account, and that for Māori, health promotion means taking control of their own health to determine their own wellbeing (Health Promotion Forum of New Zealand 2012).

SETTINGS FOR HEALTH PROMOTION

A settings approach to health promotion was advocated in the Jakarta Declaration as the 'organisational base of the infrastructure required for health promotion' (WHO 1997). A settings approach to health promotion facilitates the nurturing of human and social capital. It involves providing health promotion in the settings of people's lives, such as schools, families, workplaces, ethnic communities and regional localities – thereby taking health services to the people, and not expecting people to be entirely responsible for their health outcomes. It broadens the population approach to include organisations and systems (McMurray 2011).

Health promotion settings: schools

In 1995 WHO established the Global School Health initiative to promote and support the health and wellbeing of children. The Health Promoting Schools program strives to develop the capacity of schools as a healthy setting for living, learning and working, with a focus on: caring for oneself and others; making healthy decisions and taking control over life's circumstances; creating conditions that are conducive to health (through policies, services, physical/social conditions); building capacities for peace, shelter, education, food, income, a stable ecosystem, equity, social justice and sustainable development; preventing leading causes of death, disease and disability (e.g. helminths (worms), tobacco use, HIV/AIDS/STDs, sedentary lifestyle, drugs and alcohol, violence/injuries and unhealthy nutrition); and influencing health-related behaviours (e.g. knowledge, beliefs, skills, attitudes, values and support) (WHO

2012b). Health promoting schools foster happy, healthy, supportive and caring environments for students, staff and families (Ministry of Health New Zealand n.d.).

The Walking School Bus is an example of a health promotion initiative that is conducted in the school setting and aims to foster independent mobility in children. It comprises a group of children who walk to and from school under the supervision of one or more adults on a set route each day. Children 'board' the 'bus' at designated stops on the route. Additional outcomes include increased physical activity, knowledge of road safety, familiarity with the local area and social interaction (Commonwealth of Australia 2005).

Health promotion settings: workplace

The Jakarta Declaration identified health promotion as an investment and the workplace as a potential setting in which it could be implemented (WHO 1997). Implementing health promotion not only offers advantages to workers in the form of improved health and wellbeing, but employers also gain by reduced absenteeism and fewer worksite accidents and workers' compensation claims.

The *Ottawa Charter for Health Promotion* states that work has 'a significant impact on health' and can be 'a source of health for people' because 'the way society organizes work should help create a healthy society' (WHO 1986 p 2). Yet, despite this social framework for action provided by the charter, workplace health promotion has concentrated more on programs that aim to bring about individual behaviour change for healthy lifestyles, or the screening of 'at risk' populations, that is, illness prevention, rather than promoting health and wellbeing (Noblet & Rodwell 2010, Talbot & Verrinder 2009). This is evident in the mental health field when programs that claim to promote mental health are designed with the aim of enhancing individual skills and attitudes, or developing coping strategies, and rarely utilise health promotion methods of participation, empowerment and structural change.

Also, despite the introduction of legislation and workplace policies, structural changes have been unsuccessful in bringing about environmental modification, which fosters mental wellbeing. Bullying continues to be endemic in many work settings and research demonstrates that it affects the physical and psychological health of victims, and negatively affects their work performance (Johnson 2009). Nevertheless, while mental health promotion is appealing, there are challenges to implementing it in the workplace. These include difficulties of demonstrating the efficacy of interventions and competition for the health dollar. Additionally, entrenched institutional structures may work against change when institutions have an investment in maintaining the status quo or fear the uncertainty of change.

POPULATION HEALTH PROMOTION APPROACHES

Population refers to a group of people who are bound by a common theme. This may be ethnicity, culture, geographic location, workplace or demographic characteristics like age, gender or socioeconomic status. Disparities in health exist between different populations (WHO 2008), therefore the goal of a population approach to health promotion is to reduce difference in health status and to reduce inequities and improve the health of the whole population. This approach developed following the growing awareness that factors outside an individual's control, and drivers outside the health arena, influence health outcomes. Consequently, models and approaches to health promotion shifted from being individual to population-focused.

According to Whitehead (2007) population-wide approaches target the whole of the population through: interventions that target individual behaviour (e.g. through health information social marketing campaigns); structural mechanisms and macroeconomic policies (e.g. the provision of public housing or through tobacco taxation); or interventions that address the causes of ill health (e.g. by providing free education to all citizens). Population approaches aim to improve the health of members of the group by facilitating protective factors and reducing risk factors by addressing health inequities.

Populations in Victoria, Australia, for example, that have been identified as experiencing the greatest health inequities and therefore the greatest need for intervention, include: Indigenous people; newly arrived migrants and refugees; people with disabilities; people from low socioeconomic backgrounds; and children and young people living in low socioeconomic areas (Victorian Health Promotion Foundation 2008 p 6).

Research focus

Toft, U., Kristoffersen, L., Ladelund, S., et al, 2008. The impact of a population-based multi-factorial lifestyle intervention on changes in long-term dietary habits: the Inter99 study. Preventive Medicine 47, 378–383.

ABSTRACT

Objective

To evaluate the effectiveness of a population-based multifactorial lifestyle intervention on long-term changes in dietary habits compared with a non-intervention control group.

Methods

The study was a randomised controlled lifestyle intervention study, Inter99 (1999–2006), in Copenhagen, Denmark, using a high-risk strategy. Participants in the intervention group (n = 6091) had at baseline a health examination and a face-to-face lifestyle counselling session. People at high risk of ischaemic heart disease were repeatedly offered both individual and group-based counselling. The control group (n = 3324) was followed by questionnaires. Dietary habits were measured by a validated 48-item food frequency questionnaire and changes were analysed by multilevel analyses.

Results

At the five-year follow-up the intervention group had significantly increased their intake of vegetables compared with the control group (men: net change: 23 g/week; p = 0.04; women: net change: 27 g/week; p = 0.005) and decreased the intake of highly saturated fats used on

Cont... ▶

bread and for cooking (men: OR = 0.59 (0.41–0.86); women: OR = 0.42 (0.30–0.59)). Significant effects on fruit and fish intake were found at the three-year follow-up but the effect attenuated at the five-year follow-up.

Conclusion

A population-based multifactorial lifestyle intervention promoted significantly more beneficial long-term dietary changes compared with the control group, especially improving the intake of vegetables and saturated fat.

Critical thinking

Identify other health problems that population-focused health promotion could be applied to.

Population approach: healthy cities

Healthy Cities is a global movement that originated out of the WHO European office, with the aim of implementing the Ottawa Charter at a city level. There are now Healthy Cities in the six WHO regions, namely, Africa, East Mediterranean, Europe, the Americas, South East Asia and the Western Pacific. The movement encourages local governments to engage in health development through political commitment, institutional change, capacity building, partnership-based planning and innovative projects. Projects strive to be broad-based, intersectoral, ecological and political, are innovative and encourage community participation.

Through its Healthy Cities Project WHO identified 10 key social and political areas that influence health, namely, the social gradient, unemployment, stress, social support, early life, addiction, social exclusion, food, transport and work. The organisation's publication of *Social Determinants of Health: the solid facts* is intended 'to ensure that policy – at all levels in government, public and private institutions, workplaces and the community – takes proper account of recent evidence suggesting a wider responsibility for creating healthy societies' (Wilkinson & Marmot 2006).

Healthy Cities promotes an approach to policy and planning that is comprehensive and systematic and emphasises the importance of addressing health inequalities and urban poverty (the needs of vulnerable groups). Its approach encourages participatory governance and takes account of the social, economic and environmental determinants of health. Healthy Cities also strives to put health issues on the agenda regarding economic policy and urban development efforts such as establishing dedicated bikeways to improve safety for cyclists and to facilitate community members' engagement in physical activity. Healthy Cities is now in its fourth phase and participating cities are currently working on three core themes: healthy ageing, healthy urban planning and health impact assessment. In addition, all participating cities focus on the topic of physical activity/active living (WHO 2012a).

Classroom activity

Prior to class, access and read the journal article: Swinburn B 2009 Obesity prevention in children and adolescents. Child and Adolescent Psychiatric Clinics of North America Vol 8 No 1, pp 209–223.

In small groups in the tutorial discuss childhood obesity.

1. Identify responsibilities of the following regarding this health issue:
    » child
    » parents, family and caregivers
    » schooling and teachers
    » governments
    » national
    » local
    » private sector
    » wider society.
2. Identify and discuss health promotion initiatives that could address childhood and adolescent obesity.
3. Identify challenges to health promotion which addresses childhood and adolescent obesity.

Challenges of a health promotion approach

Despite health promotion having intuitive appeal to policymakers, health professionals and laypeople (as evidenced by colloquial sayings like 'prevention is better than cure'), and research findings that demonstrate health promotion effectiveness, there remain challenges regarding the implementation and effectiveness of health-promoting initiatives. These include blaming individuals for lifestyle and health outcomes and issues in translating research findings into healthcare practice.

Strategies that target individuals' health behaviour, such as health education and social marketing, have the potential to lead to 'victim blaming' should the person not alter their behaviour following the intervention. Attributing responsibility for the health problem solely to the individual overlooks the social and external forces that also contribute to the continuation of the behaviour and stigmatises the individual whose health problems are deemed to be their own fault. Furthermore, making the individual responsible for their own health may absolve the state and health services of responsibility in addressing the health issue or the social and political factors that contribute to it.

Population approaches, too, can be problematic. The lead time for demonstrating the effectiveness of population-focused interventions is long – often decades (Jirowong & Liamputtong 2009, McQueen 2008). Given that decisions regarding health funding allocation are made in a political environment in which the term of the governing political party that allocate the funding is only three to five years, funding decisions may consequently be made that favour initiatives that deliver shorter term outcomes and these tend to be treatment rather than prevention- or promotion-focused.

A further issue with the long lead time to demonstrate effectiveness is the range and complexity of intervening factors that may contribute to the health outcome. The breadth of contributing factors poses a challenge in deciding which factors should be addressed and which factors will or will not receive funding. Moreover, the allocation of funding may be made on the magnitude of community demand, which may only be the most vocal need rather than the most pressing one.

CASE STUDY: HEALTH FUNDING

'Southwood' is a suburb located on the outskirts of a major city. For several years a community group has lobbied the health minister seeking an intensive care unit (ICU) at the local hospital, despite such facilities being available at a university teaching hospital approximately 15 kilometres away. Meanwhile, in the same community, there is a shortage of supported accommodation for people with schizophrenia. The minister is aware of this housing shortage and of a report that identifies suitable housing as an important component for recovery following a psychotic illness; however, no formal requests have been received at the electoral office to fund supported accommodation for people with mental illness.

Critical thinking

- Imagine funding was available to fund only one of these initiatives. Which initiative would you choose, and why?
- What are the social justice implications for the initiative you did not select for funding?
- If there was to be an election in six months which initiative do you think the minister would select and why?
- What are the social justice implications for the initiative you predicted that the minister would not select?

Conclusion

Health and health outcomes are influenced by a range of factors that are located both within the person and within the contexts and environments in which people live. In this chapter health promotion was presented as an interdisciplinary field of endeavour that seeks to influence health outcomes by facilitating wellbeing, preventing illness and fostering recovery for individuals and communities, and to thereby enable people to take control of and to improve their health and quality of life. Values that underpin a social determinants approach to health promotion, such as social justice and health equity, were also identified, as were strategies for primary, secondary and tertiary intervention.

The contribution made by psychology and other disciplines was highlighted and the effectiveness of interdisciplinary and intersectoral interventions was emphasised. Finally, contemporary health promotion was located within a social justice and equity framework that sees 'health for all', as articulated in the *Ottawa Charter for Health Promotion* (WHO 1986), as a basic human right.

REMEMBER

- Health promotion is the process of enabling people to take control of and improve their health.
- The purpose of health promotion is to facilitate wellbeing and improve quality of life.
- Health promotion originated from psychological models of behaviour change and health education in the latter half of the 20th century.
- Contemporary health promotion has shifted from an exclusively individual focus to also address social determinants of health and a focus on populations.
- Effective health promotion requires input from within and outside the health sector.

Further resources

Australian Institute of Health and Welfare, 2012. Australia's health 2012. AIHW, Canberra.

Keleher, H., MacDougall, C., 2011. Understanding health, fourth ed. Oxford University Press, Melbourne.

McMurray, A., 2011. Community health and wellness: a socio-ecological approach, fourth ed. Mosby, Sydney.

Talbot, L., Verrinder, A., 2009. Promoting health: the primary health care approach, fourth ed. Elsevier, Sydney.

World Health Organization (WHO), 2008. Closing the gap in a generation: health equity through action on the social determinants of health. WHO Commission on Social Determinants of Health, Geneva.

Weblinks

Australian Health Promotion Association
www.healthpromotion.org.au

The Australian Health Promotion Association's aim is to provide knowledge, resources and perspectives to improve health promotion research and practice.

Flinders Human Behaviour and Health Research Unit
http://www.flinders.edu.au/medicine/sites/fhbhru/self-management.cfm

FHBHRU provides details of the 'Flinders Program™' for chronic condition self-management and links to research and publications.

International Union of Health Promotion and Education

www.iuhpe.org

The International Union of Health Promotion and Education aims to support everyone committed to advancing health promotion and achieving equity in health globally. The website contains information about health promotion research, publications and conferences.

Runanga Whakapiki Ake I Te Hauora o Aotearoa / Health Promotion Forum of New Zealand

www.hpforum.org.nz

The Runanga Whakapiki Ake I Te Hauora O Aotearoa/Health Promotion Forum of New Zealand is the national umbrella organisation for health promotion in New Zealand. The forum's mission is 'Hauora – everyone's right – our commitment'.

VicHealth

www.vichealth.vic.gov.au

The Victorian Health Promotion Foundation is the peak body for health promotion in Victoria. The website contains information about health promotion initiatives, publications and resources.

References

Australian Institute of Health and Welfare, 2010. Australia's health 2010. AIHW, Canberra.

Australian Institute of Health and Welfare, 2012. Australia's health 2012. AIHW, Canberra.

Baum, F., 2008. The new public health, third ed. Oxford University Press, Melbourne.

Braveman, P., 2010. Social conditions and human rights. Health and Human Rights Journal 12 (2), 31–48.

Braveman, P., Egerter, S., Williams, D., 2011. The social determinants of health: Coming of age. Annual Review of Public Health 32, 381–398.

Carter, S., Rychetnik, L., Lloyd, B., et al., 2011. Evidence, ethics and values: a framework for health promotion. American Journal of Public Health 101 (3), 465–470.

Commonwealth of Australia, 2005. Walking school bus: a guide for parents and teachers. Online. Available: http://www.travelsmart.gov.au/schools/pubs/guide.pdf 26 Sep 2012.

Commonwealth of Australia, 2009. Kids matter: how risk and protective factors affect children's mental health. Online. Available: http://www.catholic.tas.edu.au/Resources/documents/kidsmatter-1/risk-and-protective-overview.pdf 22 Jan 2013.

Garmezy, N., 1991. Resiliency and vulnerability to adverse developmental outcomes associated with poverty. American Journal of Behavioral Science 34, 416–430.

Hakama, M., Coleman, M., Alexe, D., et al., 2008. Cancer screening: evidence and practice in Europe 2008. European Journal of Cancer 44 (10), 1404–1413.

Harvey, P., Petkov, J., Misan, G., et al., 2008. Self-management support and training for patients with chronic and complex conditions improves health related behaviour and health outcomes. Australian Health Review 32 (2), 330–338.

Health Promotion, 2012. Forum of New Zealand – Runanga Whakapiki Ake I Te Hauora o Aotearoa. Online. Available: www.hpforum.org.nz 26 Sep 2012.

Hedges, T., Scriven, A., 2008. Sun safety: What are the health messages? Perspectives in Public Health 128 (4), 164–169.

Henry, M., Pasco, J., Sanders, K., et al., 2007. Fracture risk (FRISK) score: Geelong osteoporosis study. Radiology 241 (1), 190–196.

Janda, M., Kimlin, M., Whiteman, D., et al., 2007. Sun protection messages, vitamin D and skin cancer: out of the frying pan into the fire? Medical Journal of Australia 186 (2), 52–54.

Jirowong, S., Liamputtong, P., 2009. Population health, communities and health promotion. Oxford University Press, Melbourne.

Johnson, S., 2009. International perspectives on workplace bullying among nurses: a review. Journal Compilation International Council of Nurses 56, 34–40.

Kaplan, M., 2000. Two pathways to prevention. American Psychologist 55 (4), 382–396.

Keleher, H., MacDougall, C., 2011. Understanding health, third ed. Oxford University Press, Melbourne.

Kickbusch, I., Buckett, K., 2010b. Implementing health in all policies. Government of South Australia, Adelaide.

Kickbusch, I., Buckett, K., 2010a. Health in all policies: where to from here? Health Promotion International 25 (3), 262–264.

Marmot, M., Bosma, H., Hemingway, H., et al., 1997. Contribution of job control and other risk factors to social variations in coronary heart disease incidence. The Lancet 350, 235–239.

Marmot, M., Friel, S., Bell, R., et al., 2008. Closing the gap in a generation: health equity through action on the social determinants of health. The Lancet 372, 1661–1669.

McKinlay, J., 1974. A case for refocussing upstream: the political economy of illness. Applying behavioural science to cardiovascular risk. American Heart Association, Washington.

McMurray, A., 2011. Community health and wellness: a socio-ecological approach, fourth ed. Elsevier, Sydney.

McQueen, D., 2008. Self-reflections on health promotion in the UK and the USA. Public Health 122, 1035–1037.

Ministry of Health New Zealand/ Te Kete Ipurangi and Health promoting schools, nd. Online. Available: http://hps.tki.org.nz/ 6 Apr 2012.

Mittelmark, M., Kickbusch, I., Rootman, I., et al., 2008. Health promotion. In: Heggenhougen, K. (Ed.), International encyclopedia of public health, pp 225–240. Online. Available: http://www.sciencedirect.com/science/referenceworks/9780123739605 20 Sep 2012.

Noblet, A.J., Rodwell, J.J., 2010. Workplace health promotion. In: Leka, S., Houdmont, J. (Eds.), Occupational health psychology. Wiley Blackwell, London.

O'Donnell, M., 2008. The science of health promotion: editor's notes. American Journal of Health Promotion 23 (2), iv.

Planta, M., 2011. Sunscreen and melanoma: Is our prevention message correct. Journal of American Board of Family Medicine 24 (6), 735–739.

Provencher, H., Keyes, C., 2011. Complete mental health recovery: bridging mental illness with positive mental health. Journal of Public Mental Health 10 (1), 57–69.

Raine, K., 2010. Addressing poor nutrition to improve heart health. Canadian Journal of Cardiology 26 (Supp C), 21c–24c.

Rickwood, D., 2006. Pathways of recovery: a framework for preventing further episodes of mental illness. Commonwealth of Australia, Canberra.

Schrecker, T., Chapman, A., Labonté, R., et al., 2010. Advancing health equity in the global marketplace: how human rights can help. Social Sciences and Medicine 71, 1520–1526.

Slade, M., 2009. 100 ways to support recovery: a guide for mental health professionals. Rethink Mental Illness, London.

Smith, B., Tang, K., Nutbeam, D., 2006. WHO health promotion glossary: new terms. Health Promotion International 21 (4), 340–345.

SunSmart New Zealand, 2012 Online. Available: www.sunsmart.org.nz 20 Sep 2012.

SunSmart Victoria, 2012. Sun protection. Online. Available: www.sunsmart.com.au 20 Sep 2012.

Swinburn, B., 2009. Obesity prevention in children and adolescents. Child and Adolescent Psychiatric Clinics of North America 8 (1), 209–223.

Talbot, L., Verrinder, A., 2009. Promoting health: the primary health care approach, fourth ed. Elsevier, Sydney.

Taylor, S., 2012. Health psychology, eighth ed. McGraw-Hill, New York.

Toft, U., Kristoffersen, L., Ladelund, S., et al., 2008. The impact of a population-based multi-factorial lifestyle intervention on changes in long-term dietary habits: the Inter99 study. Preventive Medicine 47, 378–383.

VicHealth, 2005. Building Indigenous leadership: promoting the emotional and spiritual wellbeing of Koori communities through the Koori communities leadership program. Victorian Health Promotion Foundation, Melbourne.

Victorian Health Promotion Foundation, 2008, People, places, processes: reducing health inequalities through balanced health approaches. Online. Available: http://www. vichealth.vic.gov.au/Publications/Health-Inequalities/People-places-processes.aspx 13 Mar 2013.

Victorian Health Promotion Foundation, 2011. Health promotion. Online. Available: www.vichealth.vic.gov.au 20 Sep 2012.

Whitehead, M., 2007. A typology of actions to tackle social inequalities in health. Journal of Epidemiology and Community Health 61, 473–478.

Wilkinson, R., Marmot, M., 2006. The social determinants of health: the solid facts, third ed. WHO, Geneva.

World Health Organization (WHO), 1986. The Ottawa charter for health promotion. WHO, Geneva.

World Health Organization (WHO), 1997. The Jakarta declaration on leading health promotion into the 21st century. WHO, Geneva.

World Health Organization (WHO), 1998. Health promotion glossary. WHO, Geneva.

World Health Organization (WHO), 2008. Closing the gap in a generation: health equity through action on the social determinants of health. WHO Commission on Social Determinants of Health. Online. Available: http://www.who.int/social_determinants/final_report/en/index.html 6 Apr 2012.

World Health Organization (WHO), 2012a. Types of healthy settings: healthy cities. Online. Available: http://www.who.int/healthy_settings/types/cities/en/index.html 20 Sep 2012.

World Health Organization (WHO), 2012b. School and youth health: Global school health initiative: What is a health promoting school? Online. Available: http://www.who.int/school_youth_health/gshi/hps/en/index.html 20 Sep 2012.

Glossary

Acceptance: unconditional positive regard of another person.

Active listening: a way of engaging with the other person's verbal and non-verbal communication to achieve mutual understanding. It involves using the micro-skills of paraphrasing, clarifying and empathy.

Acute pain: pain associated with injury, disease or inflammation, generally lasting for less than three months.

Advocacy: usually means a professional representing a patient when the professional believes the patient is disempowered or unable to speak for themselves.

Allodynia: pain in response to a non-painful stimulus, such as light touch.

Ambiguous loss: a loss that is unclear, unconfirmed or indeterminate and therefore is often more difficult to deal with.

Antecedents: the stimulus events that trigger a behaviour or response.

Anxiety: an unpleasant physical and emotional reaction to a perceived threat.

Auditability: the process of ensuring rigour in qualitative research by identifying the research process and decision trail.

Authoritarian parenting: parenting that is rejecting or unresponsive while at the same time attempting to control the child and what they do.

Authoritative parenting: parenting that is accepting and responsive while trying to control the child and protect them from mistakes.

Behaviourism: a school of psychology that views behaviour as being influenced by factors external to the individual – that is, behaviours are learned depending on whether they are rewarded or not, by association with another event or by imitation.

Biological age: age in terms of physical health and development.

Biomedical model of health: a health model that holds that ill-health is caused by viruses and germs and as such there is one cause and one cure.

Biopsychological model of health: this model extends the causes of disease to incorporate the psychological aspects of illness, such as continual stress, leading to an increase in cortisol production that may have long-term physical consequences on the body's systems.

Biopsychosocial model of health: this model extends the causes of disease to social disadvantages linked to the environment and the social, cultural and political structures of a society.

Burnout: a psychological syndrome characterised by emotional exhaustion, cynicism and a diminished sense of self-efficacy that occurs as a consequence of prolonged chronic workplace stress.

Causal explanations: explanations that provide a single or sometimes multiple causes for why things occur; often formed with the word 'because'.

Central sensitisation: increased responsiveness or sensitivity of nociceptive neurons within the central nervous system (spinal cord and brain).

Chronic pain: pain that lasts beyond the term of normal healing; pain that lasts for longer than three months.

Chronological age: the number of years since someone was born.

Classical conditioning: a simple form of learning by association whereby repeated pairing of a conditioned stimulus with an unconditioned stimulus elicits a conditioned response.

Code of conduct: a statement of belief about the standard of care a profession should deliver.

Cognitive appraisal: the assessment by the individual of a situation or stressor. It can be either primary (Is the event threatening, neutral or positive?) or secondary (Do I have the personal or other resources to respond to the stressor?).

Cognitive behavioural therapy: a counselling intervention that utilises behavioural and cognitive principles to assist the person to set and achieve personal goals or change health behaviours.

Cognitive dissonance: the feeling of discomfort experienced when conflicting beliefs are held simultaneously. It is a technique used in motivational interviewing to bring about behavioural change.

Cognitive theory: a school of psychology that acknowledges the role of perception and thoughts about oneself, one's individual experience and the environment as influences on behaviour.

Collectivist culture: a culture in which the rights and aspirations of the family or group are greater than those of the individual. The smallest socioeconomic unit is the family and interdependence is valued.

Compliance/adherence: when a patient shows the behaviours and follows the treatment regimen a health professional has advised they are described by many health professionals as *compliant*. For some time, however, this term has been questioned and it has been suggested that it be replaced by *adherence*.

Complicated grief: grief that is ongoing and problematic for the bereaved person, often associated with complexities in relationships, lack of preparation for the loss and limited social support.

Concrete operational stage: when a child uses logical forms of reasoning to classify things into groups based on characteristics but only with concrete objects.

Conditioned response: the response elicited by the conditioned stimulus in the presence or absence of the conditioned stimulus such as a phobia.

Conditioned stimulus: a neutral stimulus that elicits a particular response after repeated pairing with a stimulus that naturally produces the response (unconditioned stimulus).

Consumer (of healthcare): an individual who uses health services.

Consumer (of research): an individual who utilises research evidence to inform work practices – that is, engages in evidence-based practice.

Contextual explanations: explanations that provide situational descriptions of what conditions are present when something happens.

Continuing bonds: the important ongoing connections that grievers maintain with the person who is lost, involving such activities as remembering, establishing memorials and negotiating a continuing relationship with the lost person.

Control group: the group of participants in a randomised control trial that receive either no treatment or a standard treatment.

Coping: the process of responding to and managing demands that the individual perceives as challenging or threatening.

Correlation: the degree of relationship between two or more events or characteristics.

Credibility: a measure of rigour in qualitative research. It establishes whether the results of the research are credible or believable from the perspective of the participant in the study.

Daily hassles: minor stressful events that can have a cumulative effect on health.

Deconditioning: a decline in physical fitness through a long period of inactivity.

Defence mechanism: an unconscious psychological process used to reduce anxiety and protect the conscious mind from threatening feelings and perceptions. Common defence mechanisms are denial, projection, repression and rationalisation.

Denial: an unconscious defence mechanism whereby the individual does not acknowledge an impending or actual threat or loss.

Dependent variable: the presumed effect of the independent variable in the study – that is, the outcome that results from the intervention.

Depersonalisation: an emotional and psychological state in which the person feels that self or the outside world is unreal, commonly involving feelings of strangeness, a sense that one's mind is separated from one's body or seeing oneself from a distance.

Descriptive theories: theories that do not try to explain in terms of factors but are content to just describe what appeared to take place.

Determinism: a philosophical position that views all events as being predetermined and having a cause. It also proposes that specific causal factors can potentially be known.

Developmental milestones: key events or periods of a child's development; sometimes used as a watershed to predict outcomes if the milestone is met or not met adequately.

Diagnostic and statistical manual (DSM): a reference work published by the American Psychiatric Association that provides guidelines and criteria for diagnosing and classifying mental disorders.

Diathesis-stress hypothesis: a proposition that mental illness results from a combination of a genetic predisposition and environmental stress, and that both must be present for the condition to manifest itself.

Disenfranchised grief: grief that is not or cannot be openly acknowledged, publicly mourned or socially supported. Specific types of relationships, losses, grievers, circumstances and ways of grieving may not be socially recognised.

Dual process model: a particular conceptualisation of grieving that views the grief process as the oscillation between loss-oriented work and restoration-oriented work.

Dysaesthesia: an unpleasant abnormal sensation that may be spontaneous or evoked.

Early intervention: early diagnosis and treatment of illness to minimise the impact of the illness and its consequences.

Emerging adulthood: the transition from adolescence to adulthood.

Empathy: sensing and non-judgmentally verbalising how one senses the other individual's feelings and meanings.

Endogamous marriage: a marriage in which the partners are from the same group.

Essentialism: explaining behaviour or events in terms of some 'essential' property of the person or object such as 'The tree moved because it possesses magic' or 'All African children like to dance'.

Ethics: moral principles that guide action. In health research ethical research ensures that potential benefits outweigh possible harm and that participants' consent is informed.

Evidence-based practice: using research findings to inform and establish sound clinical practices.

Exogamous marriage: a marriage in which the partners are from different groups.

Experimental group: the group of participants in a randomised control trial that receive the treatment or intervention under investigation.

Explanative theories: theories that are only satisfied when a cause or a context is given for why the events happened the way they did; description alone is not enough.

Fear appeal: efforts to increase motivation to change an individual's attitudes and behaviours by inducing fear.

Fear-avoidance: the avoidance of physical activity due to a fear of increased pain and/or (re)injury.

Fight or flight mechanism: a response to a perceived threat involving sympathetic and endocrine arousal that prepares the individual to attack or flee.

Flinders model: a cognitive- and behavioural-based intervention for self-management of chronic disease.

Formal operational stage: stage in which abstract thinking is possible and can be used in reasoning and logical processes.

General adaptation syndrome (GAS): a stress response consisting of three phases: arousal, resistance and exhaustion.

Genuineness: genuine people are 'congruent'; their non-verbal behaviour is consistent with their inner thoughts and feelings.

Gestalt psychology: a school of psychology that maintains that psychological investigation must focus on the whole individual and the context in which behaviours occur, and not just on parts of the person or on an isolated behaviour.

Grey literature: publications that are either unpublished or published in a non-commercial form such as government policies and reports, conference proceedings or theses.

Grief process: the reactions, behaviours and adaptations that grieving people experience over time in response to a loss. This process has been described using such concepts as stages, phases and tasks.

Grief work: a view of grief first proposed by Sigmund Freud that emphasises the emotional, cognitive, social and behavioural activity and effort involved in coping and making adjustments after a significant loss.

Health: a state of mental, physical, social and spiritual wellbeing; not merely the absence of disease.

Health action process approach: a theory that explains the initiation, adoption and continuation of health behaviours as a process that consists of planning, action and maintenance tasks.

Health behaviour: action by an individual that enhances, maintains or threatens health.

Health belief model: a psychological theory that predicts health behaviours based on the person's perception of the health threat and belief that engaging in a certain behaviour will reduce the health threat.

Health education: an educational approach to increase health literacy to assist individuals and communities to make informed decisions and take action regarding their health, particularly in relation to lifestyle.

Health inequities: inequalities in health that stem from differences in social status and are therefore 'socially unjust'.

Health locus of control: the individual's belief regarding responsibility for their health outcomes – that is, internal (personal), external/powerful others (e.g. doctors) or external/chance (fate).

Health promotion: the process of enabling people to increase control over, and to improve, their health. It can involve a range of educational, political, social and environmental strategies.

Health psychology: a field of study that examines how and why people stay healthy or become ill, and how individuals react when ill.

Healthy Cities: a global movement initiated by the World Health Organization that encourages local governments to engage in health development through political commitment, institutional change, capacity building, partnership-based planning and innovative projects.

Humanistic psychology: a school of psychology that emphasises the development of a concept of self and the striving of the individual towards achieving personal goals and potential.

Hyperalgesia: increased or exaggerated pain in response to a noxious stimulus.

Hypoaesthesia: decreased sensitivity, particularly with regard to touch or pressure.

Illness prevention: strategies that aim to deter the occurrence of illness.

Independent variable: the presumed cause of the outcome (dependent variable) observed.

Indigenous Australian: a person who identifies as being Aboriginal or Torres Strait Islander.

Individualist culture: a culture in which the individual's goals and achievements are valued over those of the family or group. The smallest socioeconomic unit is the individual and independence is valued.

Indulgent (or permissive) parenting: parenting that accepts what a child does and where a parent does not try to control the child.

Informed consent: an ethical principle that requires a researcher to obtain the voluntary participation of subjects after informing them of potential benefits and risks.

Interdisciplinary: an approach to healthcare practice in which different health disciplines, such as psychology, nursing, social work, podiatry, physiotherapy and other medical and allied health professionals, work collaboratively.

Intermediary determinants: the 'downstream' social factors that maintain, but can also minimise health inequalities that are caused by the structural determinants of health such as education, housing and access to transport.

Intersectoral: an approach whereby different agencies and government departments such as health, housing and transport work collaboratively on a common goal like 'health'.

Kinship: family or blood ties.

Levels of loss: Weenolsen's framework proposing that loss is experienced at five levels: primary, secondary, holistic, self-conceptual and metaphorical.

Locus of control (LOC): the individual's belief regarding responsibility for reinforcement for a particular behaviour and whether the individual believes that reinforcements (outcomes) are controlled by the self (internal LOC) or by the environment (external LOC).

Loss: separation from someone or something that has meaning for the individual and to which they feel strongly connected.

Māori: an indigenous New Zealander.

Marriage: a permanent and legally recognised arrangement between two people that includes both a sexual and an economic relationship with mutual rights and obligations.

Mechanism: a scientific philosophy developed by Descartes that rejects purpose and qualities in favour of what is quantifiable. It proposes that all natural phenomena, including human behaviour, can be explained by physical causes and processes.

Mediational/mediationism: where behaviour or concepts are mediated by something else; we see a tree and walk towards it but this is mediated by the eye and brain and these must be part of our explanation.

Medical model: the view that health and illness (including behavioural and emotional problems) have physical causes and hence are treated with biomedical interventions. It is the predominant model of care delivery in Western healthcare systems.

Micro-skills: attending behaviours that are the essence of good communication including eye contact, attentive body language, vocal style and verbal style.

Mindfulness: seeing novelty in every situation and activity, whether done before or not.

Modelling: learning by observation (also called vicarious learning).

Monogamous marriage: a marriage in which there is only one husband and one wife.

Morbidity: the frequency or occurrence of a disease and the degree to which the illness or disability affects the person.

Mortality rate: the number of deaths in a population (from a specific cause).

Motivational interviewing: a client-centred, semi-directed counselling approach that encourages an individual to change a health behaviour by focusing on reasons for and against the change. The resulting cognitive dissonance creates a state of ambivalence for the person and hence an opportunity for the person to initiate change. It is particularly suited to clients with addictive behaviours.

Multidisciplinary team (also called the **interdisciplinary team):** team composed of health professionals from different disciplines, each with their own specialised knowledge, skills and expertise, who work collaboratively.

Nature/nurture debate: the controversy concerning whether human behaviour is influenced more by genetic inheritance and biology (nature) or by learning and the environment (nurture).

Neglectful (or uninvolved) parenting: parenting that is unaccepting or unresponsive to the child and also does not try to control them.

Neo-liberal policy: policy based on the idea that the market will provide what is needed given the opportunity. Health is therefore a commodity and those who need health purchase it.

Neuropathic pain: pain arising as a direct consequence of a lesion or disease of the somatosensory nervous system.

New public health: a health movement that, prior to the 1980s, operated principally within a biomedical framework and that in the 21st century also acknowledges social and political influences on health.

Nociception: activity in the nervous system generated by a noxious stimulus.

Nociceptive pain: pain arising from injury or pathology in the tissues, for example, soft tissue sprains and strains, bone fractures or appendicitis.

Nociceptor: a high threshold sensory receptor of the peripheral somatosensory nervous system that is preferentially sensitive to noxious stimuli.

Nonfinite loss: the loss associated with experiences such as disability and dementia that unfolds throughout one's lifespan and involves awareness of having lost 'what should have been'.

Noxious stimulus: a stimulus that is actually or potentially damaging to body tissue.

Object permanence: when a child acts as if an object has permanence even when it cannot be seen.

Operant conditioning: a learning process whereby outcomes are controlled by consequences of the behaviour – that is, whether behaviour is rewarded, punished or ignored.

Optimism: the perception and belief that adverse events are a temporary challenge to be addressed and are within the control of the individual.

Pain behaviour: any behaviour that serves to indicate that a person is in pain (e.g. complaining, grimacing, limping, avoiding activity).

Palliative care: an approach to healthcare concerned primarily with attending to physical and emotional comfort, rather than effecting a cure, through responding holistically to symptoms, pain and emotional, social and spiritual needs.

Partnership: a relationship between a health professional and the recipient of care in which they both share some degree of responsibility for the treatment decisions, implementation and outcomes.

Peripheral sensitisation: increased responsiveness or sensitivity of nociceptive neurons in the periphery, which occurs in response to a noxious stimulus.

Pessimism: the perception and belief that adverse events are permanent, catastrophic and outside the control of the individual.

Phenomenology: a qualitative research methodology that examines a phenomenon or the 'lived experience' of a phenomenon. It aims to understand either the experience or the meaning of the experience for the participant(s).

Policy: a series of actions by a government that guide present or future courses of action. For example, Medicare is a government policy that provides healthcare for all Australians with funding derived from the taxation base. This enables Medicare to be classified as a universal healthcare policy based on redistribution of taxes between high income earners and lower income groups.

Polyandry: where a woman has more than one husband at the same time.

Polygyny (polygamous marriage): marriage to multiple spouses.

Population health: the health of a group of people who are united by a specific factor, for example, biological, social or geographic. A population health approach is action taken to improve the health of whole populations.

Positivism: the philosophical view that knowledge is limited to facts that are observable or obtained through scientific experiment.

Post-traumatic stress disorder (PTSD): a serious, debilitating mental illness that affects some people who experience or witness an extremely traumatic stressful event that is outside the realm of usual human experience and involves the threat of death or serious injury.

Preoperational stage: when children begin to have words for the things around them and use those words, but this stage is 'pre' operational where 'operational' refers to 'logical' operations.

Primary appraisal: the individual's judgment as to whether a particular event or situation is negative (poses a threat), positive (benign) or neutral (irrelevant).

Primary healthcare: a holistic approach to healthcare that is underpinned by a philosophy of social justice and addresses the social determinants of health in addition to biomedical causative factors for illness.

Primary intervention: the implementation of biomedical, psychosocial, political and environmental strategies that aim to foster wellbeing and prevent the occurrence of illness.

Probability: the likelihood that a research finding occurred by chance (statistical significance).

Prolonged grief disorder: a particular type of complicated grief characterised by intrusive thoughts related to the deceased, intense separation distress and/or distressingly strong yearnings for the person or thing that is lost, lasting longer than six months and causing significant impairment in functioning.

Protective factors for health: factors that reduce the likelihood that an illness will occur, for example, by being vaccinated, by having access to clean water and by having a supportive family and social network.

Proximity: the distance people place themselves from each other in different interactions such as public, social and personal.

Psychology: the scientific study of behaviour – essentially, but not exclusively, the study of human behaviour.

Psychoanalytic theory: a personality theory that asserts that behaviour is driven by unconscious processes, as well as influenced by childhood/developmental conflicts that either have been resolved or remain unresolved.

Psychological age: an individual's ability to adapt to various circumstances compared with others who might be the same chronological age.

Psychological death: a situation in which a person lacks consciousness of existence, for example, due to medical brain death, or where someone's personality or behaviour has changed so significantly, for example, due to mental illness or brain injury, that others view the person as they previously existed as dead.

Psychoneuroimmunology: the multidisciplinary study of the interrelationship between behavioural, neuroendocrine and immunological adaptive processes.

Public health: concerned with the health of individuals, communities and populations and also the identification and modification of environmental factors that impact on health.

Qualitative research: a research paradigm that is interested in questions that involve human consciousness and subjectivity and values humans and their experiences in the research process.

Quantitative research: a process that attempts to find out scientific knowledge by measurement of elements.

Quasi-experimental design: a study design in which random assignment is not used but the independent variable is manipulated and certain mechanisms of control are used.

Randomised control trial (RCT): an experimental study of the effects of a variable (e.g. a drug or treatment) administered to human subjects who are randomly selected from a broad population and assigned randomly to either an experimental or a control group.

Rational non-adherence: a person may not believe that what a health professional suggests is in their best interest and, after considering the facts, may choose not to accept treatment or choose a different therapy.

Recovery: refers to the process of making adaptations to live with an ongoing or chronic illness. The focus is on the individual's strengths, aspirations and enabling them to live a fulfilling life, regardless of any disability.

Reductionism: a philosophical approach in which concepts are interpreted with reference to simpler processes. The issue under investigation is analysed into simpler parts or organised systems, with a view to explaining or understanding it.

Refereed journal: a journal that requires its articles to have been evaluated or critiqued by expert peers before being accepted for publication.

Reliability: a statistical term for the internal consistency of a test and the extent to which it can be expected to produce the same result on different occasions.

Resilience: the ability to bounce back following adversity and to achieve good outcomes despite challenges and threats.

Rigour: the extent to which research methods are scrupulously and meticulously carried out in order to recognise important influences in the study.

Risk factors for health: increase vulnerability to illness, for example, social inequities and poor nutrition.

Sample: a group of cases or individuals studied as representatives of the population from which they are drawn.

Secondary appraisal: the individual's assessment of his/her personal (internal) and environmental (external) resources to respond to a particular stressful event or situation.

Secondary intervention: healthcare that is delivered when symptoms, injury or illness are identified. Treatment is initiated as early as possible to restore health.

Secondary source: scholarly material written by someone other than the individual who developed the theory or conducted the research. Most are usually published. Often a secondary source represents a response to or a summary and critique of a theorist's or researcher's work.

Self-actualisation: the achievement of one's potential and the mark of a healthy individual according to Maslow.

Self-efficacy: the personal belief that one can achieve certain goals and cope adequately in particular circumstances.

Sensorimotor stage: children at this stage think, as it were, through their senses and their physical movements; children explore and learn just what they physically interact with through their senses.

Social age: the social roles and expectations relative to chronological age.

Social construction: an idea, concept or phenomenon that is viewed as real because there is agreement within a social group that they will act as if the construction does exist.

Social death: the experience of sick or dying people in which they are perceived and treated by other people, such as health professionals, as if they were already dead.

Social determinants of health: the social and economic factors that impact on health outcomes such as socioeconomic status, housing and employment.

Social justice: a value base that views fairness and equity as a right for all regardless of social position.

Social learning theory: Bandura's theory of observational learning or modelling.

Social marketing: uses marketing principles and theory from the disciplines of psychology, sociology and communications to identify solutions to social and health problems and to encourage individuals and populations to lead healthy lifestyles.

Social scaffolding: having social support or help from those around you.

Sociological model of health: the view that factors that are external to the individual influence health outcomes such as social determinants.

Sociological perspective: an explanatory model for human behaviour in which the emphasis shifts from the individual to the broader social forces influencing the person.

Somatosensory nervous system: the part of the nervous system (peripheral and central) that provides conscious perception of sensory information from the skin, musculoskeletal system and viscera.

Statistical significance: the likelihood that the results of a study could have occurred by chance or not (probability).

Stigmatisation: the process of perceiving, describing or responding to a person or groups of people in such a way that they are socially discredited, devalued or isolated.

Stress: a physical, cognitive, emotional and behavioural experience of an individual in response to an event that the individual perceives to be challenging or threatening.

Stressor: the event or experience that challenges or threatens the individual's coping resources.

Structural determinants: the societal factors and components of people's socioeconomic position that generate or reinforce social and political inequalities such as class, gender, ethnicity or access to resources.

Systematic review: a literature review that examines all of the available quality literature on a research question and provides a comprehensive summary of the findings.

Tertiary intervention: healthcare delivered when the disease cannot be cured or the illness process is prolonged. It aims to assist individuals (and their family and carers) to cope with a change in their health status, to limit disability from the health problem and to promote health and quality of life.

The therapeutic triad: the three qualities considered important by Rogers: genuineness, acceptance and empathy.

Theory of planned behaviour: a psychological theory that proposes that a person's intentions and behaviour can be understood by identifying the person's attitudes to the behaviour, subjective norms about the behaviour and the person's belief regarding their control of the action.

Third force: a term used to describe the school of humanistic psychology.

Transtheoretical model: a model of behaviour change that outlines the stages a person goes through when changing a behaviour. The stages are precontemplation, contemplation, preparation, action and maintenance (or relapse).

Typology: the systematic classification of types, such as losses, that have characteristics or traits in common.

Unconditioned stimulus: a stimulus that regularly and reliably elicits a response such as salivation at the sight of food.

Validity: determination of whether a measurement instrument actually measures what it is purported to measure.

Yerkes-Dodson law: a hypothesis that predicts performance based on the degree to which the individual is aroused. The theory predicts that performance increases with arousal up to a point at which performance deteriorates.

Zone of proximal development: Vygotsky's term for the range of behaviour between what a child can do alone and what a child can do with social scaffolding.

Index

Note: Page numbers followed by 'f' indicate figures, 't' indicate tables, and 'b' indicate boxes.

development influenced by, 40–42
as milestone of adulthood, 65–69
styles, 42, 42b–43b, 65–66
partner, pain influenced by, 295
partnerships
in health
beliefs influencing, 214–215
biomedical model and, 204–207, 212
chronic illness and, 210–211
collaborative practice and, 216–217
decisions about one's health in, 212–214
disability and, 208–211
factors influencing, 211
fostering, 202–204
health professionals' challenges in, 211–212
overview of, 202, 217
PCC in, 202
PCP and, 204–205, 209t, 216
perceptions influencing, 214–215
recovery and, 205–208, 207b–208b, 209t
terminology, 203–204
as milestone of adulthood, 61–64
patient advocates, 149–150
Pavlov, Ivan, 8, 159
PCC *see* person-centred communication
PCP *see* person-centred practice
Peabody, Francis, 189
peers, 41–47, 45b–46b
perception
pain, 288–289
partnerships influenced by, 214–215
as reality, 203
peripheral nervous system, pain processing in, 286–288, 288f
Perls, Fritz, 20
permissive parenting, 42
persistent complex bereavement-related disorder, 273–274
personal control, 98–100
personality
health behaviours influenced by, 96–98
as internal coping resource, 240–242
nature vs nurture and, 17–20
resilience and, 98, 242, 243b–244b
theories, 3–17, 18t, 20
types, 96, 97b
person-centred communication (PCC), 183–186
empathy in, 185, 186t
facilitation of interaction in, 184
minimal encouragers in, 185
in partnerships, 202

reflection in, 185
skills, 184, 186t
summarising in, 185–186
person-centred practice (PCP), 204–205, 213, 216
pessimism, 241–242
pharmacotherapy, 15
phenomenology, 135–136, 136b–137b
physical effects, of stress, 235
physical reactions, in elements of grief responses, 265
physical therapies, 303
Piaget, Jean
as developmental theorist, 32–35, 32t, 38b, 55
health professionals using, 38b
policy, 114–116
political context, of SDH, 115–116
polyandrous, 62
polygamy, 62
polygyny, 62
popular media, 140–141
population approach, to health promotion, 330–334, 331b–332b
positive psychology, 11, 14
postconventional morality, 56, 57t
post-miscarriage support, 259b–260b
post-traumatic growth, 75
post-traumatic stress disorder (PTSD), 224–225, 239, 292
power imbalance, 190
preconventional morality, 56, 57t
preoperational stage, 32t, 34–35
primary healthcare movement, 89, 319
primary level of intervention, 320–323, 321t
problem-focused coping strategies, 242–245, 245t
professional boundaries, 190–191
projection, 6
protective factors, in health promotion, 317–318
psychoanalytic theory
critique of, 7
defence mechanisms in, 6–7
early lifespan and, 30
Freud and, 5–7, 30
nature vs nurture in, 19
overview of, 3, 5, 18t
in psychology, 3, 5–7, 18t
psychological approaches, to pain management, 303–304
psychological distress, from pain, 291–292
psychological effects, of stress, 237–239
psychological factors, 122